Healthcare TECHNOLOGY

Steps Toward Developing an Electronic Health Record

The HCT Project Team

Publisher
Barry Jacobs

Editor
Alexandra Wharton

Publications Director
Melissa Mumbauer

Project Manager
Brett Gajda

Account Managers
Steve Ambuul, Kelly Joseph Lemos, Jonas Tegelvik, John Watson

Art Director
Tamara Dyer

Design, Production and Graphics
Tamara Dyer

Production Manager
Christian Muncy

Copy Editor
Brian Dustrud

Proofreader
Lisa Barr

Cover and Interior Illustration
Campbell Laird

Montgomery Research, Inc.

Chief Executive Officer
Chris Trayhorn

Publisher
Nick Smith

Director of Business Operations
Kim Massey

Marketing Director
Yvonne Schellerup

IT Manager
Irene Graff

Web Production
Jill Oana

Reprint and Book Services
John Malick

Controller
Julienne Riveong

Accenture

Editor
Thomas K. Spann

Project Director
Sally E. Boyer

Project Manager
Nadia M. Leather

About Montgomery Research

Montgomery Research publishes thought leadership focusing on the convergence of technology and business. Working in partnership with leading companies and organizations, each project provides the latest thinking from the people who are shaping the future in a changing business environment.

Contributors to Montgomery Research initiatives include executives, consultants, trade groups, analysts, academicians and other key stakeholders. Montgomery Research solicits thoughtful editorial contributions from this community to create a world-class forum tailored to executive management.

Montgomery Research develops information resources for a variety of industries including: Customer Relationship Management, Supply Chain, Government, Financial Operations, Mobile Commerce and Utilities. Find out more at www.mriresearch.com.

Published By
©2005 Montgomery Research, Inc.
300 Montgomery Street, Suite 1135
San Francisco, CA 94104
Phone 415.397.2400 **Fax** 415.397.2420
ideas@mriresearch.com

This book is available from the publisher at $695.00 per copy plus shipping.

Printed in the U.S.A ISBN 1-932178-18-X

[Editorial Advisory Board]

[Editorial Advisory Board, cont.]

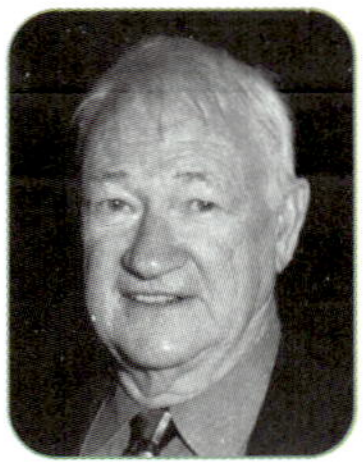

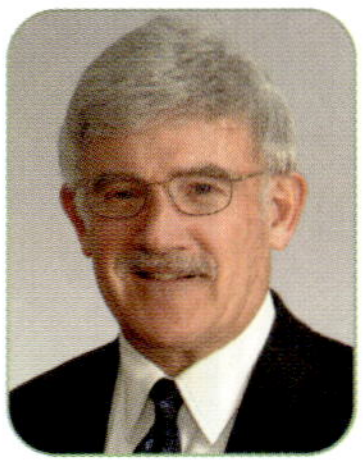

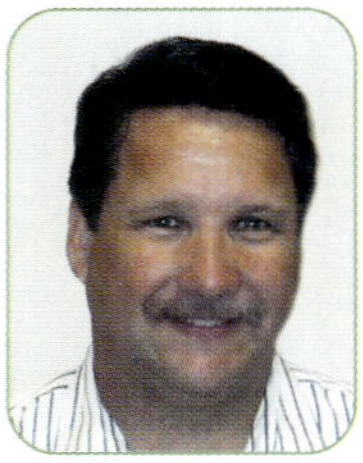

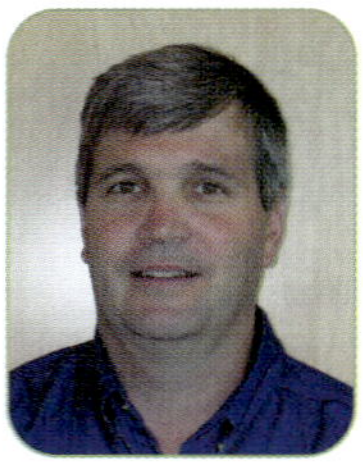

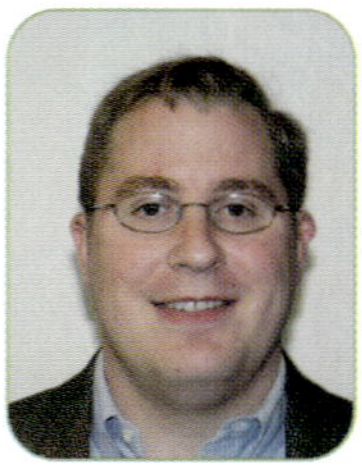

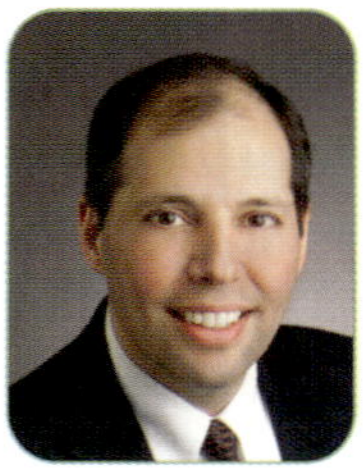

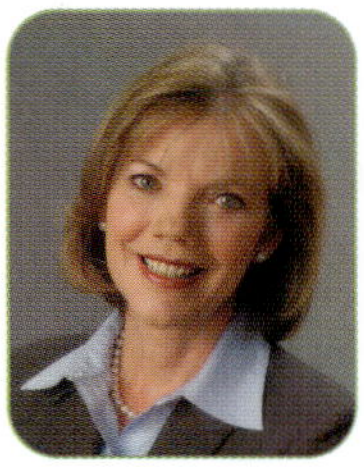

Marie Savard, M.D., is an internist, noted author and creator of a patient-centered PHR system.

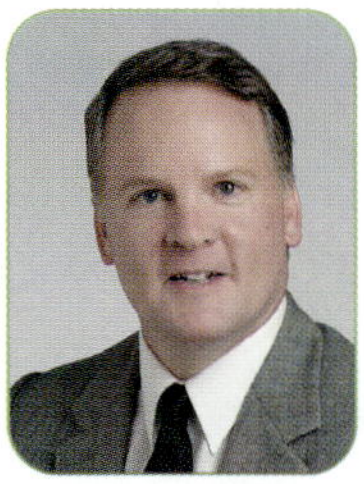

John E. Steiner Jr., Esq., is the chief compliance officer and privacy official of The Cleveland Clinic Health System and is actively involved, both internally and externally, in many of the current legal and regulatory issues presented by the EHR.

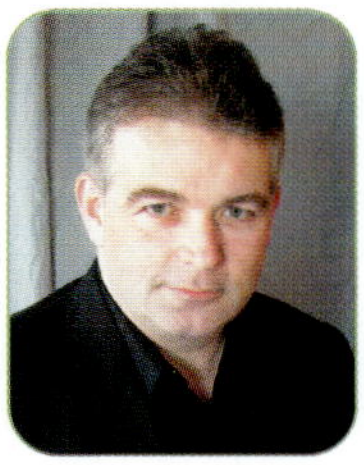

James Taylor is the vice president of product marketing of enterprise decision management for Fair Isaac. He is responsible for working with clients to identify and bring to market advanced decision management solutions that will better solve their business needs.

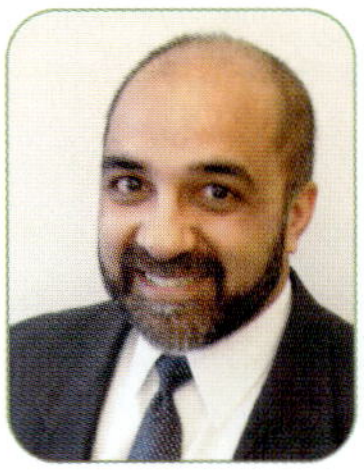

Micky Tripathi is the president and CEO of the Massachusetts eHealth Collaborative (MAeHC), a nonprofit collaboration of 34 leading Massachusetts organizations. He is also a member of the board of directors of MA-SHARE, a community utility service for statewide clinical data exchange in Massachusetts, and served as the founding president and CEO of the Indiana Health Information Exchange.

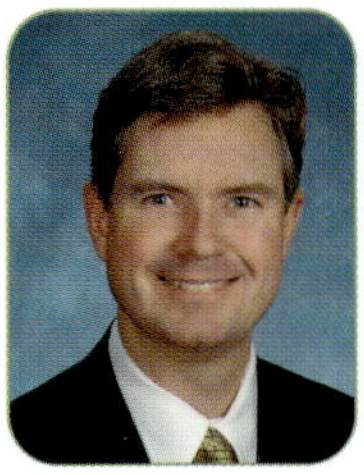

Scott Whyte is a vice president of clinical systems at Catholic Healthcare West (CHW). Prior to his role at CHW, he was vice president and CIO at Phoenix Children's Hospital and has spent over 17 years consulting with Capgemini, Siemens Medical Solutions and Ernst & Young to hospitals, health insurers and life sciences companies.

[Preface]

ACCENTURE BELIEVES THAT ELECTRONIC HEALTH RECORDS (EHRs) have the potential to transform healthcare by introducing the worldwide healthcare industry to the benefits of information technology (IT) automation. While financial services, transportation, communications and other industries have embraced IT and its advantages, the healthcare industry has been much slower to adopt IT than it has advances in clinical technologies. Now EHRs offer a fundamental building block to achieving the next-generation health system.

The topic of EHRs has become a matter of intense interest over the last three years. EHRs are a means of using computers and networks to document a patient's health and care, replacing the more limited paper records now in use. By making records electronic, they can be easily and quickly shared with other caregivers in distant or nearby locations. With improved access to patient information at the point of need, quality of care will improve while costs from unnecessary treatments, such as duplicative tests, will decline. On a broader scale, EHRs also can serve to easily aggregate anonymous clinical data that could support new medical discoveries and better public health, and could lead to a host of other benefits.

In the last two years, the momentum to move to EHRs in the United States has been steadily building. Although the industry had been slowly working toward some form of electronic records for the past few decades, a turning point came in President George W. Bush's 2003 State of the Union message to Congress, when he made EHRs part of his healthcare agenda.

Another major step forward was the presidential appointment of Dr. David Brailer as the first National Coordinator of Health Information Technology in May 2004. His express directive is to move the country's healthcare industry to portable EHRs for all individuals within 10 years.

After barely two months in office, in July 2004 Dr. Brailer laid out a framework for accomplishing this objective. He outlined four goals for national EHRs:

- Inform clinical practice: Get EHRs into clinical practice to start reducing medical errors, duplicative tests and improve patient care.
- Connect physicians both among themselves and with provider organizations so that patient health information is portable and can move with the patient through regional collaborations and a national health information network.
- Personalize care to the individual by creating consumer-centric information that helps individuals manage their own wellness through personal health records areas.
- Use EHRs to improve public health.

EHRs and the data that they contain are not just for providers. With the proper protections for a patient's privacy, they will also streamline patient-provider interactions for referrals and insurance claims adjudication. They will increase the base of medical knowledge and experience available for disease management. And they will accelerate the adoption and promotion of new medical knowledge, treatments and technology. EHRs will truly benefit all elements of the health industry.

Change will occur when processes and information flow consistently and efficiently across the "system" of care. Through integration, EHRs will offer a unique opportunity to add value to consumers and providers of healthcare.

Provider, payer and public health organizations can ready themselves for EHRs now by:

- Strategizing about how the integration of clinical data across providers, payers, government, local community, social care, volunteers and pharmaceutical companies will help each participant do a better job and then working with each other to accelerate the integration.
- Recognizing that the greatest benefits will not be derived from implementing technology per se, but from using technology to integrate information and processes across all stakeholders.
- Preparing top leadership from each organization to move forward together while each pursues their own plan and milestones for implementing EHRs.
- Starting to apply resources, including users such as physicians and nurses as well as technology experts, to define, manage and integrate data and processes.
- Beginning to prepare, involve and train people affected by the process and technology change so that when EHRs are rolled out, their full potential can be realized.

This book covers all of these dimensions and more, giving the reader a broad understanding of the state of EHRs today. It also provides readers with the information they need to start acting now. ■

[1] The Way Forward

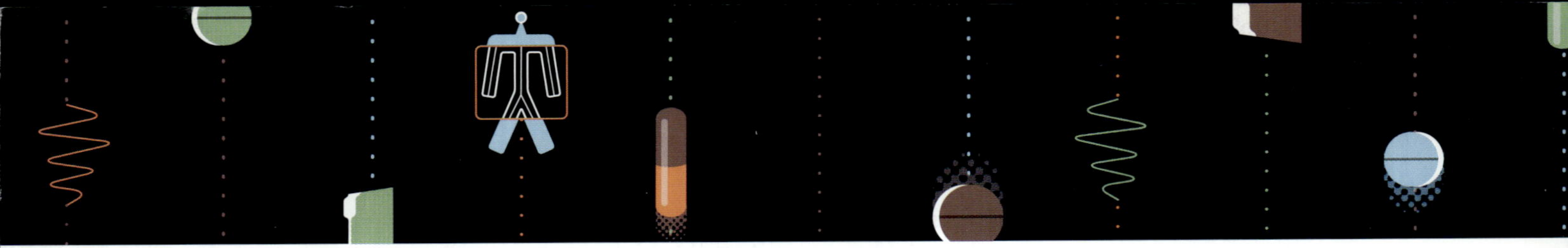

[2] Achieving Interoperability & Collaboration

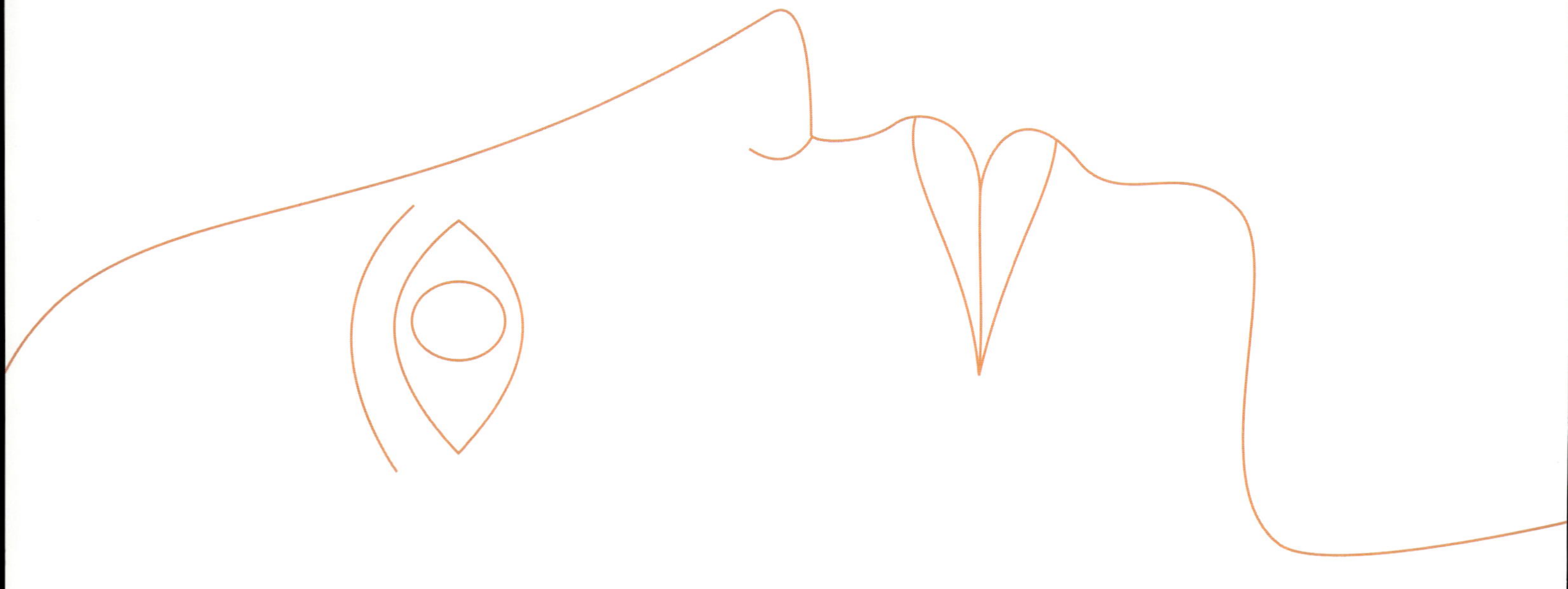

[3] Improving Clinical Outcomes

[4] Securing Physician Buy-In

[5] Increasing Efficiency & Performance

[6] Roles & Perspectives

[7] Local Health Information Infrastructure Initiatives

[Conclusion]

[Publisher's Letter]

Hurricane Katrina displaced a million people and lost thousands of medical records.

The storm made it almost impossible for physicians to attend to their patients because they had to go from memory for treatments or contact laboratories by phone for results. Health and Human Services Secretary Mike Leavitt said the chaos wreaked by Katrina "powerfully demonstrated the need for electronic health records."

EHRs will lead to safer and higher-quality patient care and provide greater efficiency. Through bipartisan support in Congress, the federal government has promised Americans EHRs over the next 10 years. Reduced medical errors, improved access to results by caregiver and decreased costs are just some of the advantages of EHRs.

Despite these tremendous benefits, many unanswered questions remain. Who will develop EHRs and the necessary technology and how? Where will the money required for implementation and advancement come from? How can we develop compelling value propositions for all stakeholders including payers, providers and employers?

The white papers, interviews and solution providers in this year's project tackle these issues as well as examine other roadblocks. Privacy and security concerns, the misalignment of downstream benefits, issues of interoperability and the lack of standards are discussed and perspectives from the visionaries and thought leaders in this space are offered.

We hope this research adds to the dialogue and contributes to the evolution of the healthcare IT system. I'd like to thank our editorial panel, authors and the Accenture team for helping us bring together this work. Readers are invited to visit www.hctproject.com for additional research and links to other resources. Feedback is essential and will be shared with all contributors so please reach out with your ideas.

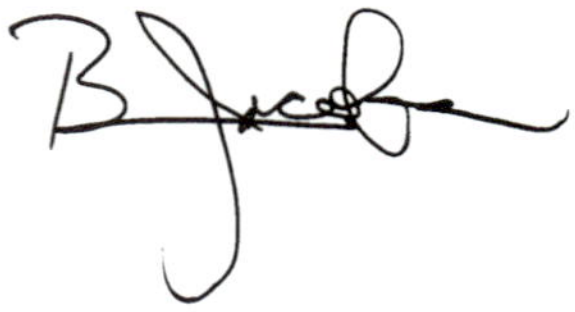

Barry Jacobs
Publisher, Healthcare Technology
b.jacobs@mriresearch.com

1

The Way Forward

The healthcare industry faces a steep climb toward the efficiencies promised by today's healthcare IT solutions. Promoting the widespread adoption of EHRs alone will require an investment of hundreds of billions of dollars, and it will take considerable resolve to settle all of the issues facing a national health IT network and develop compelling value propositions for all stakeholders. But these challenges are dwarfed by the enormous opportunity.

Building an EHR: Goals, Challenges and Tactics

Unless significant coordinated efforts are undertaken by all parties in the health industry, the ability for different providers to electronically store and exchange health-related information will not exist.

[Peter Kongstvedt, Accenture] [Lewis Redd, Accenture] [John Quinn, Accenture]

Technology in healthcare has made great progress in diagnostic and therapeutic applications. Using computers to assist in imaging, surgery and critical life support has meant lives are being saved that as recently as five years ago were being lost.

However, the application of health information technology (HIT) to clinical records has been dreadfully slow. The ability for different providers and organizations to electronically store and then exchange health-related information anywhere that a patient needs care does not exist, and looks likely not to exist, unless significant coordinated efforts are undertaken by all parties in the health industry.

Rewards for implementing electronic health records (EHRs) have proven elusive, and the expense is considerable. Confounding the progress of even this small amount of EHR implementation is the distressing fact that none of the disparate EHR systems currently in the market are capable of communicating with each other (or in most cases even themselves) in any but the most rudimentary ways, if at all.

A Universal Issue

Although the U.S. lags behind many other countries in significantly expanding the use of HIT, it is not alone in its lack of progress with EHRs. The need to enhance the quality of patient care through electronically portable clinical information is truly an international one. Healthcare leaders from across the world consider EHRs to be among the most important applications their organizations will need to invest in over the next two years. Countries that are beginning to address widespread adoption of EHRs include Australia, Canada, Finland, France, Germany, New Zealand, the Netherlands and the U.K.

In the U.S., President George W. Bush established a vision of interoperable EHRs and appointed David Brailer, M.D., Ph.D., to serve as the national coordinator for HIT. This created a focal point for action and captured the attention of both the healthcare industry and the nation. In a publication by Health and Human Services former Secretary Tommy Thompson and Dr. Brailer, four overarching goals were established. Paraphrased, these goals are: informing clinical practice; interconnecting clinicians; personalizing patient care; and improving population health, including access to care for underserved Americans.

The federal governments in the U.S. and many other countries have issued their calls for action, but many unanswered questions remain. How will HIT and EHRs be developed and by whom? Where will the money required for development and implementation come from? What are the implications for clinicians, hospitals, payers and employers?

Overcoming the Barriers

There are significant challenges facing HIT and EHRs, encompassing structural, technical, financial and social/cultural issues. Although the organizational and financial environment in the U.S. is markedly different from what is found in the other countries, many of the issues that need to be addressed are universal, and numerous lessons can be learned from the experiences abroad.

None of the challenges represent insurmountable barriers to successful national adoption, but they will need to be addressed

Peter R. Kongstvedt, M.D., is a partner in Accenture's Health & Life Sciences practice. He focuses on thought leadership, strategy and performance metrics for large health plans. **Lewis Redd** is managing partner of Accenture's Provider, Health & Life Sciences practice, responsible for all business development and service delivery to clients in North America. He has over 20 years of healthcare consulting experience, with a specialty in technology-enabled performance improvement. **John Quinn** is chief technology officer in Accenture's Provider, Health & Life Sciences practice focusing on emerging healthcare information systems technologies. He has over 29 and 32 years' experience in the healthcare and computer industries, respectively. He has participated on the HL7 board of directors since its inception 18 years ago and has served as the chair of its technical steering committee for the last 14 years.

nevertheless. First and foremost the process will need to address funding for capital outlays and financial incentives to encourage provider adoption. In the U.S., funding will need to come from private-public partnerships and include a combination of grants, loans, reimbursements, and tax and other policy incentives. And even in other countries, healthcare organizations will need to self-fund at least a portion of EHR acquisition and local infrastructure development through business process changes that yield administrative efficiencies and cost savings.

Additionally EHR adoption will require standards to facilitate accurate and easy exchange of data from one computer system to another, or interoperability. Regardless of whether the approach taken is centralized or decentralized, a national health information infrastructure of standards and privacy safeguards that restricts access only to caregivers authorized by the patients themselves will be required at some level. And the issue of patient and provider identifiers will need to be resolved so that clinical information can be connected at the patient level while ensuring individuals' privacy.

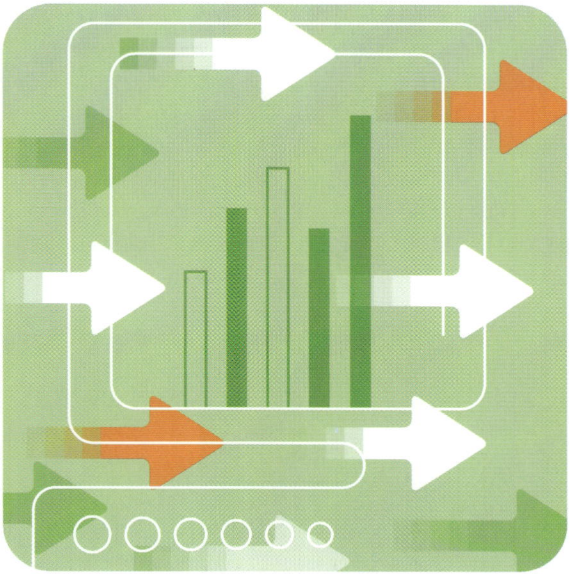

to 10 years and will continue to evolve even after that. At this early stage in the strategic formulation of a national HIT agenda, it is difficult to predict what the specific results will look like. Given the "from the ground up" approach that is being adopted, the models will certainly vary between nations; even within one country, the details are likely to vary from region to region, at least in the near term.

What is clearer is what the process will look like and what issues will need to be addressed. To accomplish the strategic goals that have been established, the process will need to address existing barriers such as funding for capital outlays, incentives to encourage clinician adoption and standards to facilitate interoperability. In the end, structural and technical challenges will need standardized solutions, while approaches to the financial and social/cultural challenges will be more variable. In truth, such variability represents an excellent opportunity for imaginative solutions.

Ultimately the widespread adoption of EHR will completely revolutionize how we measure success in healthcare. It will

In the end, structural and technical challenges will need standardized solutions, while approaches to the financial and social/cultural challenges will be more variable. In truth, such variability represents an excellent opportunity for imaginative solutions.

Broad HIT adoption most certainly will require major changes in the relationships between clinicians, hospitals, payers, employers, technology vendors and patients. All will need to participate and be invested in technology development, implementation and success. A high degree of collaboration at a local level will be necessary, and constituents will need to overcome historical animosities.

The Vision

Achievement of a national health information infrastructure is surely a long-term vision. Progress will occur over the next seven

provide an opportunity to redefine measures of quality and outcomes, and as a nation we will be able to gauge levels and improvements in patient safety like never before. There is no doubt that the EHR will come to occupy a central place in our healthcare system. What comes in the next 10 years will be the reality of how that occurs.

Taking Action

While it is early on a national level in most countries, it is not too early for organizations to take action in HIT, and ultimately take action toward implementation of the EHR. Certain actions can be undertaken now or in the near term in order to build the necessary base of support and infrastructure. Examples of such actions are as follows.

Engage the Community. No organization can be successful with HIT and EHRs by itself. Open and cooperative discussion and action must occur between hospitals, professional healthcare providers, payer or insurance executives, business leaders and consumers. In the U.S., this is frequently taking place under the auspices of a regional health information organization, many of which have been started with seed money either from the federal government or from local initiatives by payers and provider systems. The needs of all parties, the proposed benefits to all parties and the reality of the environment must all be addressed. In this way, local or regional approaches can be taken, upon which broader achievements can be built.

Redesign Processes and Workflows. No software solves problems by itself. As HIT and EHRs are implemented, organizations must redesign their processes and workflows to take advantage of efficiencies created by new technology. Failure to do so will most likely result in disgruntled clinicians and grossly suboptimal outcomes, to say nothing of a significant investment wasted. In addition, service levels must be defined and measured to ensure that improvement goals are being met.

Create a Business Case for HIT and EHR Implementation. To enter into HIT and EHRs without a well-defined business case is to risk a poorly executed and overly expensive undertaking. Organizations must define goals and investment returns associated with new technologies. Investment returns need not be strictly financial; they can be clinical (e.g., *measurable* improvements in patient safety) or service-oriented (e.g., *measurable* improvements in patient satisfaction). The first step in its creation is the creation of measures that will inform the business case; examples might include patient safety (e.g., medication errors), clinical support costs (e.g., costs of medical records), and financial improvement (e.g., improved coding and billing). The discipline of a business case provides guidance for success and cannot be bypassed

Work with Clinicians. All clinicians, but most especially physicians, must be an integral part of the process. If physicians cannot see how HIT and the EHR will improve their working lives, they will resist it. It is not sufficient to simply install new systems and expect clinicians to fully embrace it, nor will new systems necessarily achieve improved outcomes if physicians are not taking complete advantage of available capabilities. Clinical leaders must not only be deeply involved in all appropriate aspects of HIT and EHRs, they must serve to translate the organization's goals and objectives into terms meaningful to other clinicians.

Work Closely with IT Vendors. Any organization's IT vendors must be engaged, whether it's clinical support systems for hospitals, practice management systems for physician practices or e-prescribing vendors working with physicians and payers. How is the vendor looking to the future in terms of compliance with national initiatives, voluntary standards, connectivity and electronic communications, clinical support, messaging infrastructure and data analysis? It is important for the organization to make it clear what its expectations are, and for the IT vendors to make it clear what their path to the future is.

Clinical leaders must not only be deeply involved in all appropriate aspects of HIT and EHRs, they must serve to translate the organization's goals and objectives into terms meaningful to other clinicians.

Work with Patients and Consumers. Find out what is important to patients and consumers that might be part of the HIT and EHR strategy. Examples might include Web portals with health information, including access to their own health records (including test results), the ability to communicate with clinicians or the hospital, the ability to schedule visits or procedures and so forth.

Conclusion

After years of mostly ineffective talk, the forces are now aligned for the successful implementation of HIT and EHRs in countries across the world. Governmental and health industry leaders agree on the need, and if there are differences of opinion as to the degree of value, there is no disagreement that the value is positive. Given the massive size of the healthcare sector in the economy as well as the complexity of the task, there is no shortcut; success is likely to take at least seven to 10 years, or even longer depending on the country and the level of support provided. But what have served in the past as insurmountable barriers to success are now seen as challenges that can be successfully addressed by all of the individuals and organizations affected. When people of good will, supported by visionary public policy and resources, put in the effort, success will follow. ■

Achieving High Performance in Healthcare

accenture

High performance. Delivered.

Healthcare is changing significantly, bringing healthcare organizations new pressures that mount daily. Expenditures as a percent of gross domestic product have grown in most countries, and the trend shows no sign of abating. Organizations are being challenged by legislative and regulatory mandates, scarce resources, new technologies, patient safety concerns, access to data and privacy needs. Accenture understands these issues and is committed to improving the quality, access and affordability of healthcare around the world.

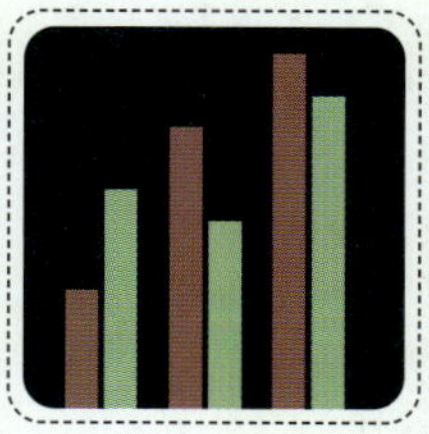

With deep industry, process, technology and change management expertise, we span the entire healthcare industry, providing our clients with insights into existing and emerging technologies and business trends.

With experienced, dedicated staff, world-class technology platforms and a proven track record, we have the expertise to transform healthcare organizations into high-performance businesses. We deliver innovative approaches – through creating and implementing revolutionary strategies for growth and savings, developing new business and operating models and coming up with new ways of using emerging information technologies. This enables our clients to transform their clinical, business, technology, processes and operations to deliver the right care at the right time to the right patient.

Accenture's clients in the private and public health sectors include integrated healthcare providers, health insurers, managed care organizations, public health organizations and pharmaceutical, biotechnology and medical products companies.

- National health services or public health departments in the United Kingdom, United States, Spain, Australia and Singapore;
- Twenty-one out of 24 health companies in the FORTUNE® Global 500;
- Four of the 10 largest healthcare providers in the United States;
- Nine of the 10 largest health plans in the United States; and
- One hundred percent of the FORTUNE® Global 500 pharmaceutical companies.

Expertise, Research And Innovation

With deep industry, process, technology and change management expertise, we span the entire healthcare industry, providing our clients with insights into existing and emerging technologies and business trends.

Our People

With more than 115,000 people in 48 countries, we are among the world's leading management consulting, technology services and outsourcing companies. Some 5,000 Accenture professionals are dedicated to our healthcare clients, and our teams include Ph.D.s, researchers, physicians, pharmacists, nurses, dentists and agency administrators, as well as senior executives from key public and private industry segments, who add their expertise to our client work.

Our Research

As part of our commitment to enhancing knowledge in the healthcare environment, we are teaming with the Vanderbilt Center for Better Health through Informatics in the United States. Together we are fielding research to define the attributes of high-performance healthcare organizations – those that are transforming the way information is used to bring better healthcare services to consumers – and to understand how collaboration will affect the future of the healthcare industry.

Innovative Technologies

At Accenture Technology Labs, the technology research and development organiza-

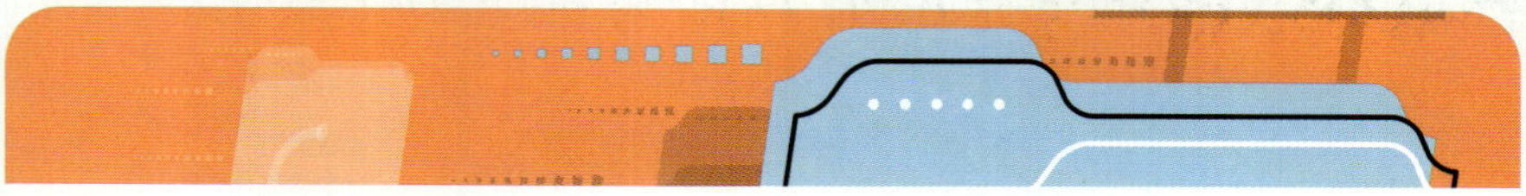

A Large United States Healthcare Provider

Formed from the merger of three organizations, this health provider called on Accenture to help it address a number of business challenges, including declining volumes, revenues and margins on its core business, and deteriorating accounts receivable performance. We helped the client develop its overall business strategies, re-engineer processes to improve cash flow and lower days sales outstanding and develop a plan for consolidating clinical and administrative systems across all clinical locations. With Accenture's help, the provider has dramatically improved its volumes, revenues and margins, leading to an eightfold increase in share price and to more than $90 million in incremental cash flow over an 18-month period. Days sales outstanding declined by 45 percent from its peak, and the client is projecting an annual net benefit stream of more than $15 million in reduced operating expenses.

tion within Accenture, we combine deep technical and scientific expertise with business know-how. By turning innovative technologies into business results, we help our clients realize a wide array of safety, quality and efficiency benefits for patients.

For example, the Accenture Digital Observations solution allows physicians to record patient observations technologically, helping them prioritize their patient rounds and optimize staff time, performance and quality of care. Additionally, the Accenture Instant Content Reporting prototype tests the uses of radio frequency identification (RFID) tags to monitor temperature-sensitive products and pharmaceuticals in hospitals and other medical facilities.

Specific Services

Healthcare organizations seeking high performance draw from Accenture's strengths across the spectrum, from idea through execution – through four key areas: strategy, clinical transformation, operations and outsourcing.

Strategy and Transformation Services

Many health systems are plagued by a myriad of financial pressures, including increasing costs, scarce labor, demanding consumers, profit erosion from competition, greater technology and physical plant requirements, and limited access to capital markets. Meeting these challenges requires a marked transformation to deliver high performance.

At Accenture we understand that the foundation of any business strategy is financial and operational security. We help our clients achieve and sustain organizational excellence by enhancing business processes, enabling technology and empowering people. Accenture can help integrate your physician community, increase staff productivity, manage return on investment and extend the life of your current systems. Through revenue and system performance initiatives, we have reduced the cost of operations by as much as 15 percent and generated a significant return on investment for some of the largest health organizations.

Clinical Transformation

Accenture works with clients in the provider and government health industry to enhance their patient care systems, reduce adverse events and improve patient/clinician satisfaction through improved clinical and health information systems. These new systems have a robust range of capabilities, such as computerized physician order entry, electronic medical record-keeping and electronic medication administration. They offer strong potential to enable high performance through reducing medical errors, fostering evidence-based medicine, giving clinicians more time for patient care, and improving financial results. But these systems cannot be implemented overnight. The investment is large, the selection process is difficult and implementation is complex.

Accenture has developed an integrated solution to directly address this need. Clinical transformation optimizes clinical operations by using information technology to help drive quality and improve financial performance. It integrates process improvements and organizational change with enabling technology and helps healthcare providers deliver the best care in an efficient environment through rapid implementation. We focus on getting physicians and nurses to adopt clinical information systems, aligning their behavior around common goals of providing high-quality care. Our approach is proven by a strong track record of quickly delivering world-class clinical outcomes that raise levels of performance. We have helped clients achieve returns on their investments as high as three to one.

Operational and IT Excellence

Top-notch operations underlie the success of our clients' strategy, and Accenture offers vast experience both in clinical and

National Health Service of the United Kingdom

For the NHS, we are designing, building and managing key information systems to improve the delivery of patient care and services in the northeast and east regions. Specifically, we are developing a system to electronically capture patients' medical histories, ultimately replacing paper records. The electronic management of patient records is designed to bring the right information to the hands of the right individuals at the right time to make critical healthcare decisions. The patient records system aims to support approximately 17 million citizens served by 370,000 members of the NHS staff, in 5,200 general practitioner practices, 167 hospitals and five ambulance trusts.

Department of Human Services of South Australia

When the Department of Human Services of South Australia needed to support care delivery more effectively, it turned to Accenture. We designed, piloted and rolled out electronic patient records, order management and clinical reporting systems. We led a change management effort encompassing complex stakeholder management, process re-engineering, online learning, classroom coaching and training materials practices. Today the program supports eight hospitals and almost 10,000 users, covering more than 2.5 million patients and more than 210 million service records. Access to patient records across multiple care facilities has been enhanced, and the improved quality of information has led to a higher standard of care.

accenture

High performance. Delivered.

National Health Group of Singapore

The National Health Group (NHG) of Singapore is on a journey to transform itself from a group of independent health services organizations, affiliated through membership in the NHG, that operate as an integrated cluster to deliver seamless, accessible, high-quality healthcare and patient centric service. Accenture is leading the first initiative in this program, which covers the design, build and delivery of harmonized processes and supporting systems across the patient management, patient accounting, finance and materials management functions of the NHG. Accenture also will provide health application management services to NHG beyond the deployment phase.

back-office healthcare operations. With a world-class understanding of technology, we explore new operating models with clients to help enhance their supply chain (including RFID) and revenue cycle operations. We integrate systems, aligning them with clients' goals and strategies, we design care processes that incorporate proven advances in managing clinical information and we provide learning and education services.

We understand that each client's needs are distinct. For some, we revamp and implement enterprisewide technology or help them select or optimize current software, ranging from order entry to advanced decision support. For others, we provide critical infrastructure support, including change management, project management, office setup/operation and privacy, security and architecture design. For still others, we create data warehouses. And for large, complex environments, we design, build and manage end-to-end electronic health records or develop predictive models of demand and utilization. In each case, excellent operations help the healthcare organization realize its strategy.

Outsourcing

When healthcare clients decide that creating clinical research infrastructures, supply chains and revenue cycles – or managing human resources, finance, learning and IT – are not core functions, they outsource them to us. As an experienced guide, we bring proven practices to our healthcare outsourcing capabilities, keeping a vigilant eye on clients' strategies and operational needs. Because we're in the business of running these operations, we know the pitfalls involved and how to avoid them. As a result, our clients can focus on delivering excellent healthcare, meeting business challenges and improving performance.

For over a decade we have been working with industry leaders to innovate and build outsourcing as an indispensable business tool. Leading organizations delegate technology-intensive processes to Accenture, which owns, administers and manages the processes, provides service according to defined metrics and continuously improves the processes over time.

At Accenture, our unique, strategicapproach to resolving client issues and our ability to deliver innovative solutions help move organizations to a higher level of performance. For more information on how we can help your healthcare business achieve high performance, go to www.accenture.com.

About Accenture's Health & Life Sciences Group

Accenture's Health & Life Sciences professionals deliver innovation and insight to both the private and public sectors of the marketplace, which includes integrated healthcare providers, health insurers, managed care organizations, public health organizations and pharmaceutical, biotechnology and medical products companies. With more than 5,000 professionals dedicated to serving the global Health & Life Sciences industry, Accenture is committed to working with clients across the industry to help them achieve and sustain high performance. We have worked with companies of all sizes, including 21 of 24 healthcare and pharmaceutical companies in the Fortune Global 500. ■

Accenture is a global management consulting, technology services and outsourcing company that collaborates with its clients to help them become high-performance businesses and governments.

William D. Green
Chief Executive Officer

Stephen J. Rohleder
Chief Operating Officer

Michael G. McGrath
Chief Financial Officer

R. Timothy Breene
Chief Strategy Officer and Group Chief Executive, Business Consulting

Accenture
Phone 312.693.5900
www.accenture.com

For more information
To discover how Accenture can help your organization achieve higher performance, call 312. 693.5900.

1

The Real Challenge in Implementing EHRs

The key to a successful implementation lies not so much in the system itself, but in the overall ability of the organization to manage the change.

[Adam J. Schreiber, RSM McGladrey Business Consulting Services] [Kate W. Galambos, R.N., M.S.N., RSM McGladrey Business Consulting Services]

The implementation of an EHR (electronic health records) system in an ambulatory care environment must be done carefully and utilize a disciplined approach. This approach should involve multiple phases and begin with in-depth planning. In planning, organizations must define the project structure, roles, responsibilities, detailed work plans, staff assignments, communications and administrative details. Ongoing administration and management of the project continues throughout and beyond the project and includes project management, status meetings, status reporting and quality assurance reviews. Components of the implementation include project management, change management with workflow redesign, technical services and end-user training. Each project phase requires planning, execution and evaluation phases. Essential to project success is a robust project team and an atmosphere of partnership among all entities involved.

Many modern practice management and EHR systems contain similar functionality, are easy to use and address virtually all aspects of the organization's requirements (e.g., registration and scheduling, billing, clinical reporting and workflow). Thus the key to a successful implementation lies not so much in the system itself, but in the overall ability of the organization to manage the change. Essential elements of change management are planning, communication, organization and resource allocation.

Planning

During the early phase of the implementation, the vendor and/or consultants work with the client project team to systematically plan the implementation, assign the needed resources, and begin work on needed tasks. At first, the client project team members will have limited knowledge of what they will be expected to do. As the project evolves, they will learn their roles and responsibilities, and become increasingly comfortable with making EHR-related decisions.

The final outcome of a well-planned implementation is the transfer of accountability for the system to the organization. By the end of the project, organizational lines of responsibility for the EHR should be well-defined and accepted. There should be a clear procedure in place for EHR support, both for technical and clinical documentation and care management issues, and also for communicating enhancement requests to the vendor. Additionally, post-implementation strategies such as monthly EHR staff meetings should be employed consistently, as should planning for training new employees.

Throughout the planning phase and beyond, it is important for the organization to have a clear vision of its purpose for making the change, and to articulate its goals for the new system. These goals should be concrete, measurable and relevant both to stakeholders and staff. The key to success is to develop shared goals that everyone understands and supports. Having a shared vision helps everyone overcome the rough spots that inevitably will occur as the project is implemented.

Goal-Oriented Project Planning

Project goals should be realistic and related to sound business practices. It is a truism that a computer system cannot improve business processes that are fundamentally unsound. It is worth the time in the beginning of the project to examine the organization's business processes and determine how the EHR will fit in. If challenges at this juncture are not addressed, they will likely

Adam J. Schreiber is a managing director in the National Healthcare Practice of RSM McGladrey Business Consulting Services, where he manages the healthcare technology consulting group. **Kate W. Galambos R.N., M.S.N.,** is the director of EMR Implementation Services in the National Healthcare Practice of RSM McGladrey Business Consulting Services, and is responsible for the implementation of EMR systems in ambulatory care organizations across the country.

be raised at a later time; during training, for instance, when the resolution will be much more problematic.

When an EHR is implemented, every employee is affected in some way. For example, front desk staff may be asked to change the way they register patients, because the new EHR system needs different information to be entered. Providers will have to change how they write a progress note in the EHR. The daily routine will be disrupted by the training schedules, the need to accommodate implementation consultants in clinic areas and having reduced access to resources and people who are newly busy with project tasks. As a result of these demands, it is natural for the staff to expect an immediate, direct benefit from their sacrifice.

Including short-term staff goals during project planning will help to address this expectation. For example, announcing the increase in the number of EHR visits per day motivates those staff responsible for the task, and helps everyone to appreciate the progress being made. Project leaders should frequently revisit the project goals and inform staff on the organization's progress. Regular reporting of progress toward goals helps everyone stay on board. At the same time, staff input should be solicited, valued and answered. Clearly, a rapid and effective response to problems is an important strategy for keeping the project progressing in a goal-oriented direction.

Planning for Change

An EHR implementation creates a significant organizational change. It is an intense process, because doctors and nurses are being asked to perform their work in a new way. Often change engenders reactions, such as fear or resistance, even anger. Thus carefully managed implementation support and effective change management are critical. Experience has shown that the most successful implementations demonstrate three key features: top-down organizational support for change; well-managed teams that share the tasks of the implementation; and support for the end users who are new to the system by providing them additional time to learn the system while not overburdening them with patient appointments.

Going Paperless

The prospect of going paperless should always be viewed as a long-term goal when adopting an EHR. Although reducing certain paper outputs may be an early outcome, several implementation criteria must be met before a paperless system can be safely instituted. For example, network connectivity must be stable and system downtime minimal, if not absent. Telecommunications, printing, scanning and electronic interfaces must be tested and reliable. Billing and workflow issues must already be evaluated and fine-tuned in the electronic environment. Lacking any one of these criteria could result in a situation in which a paperless deployment would be inconvenient and frustrating, if not counterproductive.

Achieving Full Utilization

If the organization does not achieve 100 percent utilization, the EHR implementation is not complete. Resources will continue to be split, both in workflow and in clinical output. For example, when providers create electronic progress notes and then print the notes and place them into paper charts, there is no reduction in the use of paper (in fact, there may be an increase). The new standard must be that all information is to be entered electronically.

When providers create electronic progress notes and then print the notes and place them into paper charts, there is no reduction in the use of paper (in fact, there may be an increase). The new standard must be that all information is to be entered electronically.

Without 100 percent utilization of the EHR, there are risks. For example, if one provider adds an allergy note to a patient's EHR, but a second provider does not use the EHR, there is a risk that the allergy may be missed. Also since EHRs provide automated drug alerts, providers who do not use the EHR at the point of care may inadvertently create an unsafe practice environment and could be held liable in the case of an adverse event. A top-down, consistent, focused drive toward 100 percent utilization reduces the unstable transition time during the change from the paper to the electronic record.

If going paperless is a long-term goal, 100 percent utilization of the EHR should be considered a primary short-term goal. Only

weblink

Learn how Germany is implementing its electronic health initiative in "Healthcare in Germany Today" in this book and on the Web at www.hctproject.com.

when the system is fully utilized can the expected return on investment be realized. Maintaining parallel paper and electronic systems is not a productive model. It's important to have top-down support for a consistent drive toward full utilization on the part of all users, particularly providers.

After the system has been operational for several months and the learning curve and impact of activation has settled, an assessment can be made to determine if the original objectives of productivity and accuracy have been met. Further enhancements and adjustments are often identified and could result in considerable increase in the benefits of the system.

Categories of Change

Organizing a major change process requires both structure and flexibility. While planning provides the foundation, the process itself will inevitably vary from its predicted parameters. The project team's ability to communicate effectively, provide change leadership and promote organizational goals, will be challenged by the day-to-day demands of the implementation process.

An EHR system enables change in several important areas of ambulatory care: information capture and documentation (including orders and results management); decision support; administrative support; patient support; and public health reporting and management. Most project tasks are organized around making these potential benefits become reality.

Information Capture

An EHR is only as good as the information entered into it. Project leaders must organize their current information sources such as lists, reports, flowsheets, order slips, letters and forms, and determine how the EHR will capture, store, manage and report the data automatically. Personal and departmental agendas must be put aside, and reasonable priorities must be set. Efficiency, access and documentation quality are the goals. Sometimes research will be required to determine whether associated entities will accept the new information outputs (reports, prescriptions, standard referral forms, etc.) that the EHR can produce. Categories of information to be documented in an EHR include:

- Patient information entered directly or indirectly into the EHR;
- Demographic information entered into the EHR directly or obtained via interface or integration with a practice management system;
- Clinical information entered by providers, nursing staff or associates;
- Historical information transferred from paper charts; and
- Documentation from other sources, via scanning, file transfer, interface, integration or email.

For each type of information, consider the automated capabilities of the EHR and select a preferred method for entering the information (e.g., document scanning, point-and-click, keyboard text, templates, system interface, file transfer, voice recognition, etc.). Methods selected for entering data should correspond to the methods chosen for obtaining needed reports on the data that has been entered.

In organizing the workflows needed to deliver the information to the EHR, consider the role of every department, from registration through billing, and eliminate unnecessary documents, tasks and processes.

Reorganizing orders and results management is a daunting task. Implementing an automated system may expose the degree to which the existing system is a patchwork one. However, no matter how flawed the existing orders management system may be, providers and nursing staff are often loathe to change it. Careful assessment by project leaders of the EHR's capabilities, and a consistent plan for implementing orders and results processing, will help prevent glitches.

Decision Support

Because an EHR system is designed to support clinical quality standards, the implementation forces a review of the organization's current clinical quality status, processes and leadership. Because of its capabilities to affect decision making and, ultimately, patient care quality, the new system will influence both formal and informal relationships and hierarchies within the medical

Because of its capabilities to affect decision making and, ultimately, patient care quality, the new system will influence both formal and informal relationships and hierarchies within the medical and administrative groups.

and administrative groups. Thus project management and leadership are critical to the resolution of change issues as they arise. The medical staff should be included in the definition and measurement of clinical goals, tools and resources throughout the project. Provider buy-in requires provider participation. A goal-oriented approach will help to focus the medical staff's participation when the going gets tough and when they are first using the EHR while seeing patients.

Administrative Support

Ambulatory healthcare organizations are characterized by unrelenting administrative burdens, such as insurance eligibility checking, management of paper charts and billing based upon paper encounter forms. In addition, they face clinical burdens associated with busy staff caring for an increasing number of patients per day. Last they face communication challenges such as verbal orders that are often not effectively documented and captured for billing. To cope with these challenges, real-world clinical workflows have evolved to a conglomerate of workarounds. For example, to ensure that charts are not misfiled or lost, providers hide them in desk drawers. Another example is nurses calling the pharmacy to refill a prescription before the physician has signed it, because waiting for a signature delays the patient too long.

In comparison an EHR is designed to follow simple if-then, cause-and-effect rules. Because the EHR introduces this element of logic into the clinic workflow, home-grown solutions and informal hierarchies of influence, authority and power within the organization are challenged. The organization's ability to cope with these changes determines the eventual success of the system implementation.

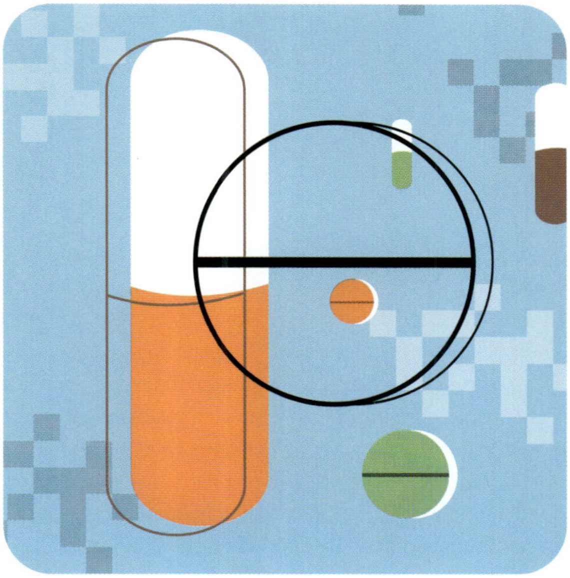

Patient Support

An important aspect of change with an EHR is the shift in the notion of data ownership. The electronic chart allows both caregivers and patients expanded access to patient data. Soon patients will maintain custody of their personal medical data via personal health records, and continuity-of-care records will be standard in EHRs. Furthermore patients will increasingly participate in the entering and viewing of medical data in the electronic chart, via pre-admission histories and chief complaint recording, and viewing of graphs, patient education and other automated features, shared by the provider in the exam room.

Organizing new strategies in the ambulatory care setting in response to these trends requires support for a more open methodology in customer service. It is worth mentioning that patients generally seem positive about their providers using EHRs. EHRs offer convenience for patients, as well as improved patient safety. Thus enlightened administrators and staff will prepare for the day when patients will enjoy extensive access to their electronic charts.

Reporting and Public Health

In the future, insurance companies and government-funded healthcare entities will require data on healthcare delivery to justify claims payments. Additionally quality standards will become linked increasingly to evidence that can be measured via widespread data analysis. EHRs are key to these initiatives because they enable the collection of massive amounts of clinical data in databases.

When preparing the ambulatory care organization to maximize its opportunities in terms of reporting, it is necessary to consider the data input as well as the data extraction. Technical planning for the storage and reporting of data must be comprehensive. On the front end, it is necessary to decide how to control the data that will be captured. Standard terminology sets (such as SNOMED, ICD, CPT or NDC) provide a foundation. However, more challenging will be the need to standardize clinical terms used by providers. Five providers may describe a fracture in five different ways, but for reporting purposes, this can produce inefficiency. Organizing for change by opting for recognized standards, such as the evidence-based criteria published by the Agency for Healthcare Research and Quality, may help.

Workflow Redesign

There are numerous resources that explain process re-engineering/workflow redesign, and the project team should be familiar with the basic tenets. In an ambulatory care organization, the redesign of workflow involves several concerns. First is the existing pattern of responsibility and authority for front-office activities. This is because the EHR system will expose inconsistencies in frontdesk operations, so change leadership falls to the leaders in these areas. Billing and medical records departments will also be affected. Often these department leaders are already swamped with work. Finding ways to organize them into effective workflow redesign teams is a challenge. Sometimes holding a brief ad hoc meeting when a problem occurs is effective. However, this is only effective if there is consistent follow-up. Department leaders deserve full respect, and their views and opinions should be solicited.

Another concern is the inclusion of staff in workflow redesign activities. A tenet of workflow redesign theory is to include the front-line workers, because they are the most familiar with how things are done. Staff opinions matter, and many of their ideas are valuable. Needed is a method for organizing their input and assigning responsibility so as to prevent negative reactions when someone's idea is not implemented. Effective communication and maintaining a goal-oriented, organized approach to change management will help structure the process. Often, in fact, one or more staff members are naturally suited to this work and become innovators or champions for change. The project leaders should take notice and empower these people whenever possible.

Making the System 'Smart'

An important aspect of the EHR implementation is helping the organization to use the new system in a "smart" way. Taking advantage of system features is key to improving overall efficiency. For example, the automation of flowsheets provides an opportunity to capitalize on the new system's capabilities. Most ambulatory care organizations rely heavily on flowsheet documents, developed by in-house experts to record and track data that was otherwise getting lost. A flowsheet must be used consistently. Yet the reality is that time constraints, lack of training or simple neglect frequently result in incomplete, outdated flowsheets.

To improve upon this process, an EHR can automate the flowsheet, so that its information is managed automatically within the EHR. The problem arises when staff cannot let go of the in-house flowsheet document and create a flat version of the flowsheet within the EHR without taking advantage of automated features. The result is a "dumb" document with limited value. A better option is to deconstruct the flowsheet, apply appropriate system features, and redefine the workflow that underlies the flowsheet to help end users obtain the same results in a more efficient manner. Helping end users let go of inefficient tools and embrace new strategies is a common challenge for implementation specialists.

Resource Allocation

The administration of an EHR system requires new responsibilities, or new challenges for meeting responsibilities already in place. For example, in the area of security, the electronic record requires additional layers of security beyond those in place for protecting the paper record. A password policy and procedure must be developed, and responsibility for maintaining and updating these procedures must be assigned. To protect patient confidentiality, user access to the EHR needs to be planned and set up. Decisions about which identifying information will be entered on each end user are needed. Procedures for adding new users, maintaining hardware and equipment, preventing theft, managing interfaces and performing regular database back ups will be required. Because most EHRs contain links to the Internet, IT support staff will have new challenges in terms of protecting the internal network from viruses and other external threats, as well as communicating to staff their role in maintaining system security. Auditing system access, protecting data integrity and data archiving are other challenges the EHR will bring about.

At the day-to-day support level of service, the IT department should undertake an annual diagnostic review assisted by an outside independent resource. The objective would be to review the presence, status and adherence of departmental policies and procedures and other professional practices. It is not necessary that an outside resource assist in the review, but it is difficult when being responsive to the day-to-day demand for continuous quality service to be objective in viewing this type of activity.

Once the formal training is finished, the burden of supporting the implementation of the EHR shifts to the organization. Many ongoing changes will occur as the system is integrated into all of the daily processes of the organization. Within a year, an administrative structure should evolve that supports the utilization of the system, provides for IT and training support and identifies the ways the system can now contribute to the overall success of the organization. ■

Because most EHRs contain links to the Internet, IT support staff will have new challenges in terms of protecting the internal network from viruses and other external threats, as well as communicating to staff their role in maintaining system security.

Readiness

As payers and providers move toward a connected EHR, each must take tactical steps to play a part in the early evolution.

[Joe Poats, Accenture]

There is so much hype about electronic health records (EHRs) that a rational and pragmatic approach is required. Many organizations have jumped in, only to waste time and money figuring it all out. A practical model for engaging in the EHR journey is the survey, align, launch (SAL) model, which describes how an organization or community implements EHR (see Figure 1).

Take Stock

The first step in computerizing health records at the community level is to take inventory of computer systems that are in place. Many physicians' offices, public health clinics, hospitals and payers have existing computerized patient records (hospitals), electronic medical records (physician practices and clinics) and e-prescribing automation. However, these systems are not typically well- connected and in many cases are not capable of being connected. This is where the EHR initiative comes into play. "In this age, we can't waste a nickel. It is very important to truly look at what needs to be accomplished from the community and organization perspective, and take advantage of the assets that exist," says Zan Calhoun, CIO for HealthCare Partners, a large healthcare organization in Southern California.

Part of this inventory step involves looking at what other groups have accomplished in converting electronic records. This includes early collaboration with payers, providers and government entities within a town, state, county and national framework – however a "community" is defined. For example, the National Health Information Network and regional health information organizations are getting established in many areas. Before beginning an EHR initiative, organizations must determine what has been accomplished and how to link to these initiatives and infrastructures efficiently.

Organizations must also evaluate current internal standards and architectures by taking stock of in-house platforms and whether those platforms are interoperable with other systems in their community.

Agree on Standards

Health Level 7 (HL7) is the leading, ANSI-accredited, international standard for data exchange between computer systems in healthcare. It enables interoperability between healthcare information systems, such as electronic patient administration and management systems, laboratory information systems, dietary, pharmacy and billing systems as well as EHR systems. SNOMED and LOINC have also been endorsed nationally for laboratory data exchange. Building upon established standards is wise, and will reduce future headaches.

At a minimum, determining if an organization will be compatible with these standards sets the stage for evaluating interoperability issues down the road. Subsequently the community of organizations will also have to standardize their definitions of processes and events within the community that trigger the sharing of clinical information.

Leverage What Is Already Going on

HIPAA forced substantial standardization. Some organizations are using HIPAA reforms as a springboard to share information and standardization practices at the transaction level. This is an excellent example of collaboration that has already occurred around sharing health information.

Another example of collaboration already in process is the work being performed around e-prescribing, which leverages demands in the Medicare Modernization Act that physicians and pharmacies work on together to dramatically streamline the pre-

Joe Poats is a partner with Accenture, responsible for provider technology services for North America. His role includes planning, designing and implementing process and technology solutions, and leading design and implementation projects for healthcare providers (hospital systems, academic medical centers and large physician groups), involving complex process and technology change.

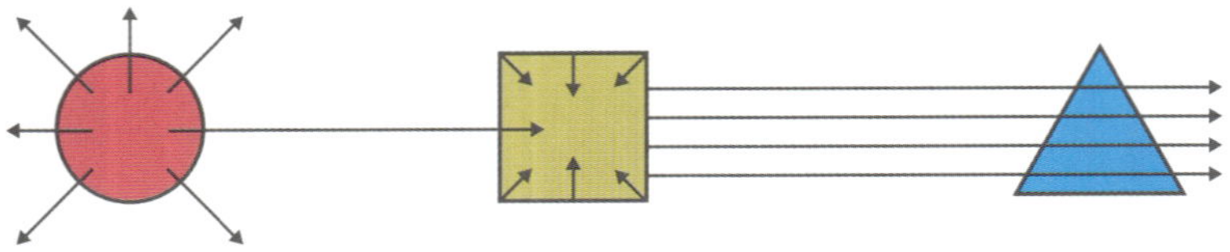

Survey

- Test true interest – is there a possible strategic alignment?
- Assess EHR readiness
- Take Stock – See what is already going on around you
- Investigate appropriate standards

Align

- Define your organization's role in and use of EHR
- Clarify expectations
- Develop organizational strategy
- Uncover and remove barriers to change
- Leverage what is going on

Launch

- Create group alignment and intention to act
- Appoint EHR czar
- Engage the community, especially the physicians
- Initiate/join in community dialogue
- Develop business case
- Form team
- Communicate

Figure 1 The SAL Model describes how an organization or community implements EHR.

scribing process. By sharing some of the interoperability and standardization issues that have already been accomplished through e-prescribing, payers, providers, physicians and patients can apply lessons learned toward EHR initiatives.

Appoint an EHR Czar

A logical strategy is to designate a leader to be the EHR "czar" in an organization. "All eyes usually go to the CIO for this role, but in a lot of situations, this role is probably better served by someone who is in the fray of relationships between physicians, hospitals, clinics, employers and payers," says Tom Martin, CIO for UW Medicine, a large academic and community-based health organization serving the Seattle area. "An EHR czar can help establish a business case for community efforts and prioritize among competing sets of initiatives that might otherwise diffuse provider efforts." This person acts as a lightning rod for EHR issues and tracks the efforts of their organization's strategic vendors.

There are many strategic and tactical options a healthcare organization can implement to begin electronic recordkeeping. However, these applications must be compatible with an organization's overall EHR system strategy. By picking one accountable person to be the expert, payers and providers reduce the risk of purchasing multiple systems that are incompatible with future EHR initiatives.

Develop an Organizational Strategy

After appointing an EHR czar, organizations must develop a strategy around community EHR implementation. Although this may seem like an organization's IT systems strategy, it is not. According to Larry Lotenero, CIO for the University of California San Francisco Medical Center, "It is all about how the electronic health record benefits the community and how each constituent views their role in that community. Return on investment is critical, but so is improving the health status of a population." A community EHR organizational strategy must encompass initiatives within communities and the state and national healthcare arenas.

A solid community EHR strategy requires careful research – both within an organization's four walls and out in the community. Payers and providers must define the value for all players, including patients. From this research, a business plan must be developed to put facts and figures around the proposed EHR investments. This solidifies buy-in and creates a clear road map for implementation.

Engage Physicians

The consumer is central to the EHR. Aside from the patient/consumer, physicians are the most important cog in the EHR wheel because they are most directly involved with using data in an EHR. For example, a physician admits patients to more than one hospital and typically participates in more than one health plan. Because the patient population is not oriented toward any one hospital, it becomes necessary to standardize information at the point of entry – with physicians.

This is an excellent example of why orchestration of an interconnected community EHR absolutely requires collaboration from the very beginning between physicians, between physicians and health systems and between physicians and payers. Collaboration among physicians creates an excellent forum for sharing best practices.

Begin a Community Dialogue

The EHR czar must initiate a community dialogue as early as possible. This brings different groups together to clearly identify collaboration partners who will share knowledge around electronic patient recordkeeping and establish common objectives.

Although EHR initiatives can be technically challenging, the greatest difficulty is to align the objectives of players with radically different perspectives. For this reason, all community EHR objectives should revolve around consumer and community health. Because a community EHR initiative cannot possibly deliver the same ROI for each participant, setting the goal of improving community health is a logical strategy to move everyone forward.

For example, patient safety is increased by computerized physician order entry (CPOE) in the inpatient setting and by use of an electronic medical record (EMR) system in the physician office/clinic setting. CPOE systems and EMR systems are used by clinicians to order medications/prescriptions directly in computer systems. Such systems have been shown to help dramatically reduce medication errors and should be seamlessly integrated for physicians regardless of where in the community they are using a system. Therefore, EMR and CPOE initiatives are important building blocks in an EHR, but they must be linked at the patient, consumer and physician levels.

Develop a Business Case

After creating a community dialogue and establishing a framework for collaboration, the next step is developing a business case that outlines benefits by constituent. For example, a hospital might make a case for standardizing the interconnection of patient records to improve accuracy and reduce the rework that occurs when patient data are re-entered multiple times.

For a laboratory, the business case might be reducing the number of redundant tests ordered per patient by different physicians. For a payer, improvements in claim submissions due to electronic standardization could lead to fewer pended, rejected and resubmitted claims, resulting in reduced rework, lower processing costs and improved satisfaction.

In addition, overall benefits for a healthcare community must be part of the business case. Examples might include decreasing infant mortality or improving the rate of immunization in the community. By establishing micro- and macro-level benefits, all organizations involved in EHR implementation have a business case to support the necessary time and effort.

The business case must also outline overall cost projections and short-term and long-term sources of funding. This section of the business case is particularly important as it will carry the project forward.

Start Now

Many organizations are intimidated by beginning a community EHR initiative, perhaps because of the sheer magnitude of the project. Others are stalled by lack of funding or buy-in from members of their organizations. These, however, are short-term views. To reap the early benefits, organizations must take the following steps now to leverage a linked EHR system as it begins to deliver value:

- Build a community architecture plan. The best place to start is with infrastructure that already exists. Determine what exists on a regional, statewide and national basis so organizations can tie into these systems and follow established standards.
- Establish a delivery and support model. Payers, providers and other stakeholders must collaborate to decide how to deliver and support a community EHR before addressing individual systems. Questions that must be resolved include where the data will be housed, how the data will stay "clean," who will address security concerns and how the network will be supported.
- Keep it simple. A community EHR is a massive undertaking, so health executives should carve up implementation into small, manageable projects. Unless participants see early wins it will be hard to gain momentum to tackle more difficult issues later.
- Integrate EHR standards and requirements into clinical design. Once all participants agree on how EHR will be implemented communitywide, introduce these standards and requirements for sharing information in-house and incorporate them into clinical design. An example can be seen in the way that HIPAA was addressed. Payers and providers communicated individual system needs and requirements through a HIPAA coordinator. From this information, standards and requirements were developed and incorporated into individual information systems to uphold HIPAA regulations.
- Monitor and communicate success. Establish metrics early on to measure the success of community and local EHR initiatives. This will hold all players accountable and will communicate early wins within each organization and within the healthcare community.

Summary

As payers and providers move toward a connected EHR, each must undergo a tremendous shift in culture, process and technology. Each must explore the current state of electronic recordkeeping within their individual organizations and within the healthcare community. Selecting a person within each organization to champion the community EHR movement will aid the development of an organizational strategy. This person must reach out to physicians to streamline efforts around a patient-centric system that aids physicians. Early steps also include taking an inventory of current technology and processes to provide stepping stones to early local and then community EHR implementation. Payers and providers must also initiate a community dialogue consistent both with individual and group strategies. As part of this collaboration, the group must establish community goals at the heart of the effort and communicate these goals through a business case. The business case must also provide overall cost projections and potential funding sources. The most important thing is to get started. By coming together now to establish proposed architecture, delivery, standards and requirements, all players will be ready to embrace an evolving community EHR model as it unfolds. ■

weblink

Learn more about local health infrastructure initiatives in the interview with Micky Tripathi in this book and on the Web at www.hctproject.com.

Take Control With Healthcare Document Solutions From FedEx Kinko's

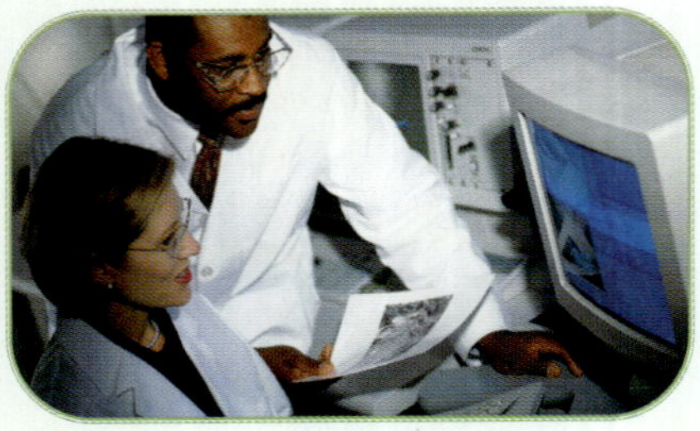

In order to meet the growing demands placed on today's healthcare systems, processes and people, healthcare organizations are constantly looking for simple ways to improve efficiencies and streamline operations.

With resources, facilities and funds growing scarcer, and governmental mandates and regulations on the rise, more and more healthcare organizations are turning to outsourcing providers for a broad range of services, such as document production and management to help meet these new demands.

Whenever a gurney rolls down the hospital hallway, a doctor picks up an instrument or a nurse tends a patient, a paper record results. The central role that these documents play in healthcare is best captured in a single statistic: According to the American Hospital Association, every 30 minutes to one hour of patient care results in one hour of accompanying paperwork that must be properly documented and communicated.

Along with being a big-budget item for hospitals, documents can also be a big headache. With increasing paperwork comes greater potential for human mistakes. And lost paperwork can lead to non-reimbursed services, with hospitals and other healthcare organizations absorbing the cost. In recent months, the issue of electronic health records (EHRs) has captured considerable attention as a way of alleviating this increase in paperwork. EHRs are being adopted with the goals of improving patient safety, reducing human error and lowering document costs.

According to a 2003 study by CAP Ventures, the healthcare industry prints more than 100 billion pages each year. Of these documents, 75 percent are primarily black-and-white forms such as standing orders, preprinted orders, patient care maps and hundreds of other documents vital to tracking, scheduling and administering patient care.

In addition to forms used for tracking patients and treatment, as well as those used to meet administrative and regulatory requirements, other document types in the healthcare setting include:

- Publication documents – Directories, manuals, user guides and newsletters;
- Transaction documents – Invoices, statements, evidences of coverage, contracts and policies;
- Utility documents – Forms, labels, stationery, envelopes and business cards;
- Office documents – Memos, reports and presentations;
- Promotional documents – Brochures, catalogs and direct mail; and
- Patient-specific materials – Educational, correspondence and identification materials.

These documents have a significant financial and operational impact on the stability of a healthcare institution. Too often, valuable resources are wasted dealing with things like printing costs and logistics – redirecting their focus away from more critical operational or patient care issues.

Healthcare's Variable-Cost, On-Demand Printing Solutions

As healthcare organizations continue to implement print-on-demand solutions, print service providers such as FedEx Kinko's become valuable partners in analyzing document workflow and identifying areas for improved efficiencies and cost reductions.

Replacing the costs and inefficiencies of the in-house print shop with the print-on-demand capabilities of a document service provider can provide healthcare organizations with an array of benefits. Instead of producing and storing large quantities of documents that ultimately become obsolete and go unused, organizations can employ online catalogs, centralized content management and other service provider capabilities to create, manage and maintain a broad range of document types. Forms, training manuals, marketing brochures and other documents can be produced in whatever quantities needed, with significant savings in paper, printing and storage.

Healthcare Document Solutions from FedEx Kinko's delivers variable-cost document outsourcing solutions that can remove fixed printing costs from a healthcare organization's balance sheet.

Changing the Rules of Document Services in Healthcare

Traditional document solutions cost time, space and money due to expensive print overruns, documents that eventually become obsolete, warehousing and fulfillment. Together, these costs can eat away at a healthcare organization's bottom line.

What's more, traditional document solutions have historically required healthcare organizations to lease copiers, printers and other devices for use in centralized reproduction, at the department level. These systems generally come with rigid requirements, such as three- to five-year contracts for equipment and service that dictate minimum usage fees. Even worse, they place fixed costs on the books. Supply contracts and maintenance agreements have compounded the problem, as have rapid technological advancements that render equipment obsolete.

Organizations also tie up human capital in running on-site print shops. Fixed costs for training employees and keeping them in jobs not related to the facility's core business, coupled with the expense of real estate dedicated to noncore activities, contribute to inefficiency as well.

Additionally traditional solutions only offer a limited scope of print technology, depending upon a vendor's equipment and service offerings.

That is why FedEx Kinko's has introduced Healthcare Document Solutions: a simpler, more cost-effective way to produce medical documents and forms.

FedEx Kinko's: The Total Document Solution For Healthcare Providers

FedEx Kinko's unique variable-cost model has made standardized printing packages and costly contracts extinct. Healthcare Document Solutions from FedEx Kinko's delivers variable-cost document outsourcing solutions that can remove fixed printing costs from a healthcare organization's balance sheet. This model can dramatically reduce a healthcare provider's costs of labor, shipping, real estate and inventory. FedEx Kinko's customers have reported savings of up to 25 percent or more.

The partnership starts with FedEx Kinko's analyzing the costs associated with an organization's existing document workflow. These include machine utilization rates, monthly document production volumes, supplies consumption, manpower and billing procedures.

By eliminating fixed costs for property, equipment and labor, healthcare institutions only pay for the documents that are produced. The result is simple, predictable pricing and substantial savings in document-related expenses.

What Can Healthcare Document Solutions From FedEx Kinko's Do for You?

Lower costs:

- Eliminate equipment leasing and operating cost;
- Eliminate document obsolescence and waste;
- Take advantage of easy-to-understand pricing;
- Reduce warehousing, distribution and fulfillment costs; and
- Eliminate nonessential vendors and suppliers.

Increase productivity and workflow:

- Access state-of-the-art technology;
- Reduce downtime;
- Redeploy staff to perform critical tasks;
- Improve speed of document production; and
- Reinvest capital in what's really important – your patients.

On-Demand Opportunities For an On-Call Industry

Print-on-demand solutions from FedEx Kinko's harness the power of electronic storage and distribution capabilities to create significant value for a healthcare organization, a concept that healthcare providers are already embracing with electronic health records management. The ability to create, revise, update, order, distribute and print forms online and on-demand with FedEx Kinko's offers significant cost and productivity improvement benefits, including:

- Electronic document storage;
- Elimination of the need for expensive warehousing programs.
- Quick and easy revision and updating of printed documents; and
- Reduced inventory waste and obsolescence.

The pressures on the healthcare industry to contain costs while delivering quality care show no signs of abating. Instead providers are challenged to wring even greater efficiency out of their operations. By capitalizing on the opportunities of variable-cost on-demand printing solutions, healthcare institutions can take a major step toward that goal, all while maintaining their focus on healing and health. ■

FedEx Kinko's
Office and Print Services

FedEx Kinko's Office and Print Services is the world's leading provider of document solutions and business services.

Gary Kusin
President and
Chief Executive Officer

Ken May
Executive Vice President and
Chief Operating Officer

John McDonald
Executive Vice President
Commercial Document
Solutions

Bill Keffeler
Regional Vice President
Healthcare and Strategic
Accounts

FedEx Kinko's
13155 Noel Road, Ste. 1600
Dallas, TX 75240
Phone 888.546.5671
www.fedexkinkos.com/commercial

Business Contact
Phone 888.546.5671
business.development@
fedexkinkos.com

Toward the Future of Healthcare Information Work

IT tools for healthcare information workers are now converging in the direction of the workers' natural skills and practices, which give people the tools to manage information effectively in a complex environment.

[Bill Crouse, M.D., Microsoft]

According to a report from Boston University, 50 percent of the $1.9 trillion that will be spent on healthcare in the United States in 2005 will be lost to waste, excessive pricing and fraud. That makes improving productivity and efficiency in healthcare a critical priority for patients, providers and payers. But improving efficiency cannot come at the expense of two of healthcare's most important goals: improving outcomes and extending access – objectives that almost always come with added costs.

IT will play a vital role in any effort to tackle the issues that the industry is grappling with today while ensuring that it continues to meet the goals and expectations we have as a society for healthcare. Technology innovations have been the catalyst for a new generation of IT solutions that have delivered new levels of efficiency and productivity for a broad range of industries. Because healthcare is so information-intensive and collaborative, the same innovations that have transformed other industries by targeting the information needs of "information workers" offer great promise for the healthcare field.

Information worker technology is especially critical because nearly everyone employed in healthcare is fundamentally an information worker. Physicians, nurses, administrators and support staff all depend on having access to the right information at the right time in the optimal format in order to make the decisions that are critical to their jobs. But the healthcare industry has been among the slowest to adopt the kind of IT solutions that have driven efficiencies and productivity improvements in so many other sectors.

There are many reasons that adoption in the medical field has been so slow, including the high cost and complexity of IT infrastructure, the limitations and difficulty of proprietary applications and the lack of standards. Habit plays a role as well. Traditional practices based on paper records, handwritten notes, informal meetings and face-to-face conferences and consultations are deeply entrenched. Unfortunately the combination of paper-based, manual information management methods and increasing complexity has given rise to a seemingly never-ending spiral of rising costs, narrowing access and increasing inconsistency in care quality across the industry.

The lack of a standard for electronic health records (EHRs) is clearly one of the key bottlenecks that impedes the industry's attempts to reign in rising costs. According to an article in *Medical Economics,* the widespread use of electronic records could save 20 percent of the total of all healthcare costs, while reducing medical mistakes and drastically improving healthcare quality.

The Foundation for Successful Healthcare Information Technology Adoption Today

What will it take to enable healthcare organizations to move away from outdated and inefficient modes of information management and begin to more fully take advantage of EHRs and other technology solutions that streamline patient data creation, storage and access?

The starting point is tools that are matched to both business requirements and information worker skills and practices. Good, effective tools are those that provide easy access to data, processes and people, anywhere and anytime. In healthcare, where timely delivery of correct information can spell the difference between life and death, information workers place a premium on data that can be communicated clearly and succinctly using the simplest available interface and is mobile enough to keep pace with the fast-moving clinical environment.

Before it can replace traditional practices, an EHR solution must meet this need for simplicity, speed and portability. That means interfaces must be intuitive. Because keyboard input

Bill Crouse, M.D., is global healthcare industry manager for Microsoft's Healthcare & Life Sciences Industry Group. He is responsible for working with industry partners and healthcare organizations to help them benefit from using Microsoft technologies and solutions as an essential platform for line-of-business applications in the healthcare industry.

is neither comfortable nor practical in many clinical scenarios, tools that allow natural input via digital ink, voice, touch-screen or point-and-click are essential. Applications also need to run on mobile devices and must provide easy ways to connect to central data stores.

Ease of use and access are not the only requirements. Many first-generation healthcare IT products were based on closed, proprietary technology, accessible only through dedicated applications with difficult, inflexible interfaces. Today's solutions must be able to integrate with these systems in meaningful ways. Newer architectures should be interoperable and interconnected, using open standards and a highly distributed model to share information not only among hospitals, clinics and physician offices, but with insurance providers, government agencies and patients.

The final requirement for EHR systems and other IT solutions is low cost of ownership. There are many high-cost components of the healthcare system – for example, expertise, equipment and insurance – that are perceived as more central to the core mission of providing care than computers and software. The IT tools that can drive better outcomes, greater efficiency and wider access to healthcare must be based on a proven, standard and affordable platform for information work.

Current tools based on Microsoft® products such as Microsoft Office InfoPath®, Microsoft SharePoint® Team Services, Microsoft Office Live Meeting and Microsoft BizTalk® Server provide the foundation for comprehensive electronic record systems that meet all of these requirements. Today these products are delivering enormous benefits across the healthcare system, from clinical care to billing and compliance.

The Future of Healthcare Information Work

More widespread adoption of standard EHR systems is an important near-term priority across the healthcare industry. At the same time there are other innovations in information worker technology on the horizon that will extend the power and value of EHRs, driving better outcomes, greater access and lower costs that are consistent with the priorities of the healthcare industry and its customers.

Currently Microsoft is working on a number of emerging technologies that promise to optimize today's EHR solutions by making them more pervasive and less intrusive. These new technologies will add greater automation of low-value activities; smarter, simpler interfaces that can anticipate user needs based on context and observed behavior; improved security that provides more control over sensitive information; ways to model and present complex data in real time; and features that capitalize on lighter, more powerful mobile devices, new form factors for digital devices and new ways to interact with data in the physical world.

These are just a few of the emerging innovations that offer the promise of new approaches to the way patient information is created, stored and accessed through EHR systems in the coming decade and beyond.

> Innovations in information worker technology on the horizon will extend the power and value of EHRs, driving better outcomes, greater access and lower costs that are consistent with the priorities of the healthcare industry and its customers.

Pattern Recognition Technology

While the problems of searching through multiple file systems and formats is being addressed through EHR systems, the task of navigating databases and forming queries to produce relevant results remains a challenge. Pattern recognition technology that simulates human decision-making processes will make the next generation of information worker tools much more context-sensitive. This technology will automate many of the mental steps that workers themselves must now perform, yielding greater speed and better quality of information while enabling healthcare workers to base their decisions on the most solid foundation of data.

Smart Documents

Pattern recognition provides the first layer of efficiency in information management. But often, even well-chosen documentary information is not sufficient to answer the question at hand. Access to the people who authored a document can be critical to getting the information needed to take action. Today locating the right people involves phone calls, leaving messages and waiting to hear back. At best the process is uncertain; at worst there is no way to identify the author of a document.

"Smart documents" provide the solution. Smart documents contain metadata that dynamically tracks authorship and provides tags to assist in search and retrieval. Author information will communicate with collaboration applications such as contact managers, email, instant messaging and presence detection, providing the information necessary to follow up with the author and even determine whether the author is available immediately to respond to questions.

RFID

New technologies will also provide new and better streams of critical information in real time. Radio frequency identification (RFID) chips – tiny transmitters that broadcast a data signature to land- and satellite-based receivers – are already being used to track inventory in the manufacturing and retail industries. For healthcare, RFID has the potential to introduce dramatic new efficiencies in patient care by providing rich real-time information on patient health, regulating the release of medication and communicating with other devices to reduce errors, assist nurses and clinicians and provide data for more accurate diagnosis and treatment.

Using RFID-based technology, a single nurse can monitor an entire ward with precision and real-time responsiveness from one workstation. Subcutaneous RFID devices for patients could communicate with similar devices embedded in medication labels to alert caregivers to potential allergies or errors in dosage. Outpatients could be monitored remotely, with care dispatched automatically in the event of an emergency.

In reports created from multiple documents, confidential content that compromises privacy or security would be automatically removed. And individual fields of medical records could be easily shared for research or compliance purposes.

Adaptive Interfaces

For physicians and nurses, easily comprehensible information display is essential. Interfaces that are counterintuitive and complex can be worse than useless in critical situations. Today many computer applications allow users to customize the way information is presented, but this is a static rather than dynamic process. Using pattern recognition and machine-learning technology, the next generation of information worker applications for healthcare will feature adaptive interfaces that provide clearer, simpler access to relevant information without the need for the user to learn complex features or continually reconfigure applications depending on the circumstance.

Information Rights Management

Maintaining control over who has access to documents is one of the most important problems that the healthcare industry faces. Microsoft Office 2003 includes information rights management (IRM) features for setting permissions on access and transfer of documents. This is an enormous step forward in the protection of intellectual property and confidentiality.

However, current IRM schemes work only at the document level. Evolving IRM technology will enable rights management of content at a more granular level, allowing individual words, lines or paragraphs of documents, cells and formulas of spreadsheets, fields in data records, or slides in a Microsoft PowerPoint® presentation to be tagged as hidden to users who lack proper security credentials.

In healthcare, this means that providers, administrators, payers, regulators and patients could all have access to the same document, but with different views based on their roles and security level. In reports created from multiple documents, confidential content that compromises privacy or security would be automatically removed. And individual fields of medical records could be easily shared for research or compliance purposes without disclosing private patient information.

Conclusion

Today, the healthcare industry faces a steep climb toward the productivity gains and efficiencies promised by healthcare IT solutions that are available now. Promoting the widespread adoption of a standard EHR alone will require an investment of hundreds of billions of U.S. dollars.

Organizations facing this kind of commitment can be excused for having some trepidation about the impact of all this new technology on an industry that has always run on human expertise. How will new information worker software affect the ability of doctors, nurses and administrators to do their jobs? Will busy professionals need to learn new skills and adapt to uncomfortable new procedures to realize the productivity and efficiency benefits that are so urgently needed?

These are reasonable questions. But the fact is that IT tools for healthcare information workers are now converging in the direction of the workers' natural skills and practices, giving people the tools to manage information effectively in a complex environment. ■

Streamline Information Flow, Control Costs and Improve Patient Care

Microsoft®

The healthcare industry faces rising costs, declining profitability and widespread inefficiency. Meanwhile, a fast-changing regulatory environment and pressure to improve quality, safety and access are driving industry transformations. Microsoft Collaborative Healthcare solutions are helping healthcare providers meet the challenges. As a pioneer in the field, Microsoft understands how people use digital information technologies and has applied that knowledge to the challenges of healthcare providers, health plans and life sciences organizations. Microsoft launched the Collaborative Healthcare initiative to help streamline information flow, control costs and improve patient care.

Patient Information Access: Healthcare Portals

Microsoft healthcare portal solutions provide the foundation for information sharing, enabling physicians, clinicians, nurses and administrators to work together more effectively, respond more quickly and deliver higher-quality care at a lower overall cost. Healthcare portals also provide the infrastructure for better collaboration between caregivers to enable healthcare professionals to access all appropriate clinical and administrative information.

Electronic Health Records

Electronic record management systems built on Microsoft Windows Server™ 2003, Microsoft SQL Server™ 2000, Microsoft Windows Mobile™, the Tablet PC and other Microsoft products and technologies give clinicians instant access to patient data from across a healthcare organization's systems. Microsoft industry partners, such as Eclipsys and Allscripts, use the Microsoft platform to offer EHR solutions that provide intelligent guidance and enable physicians, nurses and administrators to access crucial information wherever and whenever they need it.

Through Online Training, Education and Team Building

Microsoft Office Live Meeting is a communication and collaboration tool that allows healthcare workers to meet from their various locations and conduct grand rounds presentations, clinical case conferences, medical staff meetings, staff training, patient referrals and case consultations using just a computer with an Internet connection and a phone. With Live Meeting, hospitals can ensure that medical staff stays up to date on regulatory compliance, medical data and other critical information, and it makes it easier to form virtual teams of specialists in real time.

Clinical and Administrative Forms Automation

Microsoft clinical and administrative forms automation solutions allow healthcare providers to replace paper forms with digital information processes that automate the way healthcare workers collect and share patient information. Based on InfoPath 2003, BizTalk Server 2004, Windows SharePoint Services and SQL Server 2000, a new Reference Implementation for Clinical Forms consists of downloadable forms, code samples and documentation that automate the collection, retrieval and sharing of patient information.

Business Intelligence

Microsoft offers a set of business intelligence (BI) solutions that deliver insightful analysis to management and healthcare workers alike. Created to provide the building blocks for end-to-end solutions that link systems and data across departments and organizational boundaries, BI solutions from Microsoft and its partners automate manual data analysis processes and ensure that decisions are made based on a complete view of the available data.

Integration

With a typical hospital running dozens of disconnected systems, the difficulties that healthcare workers face in accessing the information they need can be immense: The need to link a wide range of applications running on different platforms is critical. Microsoft Collaborative Healthcare gives healthcare organizations an easier way to manage integration, more cost-effective methods to communicate information back and forth and faster methods of developing and implementing new interfaces among systems. ■

Founded in 1975, Microsoft (Nasdaq: MSFT) is the worldwide leader in software, services and Internet technologies for personal and business computing. The company offers a wide range of products and services designed to empower people through great software – any time, any place and on any device.

Steve Shihadeh
General Manager
Healthcare and Life Sciences

Tim Smokoff
Managing Director
Healthcare and Life Sciences

Microsoft Corp.
One Microsoft Way
Redmond, WA 98052
Phone 425.882.8080
Fax 425.936.7329
www.microsoft.com/healthcare

Business Contact
Laura Bridenback
Industry Marketing Manager, Healthcare
laurab@microsoft.com

The Government Perspective: Public Sector Value and EHR

Understanding how public entities are able to deliver healthcare benefits to their users is important in determining appropriate future spending priorities.

[Rick Wheeler, Accenture] [Janhavi Bonville, Accenture]

The public sector value (PSV) framework appropriates tenets of the private sector's method of evaluating "shareholder value," applies them to government organizations in order to determine the value they create for citizens and evaluates how the maximum benefits from investments in health-related technologies can be achieved.

Definition of PSV

As part of a major research program to identify the characteristics of high-performance businesses and governments, it became clear that a way to identify high performance in the public sector was needed. To address this need, a more holistic approach to measuring value was developed. Designed to work in conjunction with existing performance measures, and flexible enough to be applied globally, the PSV model is a disciplined approach to defining public sector outcomes and quantifying results (see Figure 1).

PSV involves a rigorous approach for measuring and driving value. It uses a quantitative methodology to define an agency's intended results and outcomes, which are a combination of strategic goals and stakeholder expectations. A structured and balanced framework quantifies results by linking achievement of objectives to cost-effectiveness.

In the current political environment, governments must allocate scarce resources in order to perform more services. The PSV mindset requires an agency to prioritize goals by assigning weights to targeted factors in its organization. Historical performance trends are analyzed to establish a baseline. Future performance is then projected from the baseline.

Agencies can make decisions by comparing their performance results from year to year, learning from historical performance, evaluating trade-offs and understanding the impacts that investment decisions will have on their overall performance. PSV reinforces a "good governance" mindset that continually balances outcomes and cost – and enables policy and budget decision making grounded in a metrics-based rationale.

Using PSV to Evaluate Investments in Healthcare

The public sector traditionally has evaluated discrete operational process measures with incomparable units, such as changes in satisfaction levels. The day-to-day operational perspective in a single agency department provides a limited snapshot that may give a false sense of agencywide performance. PSV evaluates how well a government agency is able to attain its objective in delivering healthcare by aggregating multiple outcome-driven, agencywide metrics to assess the overall value the agency's care creates for citizens – its stakeholders. It pinpoints areas within the healthcare agency which indicate underperformance in healthcare cost, effectiveness and efficiency. The tool enables comprehensive benchmarking and decision making, by allowing agencies to compare care methods and performance over time within themselves as well as with peer organizations.

Results of such an analysis can be used in multiple ways, including, for example, to provide justification for targeted and detailed budget requests to legislatures. A state Medicaid agency preparing to testify regarding a budget request can, for example, use the PSV framework first to decide how to allocate its scarce resources, then to create details for its state Medicaid performance story in order to legitimize its request to the legislature. Agencies have also explored PSV as a decision-making tool for project approvals and continual resource allocation.

Rick Wheeler is the global managing partner for Accenture's Health & Life Services practice. In this role he sets strategic direction for the industry and is responsible for specific clients, including Texas and Kentucky Medicaid clients, as well as industry relationships, including the International Social Security Association. **Janhavi Bonville** is in Accenture's Health & Life Sciences and Government Health practices and is responsible for the Public Sector Value Model health asset. She comes from a background of public policy and international public health and has worked with health plans, public and private hospitals and government systems.

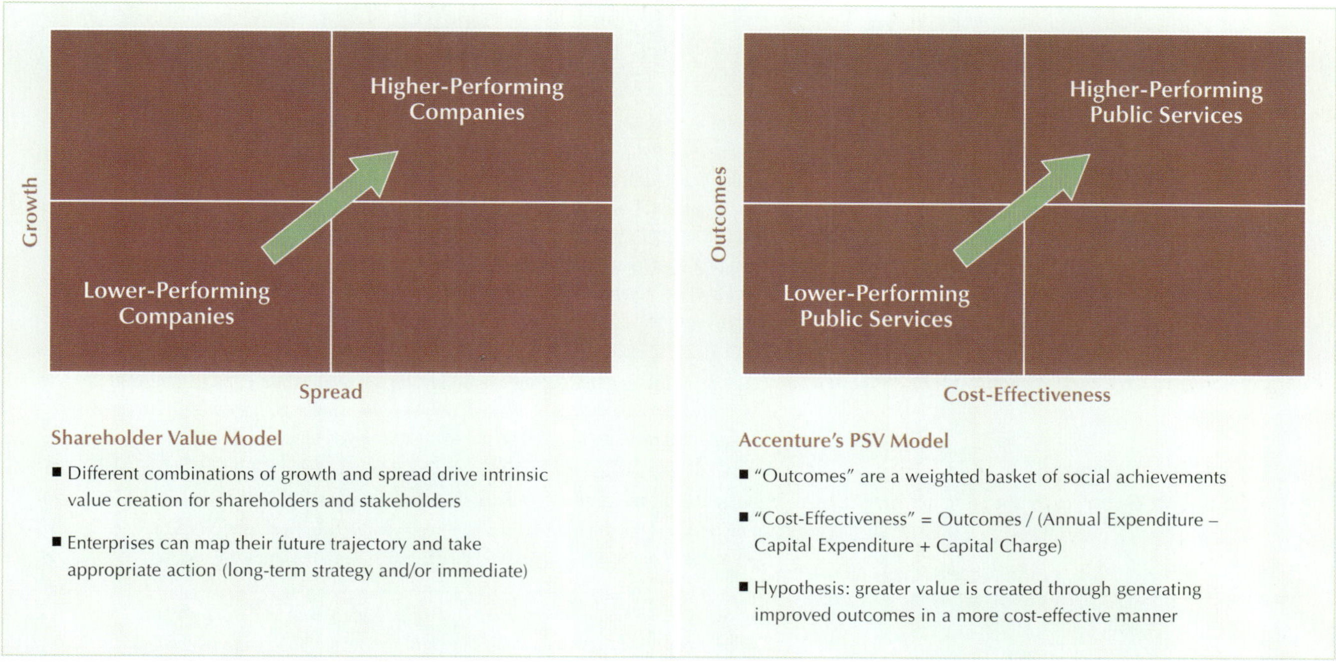

Figure 1 The PSV model applies the key tenets of shareholder value analysis to the public sector.

PSV Metrics and Analyses

A typical PSV analysis includes the following five steps:

- Developing an agency outcome model and selecting metrics;
- Assigning weights to the factors involved;
- Calculating the overall outcome score;
- Calculating the cost-effectiveness score; and
- Analyzing results and developing recommendations.

PSV requires that an agency determine the end results they want to deliver to key internal and external stakeholders. This often entails defining and delineating the objectives or raison d'etre, in as quantitative and measurable a manner as possible. The next step is to prioritize objectives and identify raw metrics for determining successful achievement of this *raison d'etre*. Finally, the raw metrics must be filtered through multiple screens of feasibility and validity to decide which will drive results most effectively, and which are most critical to include in aggregate measures.

Developing PSV analyses requires close collaboration of PSV-trained practitioners with the agency in question. Assigning quantitative value or measures to health-associated measures is always challenging. However, general objectives such as "improving the quality of healthcare" are too broad and vague to measure – and the goal of PSV is to get the agency to a stage such that it is able to measure performance and value delivered. An intense workshop-style forum is often required to determine the agency's key goals and desired outcomes – and then drill down into sub-outcomes, metrics and sub-metrics to determine how to measure those agency outcomes. While most goverment health agencies have similar goals, priorities may differ as may availability of metrics and information.

> To measure outcomes, a large pool of eligible metrics is often explored. This may include industry best practices and currently tracked data. However, many health organizations have many metrics, or metrics that are too general, irrelevant or vague for use.

The Government Perspective: Public Sector Value and EHR

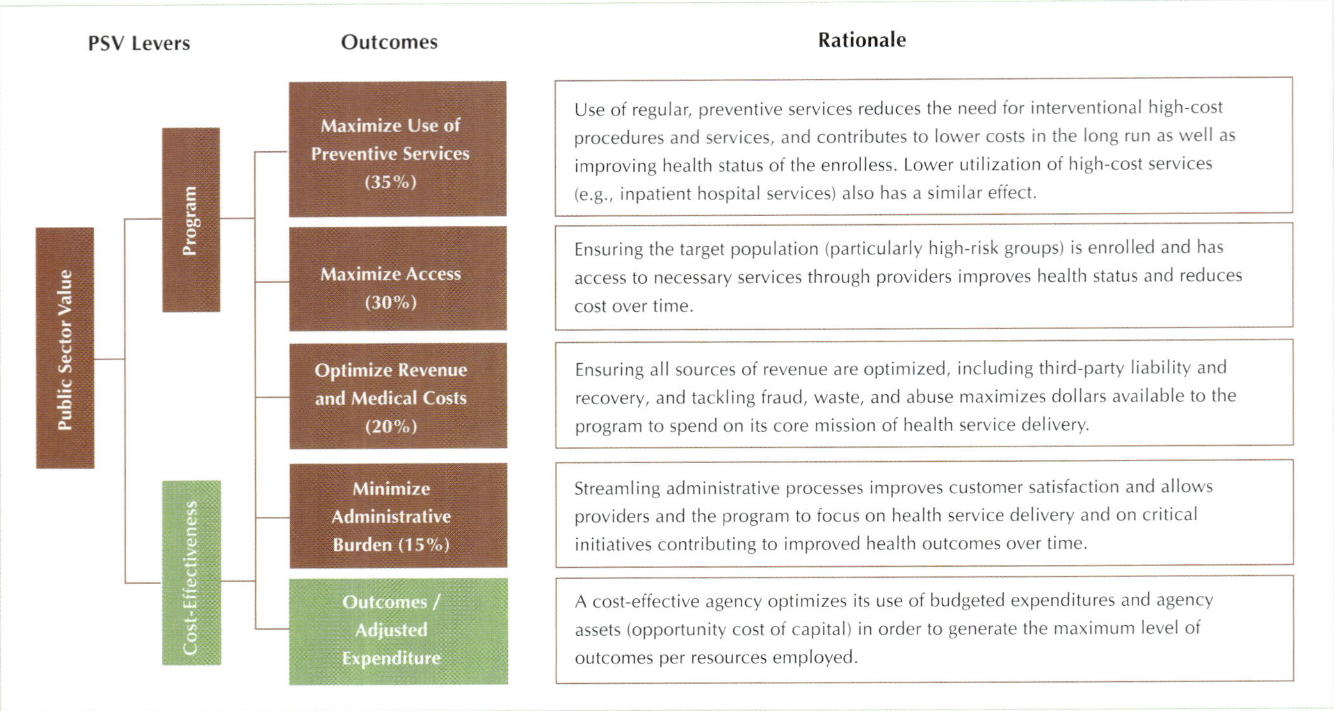

Figure 2 Examples of Stated Outcomes for a State Medicaid Agency

To measure outcomes, a large pool of eligible metrics is often explored. This may include industry best practices and currently tracked data. However, many health organizations have many metrics, or metrics that are too general, irrelevant or vague for use. Metrics are thus passed through two filters: a) the intentions filter; and b) the feasibility filter.

The *intentions* filter locates metrics that are outcome-focused, customer-focused, measurable and actionable; and

The *feasibility* filter determines the metrics that are affordable to measure, aligned to resources, comprehensive and meaningful.

Once metrics have been determined, it is critical to weight them. The weighting exercise is telling in requiring agencies to prioritize key areas according to availability and quality of data as well as importance to mission.

For example, a state Medicaid agency can use PSV to rank desired outcomes that increase program results and cost-effectiveness. Its outcomes can be illustrated – along with the respective weights assigned to each according to the filtering method described above. The agency can filter metrics over four years to create a PSV analysis that shows its performance over time (see Figure 2).

Results of a PSV analysis can be demonstrated graphically. Outcomes are graphed on one axis, cost-effectiveness on another and a trend line is drawn to indicate performance. Movements in different directions indicate where the agency has either under- or over-performed with respect to its own average performance over time (see Figure 3).

When such an analysis is complemented by qualitative information on key investments and key policy directions, it tells a powerful story regarding an agency's performance and direction over time. An agency can thus use such analysis to justify its budget, spending decisions and policy decisions going forward.

For one specific agency for which a PSV was conducted, analysis indicated that outcomes improved despite the overall reduction in adjusted cost per enrollee. The story the agency chief was able to tell was compelling, indicating ability to use technology effectively to increase revenue and customer service, maintaining enrollment in Medicaid and improving utilization of preventive care, such as prenatal care and community care-based services, has improved, while slowing utilization of inpatient hospital services.

PSV Use for EHR

EHR can have an integral relationship with PSV. Government agencies can use PSV to evaluate, prioritize and justify investments in clinical information technology and development of EHR systems. Conversely EHR can also be used to support PSV analyses, since it is an outstanding tool for measuring care performance and values. As a method for delivering records

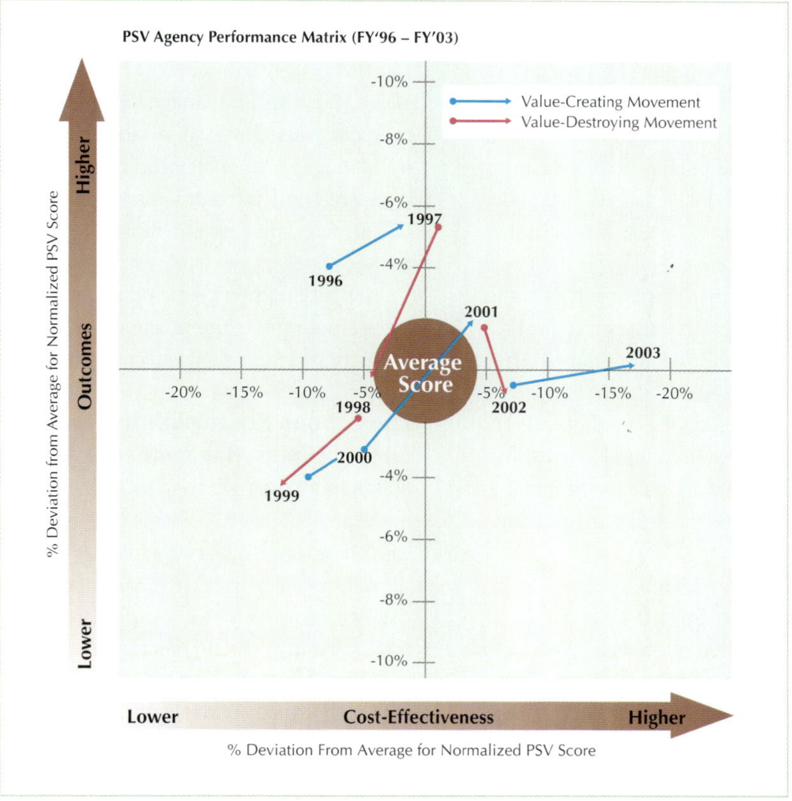

Figure 3 The PSV analytical methodology is a framework that can help governments allocate scarce resources so they can do more with less.

effectively and efficiently, EHR is an important factor in the public agency's process and overall outcomes.

EHR gathers data about the agency's stakeholders to effectively provide seasoned case management, which aids in the mission of effective and efficient governance. It minimizes an agency's administrative burdens by reducing the time spent to gather and input the stakeholders' data and allowing management to focus on the more critical task of maximizing effective utilization of those data.

EHR "improves patient safety," but healthcare agencies must first determine what the phrase ultimately means to their organizations. Does it mean ensuring drugs are prescribed appropriately, the right diagnostic tests are performed, patients requiring care from specialists see them promptly? The agency must define the phrase on its own terms, and then develop its patient safety metrics and expected outcomes so that they can be integrated within the PSV framework for credible and quantitative results.

Multiple countries and localities are adopting EHR, but because their purposes and methods of use vary due to different objectives and values, EHR design must also be modified to reflect multiple systems. PSV can be used to quantify the different data and specifics from locale to locale, and its overall framework need not be altered to produce targeted results and outcomes. An important key to success for this issue occurs in initial meetings with public sector clients, when they must determine their priorities and outcomes objectives.

Many public agencies must make major decisions in healthcare policy and spending on a regular basis, and they must subject those decisions to detailed scrutiny by government legislatures. Rigorous examination of EHR usage is also to be expected by officials. If an agency invests in EHR, how can it justify that decision unless it shows that EHR has improved care performance and by how much? Traditional methods used by healthcare agencies are inefficient for drawing correlations. Granular metrics are needed to produce graphs showing how outcomes and costs have changed over time. Those must be supplemented with qualitative and historical information, which the PSV framework provides.

Key for Success

A critical factor in successful PSV usage is the involvement of the key stakeholders from all departments participating in the process. These include administrators, IT departments, nurses and physicians, who must be given the opportunity to offer opinions about desired outcomes, factor weighting and metrics. Decisions must not be made in a vacuum; otherwise, stakeholders will reject utilization of PSV.

Conclusion

PSV provides government agencies with a credible tool for determining if performance is improving or deteriorating over time, and pinpointing areas within the organizations that are underperforming. Results offer a high-level perspective on how agencies compare to their peers in benchmarking analyses. How they compare to their own average and best performance can provide justification for budget requests to federal, state and local legislatures, and can be used to inform policy direction and decisions in the long term.

As the current economic climate in the public sector increases pressure on time and resources, agencies can use PSV to determine how to allocate their resources for patient care more effectively and efficiently. At the same time, EHR is an integral part of PSV, because its data-gathering procedures are an important factor that drives the public sector in its quest to achieve an overall effective healthcare model. ■

Oracle Healthcare Solutions

Improving the Prognosis

Healthcare organizations confront enormous challenges: spiraling costs, staffing shortages, increasingly strict regulatory requirements, rising patient expectations, constrained reimbursements and more. Most of the challenges organizations face are permutations of one basic dilemma: How do you provide the highest-quality care and fulfill regulatory requirements while contending with rising costs and limited resources?

Healthcare organizations are seeking solutions that can automate and integrate business processes, accelerate staff hiring and training, lower supply chain costs, improve financial information, enable information sharing across the organization, enhance service to consumers and ensure the security and privacy of patient information. The challenge is to do all this while still increasing the quality of care. Sound like an impossible order to fill? It's not. Thousands of the world's most successful companies are already relying on Oracle products and services to accomplish precisely that – and they're saving millions of dollars. Oracle delivers scalable, reliable and secure database software and integrated business applications that can provide quality information and transactional efficiency – at a lower total cost of ownership.

Data security and privacy are paramount concerns in the healthcare industry. Oracle understands these concerns and develops features and solutions to help organizations across the healthcare and life sciences spectrum ensure the security and privacy of sensitive data. Only Oracle offers a unified data model, so you can manage huge volumes of patient and insurance information, ensure regulatory compliance, and procure and manage materials as economically as possible. Oracle Healthcare Transaction Base integrates critical data from all source applications, to give you a true 360-degree view into your healthcare organization. And when Oracle for Healthcare runs on Oracle technology, you speed implementation, optimize performance, streamline support and maximize ROI.

World-Class Leadership

Oracle is a leader in developing information technology solutions for the healthcare industry. Oracle's healthcare presence spans the globe and encompasses institutions in both the public and private sector. Ten out of 12 of the Fortune Global 500 healthcare organizations and four of the top five AARP-ranked hospitals run Oracle applications. One of the company's highest-profile healthcare initiatives is its work with the United Kingdom's National Health Service, which selected Oracle to provide database technology for a nationwide IT project involving 50 million patients. The 10-year project could save the National Health Service as much as $182 million.

How to Know More, Do More and Spend Less

In an industry that relies on the sharing of data across a labyrinth of departments, geographies, disciplines and delivery settings, information is the lifeblood. You need to understand how your organization is performing in real time and across all functional areas. To achieve this holistic view, you can spend millions of dollars attempting to integrate numerous "best of breed" business applications and still not get the desired results. Data will remain fragmented, and you will actually be paying more to know less. Data fragmentation is the No. 1 IT problem plaguing healthcare organizations today. With Oracle, you can benefit from an integrated architecture that provides consolidated information. Only Oracle uses a single, unified data model that stores information for all applications in one place, giving you a single version of the truth.

Streamline Your Human Resource Processes

With Oracle Human Resources, you can improve the efficiency of HR processes by sharing workforce data across the entire organization. Oracle Human Resources can meet the most complex needs of healthcare organizations, such as managing differential staffing by shifts and managing a contingent workforce.

Oracle iRecruitment simplifies the process of recruiting, reducing the time to hire and cutting the number of open vacancies. It allows you to manage the entire recruiting cycle via a self-service interface:

- Managers can open job vacancies, search for candidates, manage the interview process and more.
- Recruiters can extend recruiting functionality to managers and focus on promoting the organization's employment brand to a target candidate pool.

Lower Your Costs With Integrated Supply Chain Management

Making sure the right supplies are available at the point of care at the right time is critical. Oracle Supply Chain Management is the only completely integrated solution that delivers value in five critical operational areas: planning, procurement, sourcing, order fulfillment and supplier relations. With Oracle Supply Chain Management, you can:

- Maximize efficiencies by automating and streamlining procurement processes;
- Introduce more control into the procurement process, including budgetary control, contract enforcement and best practices;
- Save money by collaborating more effectively with suppliers and lowering the cost of each transaction;
- Track critical performance indicators via personalized views of purchasing portals;
- Allow your suppliers to access their accounts via the Web for improved supplier relationships; and
- Manage purchasing contracts and compliance.

Take Control of Your Finances

Oracle provides an integrated solution that can give you complete visibility into your finances while increasing the efficiency of your operations. You can close your books faster, make better business decisions based on real-time data and reduce the overall cost of running your organization. Plus, increased speed and transparency in your financial reporting can help you meet today's corporate-governance demands. Part of the Oracle E-Business Suite, Oracle Corporate Performance Management is an integrated solution that provides the following key capabilities:

- Financial management;
- Cost structure modeling;
- Analytical reporting; and
- System integration.

Share Information Across Business and Clinical Functions

The Oracle Healthcare Transaction Base is a service framework that helps you integrate, develop and operate healthcare applications across the healthcare continuum. It enables you to capture information from multiple stand-alone and disparate applications into a common database, with a common nomenclature. This allows you to access one repository for a single, complete view of information that previously resided in separate applications.

Oracle Healthcare Transaction Base consists of a comprehensive, healthcare-specific data repository and HL7 Version 3 standard-based information model coupled with a set of integrated services for data normalization, customer-defined security and auditing and business process/workflow. The platform is designed specifically for the healthcare industry and supports meaningful data consolidation, rapid application development and genuine interoperability among different systems.

Empower the Healthcare Community

Oracle Application Server Portal, in conjunction with Oracle Collaboration Suite, gives you secure, reliable connectivity. Whether for employees accessing their email, staff submitting hours and schedules, providers reviewing critical patient data or patients and plan members accessing their claims or benefit information, Oracle Application Server Portal provides a secure means for sending, receiving and sharing information. Used with Oracle Healthcare Transaction Base, Oracle Application Server Portal allows your community to access information across disparate clinical, financial and administrative systems. Oracle provides a complete, integrated, low-cost business intelligence infrastructure delivered through our Oracle Application Server Portal.

Unbreakable Security

Oracle is the industry leader in providing unbreakable security. In fact, Oracle has 17 independent database security evaluations, including certifications from the U.S. Central Intelligence Agency and the National Security Agency. No other vendor can make this claim. Oracle protects data itself, where it is stored – in the database – and protects it at a more granular level than any other vendor. The Oracle Database provides a variety of security features, from user authentication to privilege management and row-level access control. Recently Oracle completed the International Common Criteria (ISO 15408) security evaluation at Evaluation Assurance Level 4, the industry's most rigorous assessment for commercially available software. Security has been built into all Oracle products from the very beginning, not just retrofitted or bolted onto products already on the market.

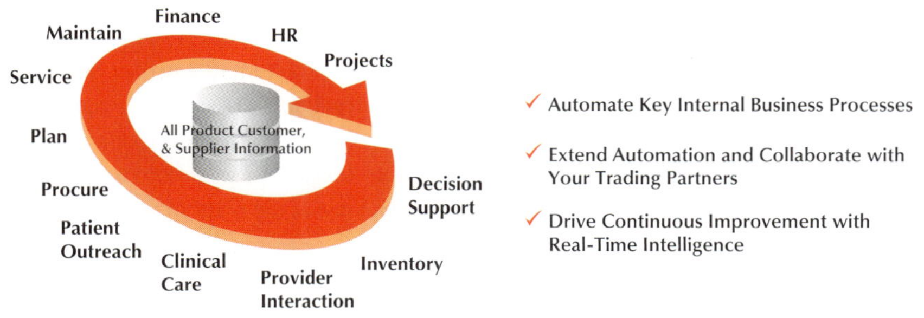

The Right Prescription

Oracle understands the challenges that healthcare organizations face in today's competitive environment. We provide focused expertise and innovative products to successful healthcare organizations around the globe. Let us help your organization achieve its objectives. ■

Larry Ellison
Chief Executive Officer

Charles Phillips
President

Gregory B. Maffei
President and CFO

Safra Catz
President

Oracle Corporation
500 Oracle Parkway
Redwood Shores, CA 94065
Phone 650.506.7000
www.oracle.com

For more information
Please contact your Oracle Healthcare Representative at 1.800.633.0676.

The Pivotal Role of Government in Transforming U.S. Healthcare

A national healthcare IT network would enable the electronic exchange of health data among patients and clinicians as well as with the public health sector and life sciences industry.

[Rick Wheeler, Accenture] [Jon Kaplan, Accenture]

Like the other 60 percent of the U.S. healthcare system, Medicare and Medicaid are at a critical crossroads. Budget pressures are escalating as costs far outpace state and federal revenues, with the National Association of State Budget Officers predicting Medicaid cost increases will exceed 12 percent a year compared to annual revenue growth among the states of 5 to 7 percent. Moreover, government health programs as well as providers across the country are facing growing scrutiny over quality, safety and access to care.

As a result, momentum is rapidly building within the public and private sector to embrace information technology as a component of the means for healing healthcare. In particular, the U.S. Department of Health and Human Services is leading an ambitious public-private sector effort to map out plans to build a U.S. healthcare IT network.

This network offers a singular opportunity to reach a new level of high performance that could change the practice of medicine in America. At this point, though, the United States is playing catch-up with some other nations. The United Kingdom, Australia, Canada, France, Spain and Germany already have moved aggressively to develop interoperable EHR systems.

As plans are being laid, state and federal government health programs could seize the opportunity to use their enormous clout as massive payers and purchasers of American healthcare to ensure the creation and widespread use of such a vital network. This opportunity is not a case of HIPAA, Part II. Rather than looking to Congress to pilot programs, fund initiatives and legislate how a healthcare IT network would work, government programs can assert their leadership by taking steps to establish de facto standards that encourage the pervasive adoption and use both of electronic health records (EHRs) and a national health IT network. In the process, they would dramatically lay the groundwork and infrastructure to improve the cost outlook, efficiency and quality of U.S. healthcare.

Improving Care While Cutting Costs

A nationwide electronic health network would greatly ameliorate one of healthcare's most costly problems: the lack of timely access to critical patient information. With the vast majority of patient health information kept in paper records that are scattered among doctors' offices, hospitals and other providers, crucial information often is not available at the point of need, especially in emergencies.

A national healthcare IT network would enable the electronic exchange of health data among patients and clinicians as well as with the public health sector and life sciences industry. Having accurate electronic patient records rapidly available would significantly reduce medical errors, lower the cost of care, reduce redundant healthcare procedures and improve the quality of healthcare delivery. With the ability to aggregate and sort data, a national network also would facilitate medical research and the handling of public health issues and potential outbreaks of disease.

Although the potential benefits are far greater, if a national health IT network only reduces redundant and unnecessary treatment, it would more than pay for itself. A recent study by the Center for Evaluative Clinical Sciences found that "close to one-third of the U.S. health spending goes to care that is duplicative, fails to improve patient health or may even make it worse." That's the equivalent of $3.1 trillion wasted each year, with the

Rick Wheeler is the global managing partner for Accenture's Health & Life Sciences practice. In this role he is responsible for setting strategic direction for the industry and is responsible for specific clients, including Texas and Kentucky Medicaid clients, as well as industry relationships, such as the International Social Security Association. **Jon Kaplan** is a partner in the Health & Life Sciences practice of Accenture. His focus is large-scale transformation for clients in the payer, provider and life sciences industries, and he has worked with a variety of clients from large health plans to academic medical centers.

public sector paying 46 percent of the total waste and the private sector accounting for the balance.

Electronic information sharing could eliminate a huge portion of that waste. Health and Human Services estimates that standardized healthcare data exchange would deliver national savings of $86.8 billion annually after full implementation. Significant direct financial benefits would accrue to providers, payers, companies with employee health plans and patients, who are shouldering an increasing share of their healthcare costs.

Structuring the Network

A monolithic system with central control of patient data would prove unwieldy, rigid, costly and inefficient. Rather, a distributed data and services model composed of hundreds, or perhaps thousands, of smaller networks, offers the best structure for building a robust and flexible IT network that is:

- Patient-centric;
- Standards-based;
- Secure and private;
- Focused on supplying accurate and timely information that improves clinical outcomes;
- Large enough to ensure patient coverage and assure an appropriate return on investment;
- Built to complement and integrate with existing IT investments; and
- Designed to allow incremental improvements.

Because care is delivered locally, regional health information organizations (RHIOs) are the ideal, patient-centric building blocks of a national network.

Because care is delivered locally, regional health information organizations (RHIOs) are the ideal patient-centric building blocks of a national network. With an RHIO, diverse healthcare stakeholders voluntarily band together, usually within a specific geographic area such as those in Santa Barbara County, Calif., and regions of Tennessee or Massachusetts. RHIOs would maintain critical clinical information for each patient, representing a subset of the patient's full EHR. The RHIOs would provide instant access to data across the interoperable national network.

This approach would enable providers to aggregate and retrieve clinical data faster and more reliably than in a non-centralized system where data is stored in individual doctors' offices. Regionalized systems also could more easily accommodate clinical decision support queries, which facilitate the use of best practices, also known as evidence-based medicine, and thus reduce errors. At the same time, RHIOs would keep governance, organization, deployment and interaction, including the control over access to patient data and physician involvement, at the local level.

This information could also be the basis of information sharing that could support regional disease management initiatives. Clearly the access to more complete and timely information for a patient, during a time of illness, will help to integrate care and allow for care to be more effectively managed. This will benefit the patient and the provider of care, while at the same time decreasing the overall cost of care.

The Role of Government

State Medicaid programs are extremely well-positioned to create RHIOs and ensure use. As single payers covering large, diverse populations, Medicaid programs could make part of their reimbursements contingent on using an EHR and, when appropriate, a regional health IT network, for instance. Of course, there are times when multiple states may need to come together to support regions of the country (e.g., cities and communities which are near state borders). Also Medicare could stimulate demand for EHRs and RHIOs, and thus help create a de facto standard along with Medicaid, by tying reimbursements to their use.

So far though, Medicaid programs have been conspicuously absent from almost all of the more than dozen RHIOs in various stages of development and implementation. Tennessee is an exception. With estimates showing its Medicaid program would absorb 91 percent of all new revenues coming into the state by 2008, Tennessee teamed up with the Vanderbilt Center for Better Health and Accenture to plan a statewide infrastructure for sharing clinical data among all healthcare users, including hospitals, payers, commercial labs and doctors' offices. With a $5 million grant from the Agency for Healthcare Research and Quality, Tennessee will pilot its Volunteer eHealth Initiative in a three-county region that includes Memphis. But even in

weblink

Read about how Massachusetts implemented a system that shares all of the clinical data in an entire region in the interview with Dr. John Halamka in this book and on the Web at www.hctproject.com.

Tennessee, the Medicaid program itself is not driving the initiative, although they are heavily involved.

Besides using the might of Medicare, the federal government can offer carrots to drive development of a national network.

Ongoing funding has to come from operating sources. Examples of this may come from a tax-like cost associated with claims processing that does not support the sharing of clinical information with an RHIO in that region, or

While the U.S. is unique in its healthcare structure compared to the rest of the world, there are also many of the same issues facing the U.S. health system as it moves toward RHIOs and interoperable EHRs.

While the U.S. government's fiscal situation precludes it from financing the entire network, it has a crucial role to play in funding at three levels – providers, RHIOs and national. Funding is necessary for the development of these RHIOs as well as the ongoing cost of operations.

Funding could include:

- Grant funding from public and private entities. This has even been seen from certain Blue Cross plans in a number of states that have made grant funding available to support RHIO-type initiatives (e.g., Massachusetts);
- Tax incentives and low-interest loans for participating in the formation of the national network;
- Grants for developing RHIOs, possibly requiring matching funds from other sources; and
- Contracts awarded to third parties for providing national network services to RHIOs such as patient identification, access and security management, authentication and patient consent management services.

While federal and state funding is needed to overcome the initial financial barriers associated with creating the national healthcare IT network and having clinicians use it, the national network should become self-sustaining after a start-up phase of three to five years.

from participants in the region of the RHIO that benefit from the shared information (e.g., payers).

Conclusion

As we move forward with implementing the EHR and look at the role of government, we need to be mindful of the design, implementation and adoption of innovative EHR systems for Australia, the United Kingdom, France, Spain and even Tennessee and California in the United States. While the U.S. is unique in its healthcare structure compared to the rest of the world, there are also many of the same issues facing the U.S. health system as it moves toward RHIOs and interoperable EHRs.

It will take considerable resolve and creativity to settle all the issues facing a national health IT network and develop compelling value propositions for all stakeholders, but these challenges are dwarfed by the enormous opportunity.

A national healthcare IT network that links the efforts of RHIOs and facilitates the electronic exchange of patient data will serve as the much-needed catalyst for attaining new standards in effectiveness, quality, safety, access and costs. The government, both at the state and federal levels, can be a strong force for fostering and implementing required change. ■

Build Business Value Through the Use of IT and Management Consulting

RSM McGladrey

The Information Technology Group of The National Healthcare Practice of RSM McGladrey Business Consulting Services provides consulting services that enable our clients to build business value through the creative, innovative and strategic use of information technology and management consulting. We are dedicated to aligning information technology, business processes and organizational resources to help our clients achieve higher levels of performance. We deliver on our commitment to clients with project teams as knowledgeable and specialized as they are dedicated. Our management consultants, implementation specialists, software designers, programmers and network engineers work in conjunction with our clients to provide seamless services that uniquely address the needs of not-for-profit healthcare services organizations. These services involve taking our clients through the entire systems development life cycle and include offerings around:

- Information technology strategic planning;
- Business analysis;
- System selection;
- Solution design;
- System implementation;
- Change management;
- Workflow redesign; and
- Technology related regulatory compliance.

We provide consulting services to community health centers, free clinics, substance abuse and mental health clinics, Healthcare for the Homeless Programs, HIV/AIDS services providers and Indian health clinics, as well as primary care associations, regional networks, managed care organizations and public health departments. Our staff members are regularly asked to present at major industry conferences on issues such as information technology and electronic health records (EHRs) implementation, and to serve on federal, state and industry committees and task forces. Our offices are located in New York, Chicago, Los Angeles, Baltimore, Cleveland and Boston, and we serve a client base spread across all 50 states. Our staff consists of healthcare industry experts and includes clinicians and other healthcare informatics experts.

Understanding that an EHR system implementation represents a major organizational change, our implementation methodology incorporates tools and processes specifically designed to support change management throughout the project.

Since 1998, RSM McGladrey Business Consulting Services has worked with healthcare organizations on full life-cycle EHR implementation projects. Working in close partnership with our client organizations, we have employed our proven methodology for EHR implementation, addressing all aspects of the project, from pre-implementation support to final project evaluation and knowledge management. Understanding that an EHR system implementation represents a major organizational change, our implementation methodology incorporates tools and processes specifically designed to support change management throughout the project.

EHR Implementation

Analysis and Planning

We believe that the success of an EHR implementation is contingent on an organization's ability to carefully plan and provide stable ongoing management processes. As part of the initial analysis and planning phase, we evaluate the existing management structure and processes in light of the current status, strengths, weaknesses and barriers. From that assessment, we will suggest strategies for managing the project going forward.

Our goal is to attain consensus on the implementation plan by supporting a common base of knowledge and understanding among the healthcare organization's staff. We facilitate discussions among the administrative and clinical staff to identify strengths, weaknesses and barriers, and support them in developing plans for attaining their priorities.

Areas addressed during analysis and planning include technical environment, current applications requirements, staffing, workflow, clinical requirements and management processes. These findings are incorporated into our discussions with the project team as part of the process of

weblink

Learn how organizations can manage change in "The Real Challenge in Implementing EHRs by Adam J. Schreiber and Kate W. Galambos, R.N., M.S.N., RSM McGladrey Business Consulting Services in this book and on the Web at www.hctproject.com.

planning the short- and long-term goals of the project.

We expect that the organization will make a consistent commitment to the EHR implementation project, from the top down. Executive commitment to the EHR project is critical. We offer expert support to the organization's leaders as they manage the many changes incurred by bringing in the new system.

Implementation Support

Implementation support includes project management and process redesign support. Because an EHR project typically requires several months to complete, our project management methodology is employed to help the project team achieve consistency and control during that time. In our role as advisors to the project team, we assist in the transition of accountability for the EHR. Our professional support for change management, and specifically workflow redesign, is also designed to result in the eventual success of the implementation.

Project Management

RSM McGladrey project managers are experienced in EHR implementation and dedicated to the organization's success. Our project manager oversees the project as it unfolds, working closely with the in-house project team. The in-house project team should include representatives from both administrative and clinical areas. Recommended job titles for the project team include: CEO, CIO, IT director or staff, medical records director, billing director, medical director, nursing director and QA/QI director. Other participants might include EHR champions from the clinical or front desk staff.

Our role is to inform and support the project team's activities in leading the EHR project. We schedule regular meetings with the project team and provide our standard proven tools, such as agendas, minutes, spreadsheets and schedules, to help them achieve their task assignments. We also develop and maintain the project plan, which is regularly updated and serves as the backbone for the team's activities. We provide structure to a process which may appear confusing or overwhelming at times, as well as giving feedback or guidance when needed. We assist the organization in balancing the need for stability (planning) with unpredictability and change ("real life" in a healthcare organization).

During an EHR implementation, staff from nearly every department is affected.

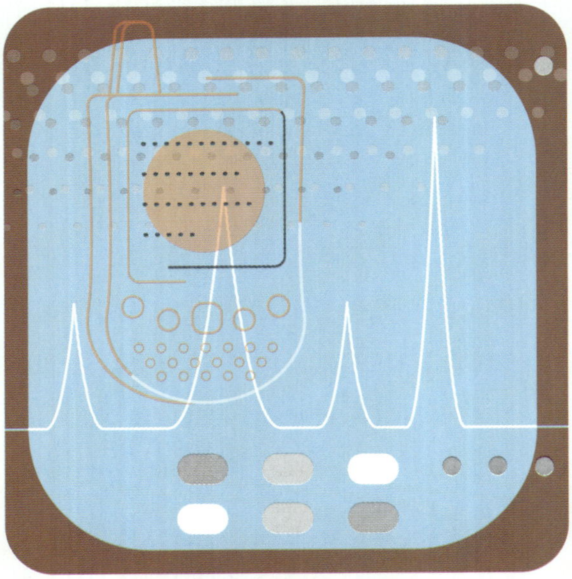

We help coordinate the different program units and develop the infrastructure required to plan for, carry out and monitor the EHR implementation. We work with the organization to plan the timing and sequence of the implementation, as well as identify areas in which the workflow may require redesign. All project management activities are documented using standard forms and updated regularly.

Change Management And Workflow Redesign

The implementation of an EHR system creates significant organizational change. It is an intense process, because providers, nurses and staff are being asked to do their work in a new way. Often change engenders reactions, such as fear, resistance, even anger, so planned change management is essential to the success of the implementation project. Our experience has shown that the most successful implementations demonstrate three key change management characteristics: top-down support for change; well-managed teams that share the implementation tasks; and support for new system end users by providing them additional time to learn the system while not being swamped with patient appointments.

We can begin to assist the organization with the redesign of work processes before the system is even installed. We work closely with the team to analyze the current workflows and help with identifying processes and documents that the new system may automate. We encourage the project team to include staff in workflow redesign efforts. Our experienced project managers often add value to these discussions by describing best practices in workflow redesign encountered in previous EHR projects.

As the project progresses through installation, configuration and end-user training, we weave the concepts and strategies of workflow redesign into all aspects of our project work. In project management, change management and even in the training, we work to help the organization to incorporate workflow redesign. Our goal is for every staff member to understand their important role in improving efficiency and, ultimately, in providing better patient care, through the reworking of old processes into the new system's capabilities.

Once the training is finished and the project plan complete, the organization becomes fully accountable for maintaining the ongoing success of the EHR. Yet many changes will continue to occur as the system becomes integrated into all of the daily processes of the organization. Within a year, an administrative structure should evolve that supports the utilization of the EHR, provides for IT and training support, and identifies the ways the system can now contribute to the overall success of the organization. Partnership with the vendors and consultants is of critical importance during this period.

Technical Services

RSM McGladrey offers a full range of technical expertise related to EHR implementation. Our network assessment is fundamental for an EHR project. Using standard tools and processes, our technical experts evaluate the organization's current technical environment in light of the requirements of the proposed new system, and develop recommendations for infrastructure upgrades or reconfiguration necessary in order to ensure network stability with no downtime during clinical hours. Our network assessment evaluates the hardware, software, network, Internet access, databases, clinical data management tools and IT support staff, as well as specific issues in the areas of data conversion, printing and document management, and the need for system interfaces. If interfaces are required, we have interface project plans and other tools to employ for coordinating the technical and programming work needed to bring an interface live.

If needed, RSM McGladrey will install and configure the EHR system. Additional services include in-house IT staff training and technical support throughout the implementation project. We solicit a comprehensive evaluation of our services upon the completion of the technical phase.

End-User Training

RSM McGladrey is convinced that good end-user training is essential to an EHR's success. Accordingly we have developed a comprehensive, proven training methodology. We hire clinically prepared health professionals, with experience in the provision of care, to provide top-notch EHR training for all levels of staff. Our EHR trainers are expected to teach more than the application itself; they also must understand process redesign, change management and adult education and training concepts, as well as the requirements of an ambulatory care IT system. Our trainer preparation includes one-on-one physician training. A trainer must demonstrate training proficiency before being assigned to work with clients. Lesson plans, handouts and guided exercises are used for every class.

We work intensively with the project team to prepare for the end-user training. Prior to training, schedules must be developed, coverage arranged and materials such as coding reports obtained. The organization should evaluate its staff on computer competencies, and provide any assistance needed to prepare them for training on the new system. The organization must commit to the training schedule, and ensure that staff attends training.

We hire clinically prepared health professionals, with experience in the provision of care, to provide top-notch EHR training for all levels of staff.

End-user training is designed to prepare the staff with the basic skills they need to use the EHR system independently. The categories of staff needing EHR training are providers (physicians, nurse practitioners and physician assistants), clinical staff (RNs, LPNs, NAs and MAs), technicians (lab, radiology, pharmacy), associates (counselors, nutritionists, etc.), and administrators (medical records, billers, administrators). Trainees in each category learn how to use an appropriate set of EHR features. We organize the training sessions in a specific sequence, beginning with simple skills and progressing to more complex skills and concepts.

We distribute training evaluations at the end of every training session and provide a formal performance review for every learner at the completion of training. One-month and three-month post-training evaluations are also obtained to measure end-user performance and utilization of the system.

This detailed and comprehensive process is meant to ensure the successful implementation of the EHR and, in turn, the realization of the ultimate goals of increased efficiency, reimbursement and quality of care. ■

RSM McGladrey

The National Healthcare Practice of RSM McGladrey Business Consulting Services is a recognized leader in healthcare consulting. We help our clients achieve results by providing them with specialized knowledge – our term for relevant, practical and strategic business and financial information – delivered by experienced, knowledgeable and responsive industry professionals.

Randall Siemsen
Executive Vice President,
National Consulting

Eric S. Holzberg
Lead Managing Director,
National Healthcare Practice

Adam J. Schreiber
Managing Director, Healthcare
Technology Consulting

RSM McGladrey, Inc.
1185 Avenue of the Americas
New York, NY 10036
Phone 212.372.1000
Fax 212.372.1001
www.rsmmcgladrey.com

Business Contact
Adam J. Schreiber
Phone 212.372.1487
Fax 646.885.1487
adam.schreiber@rsmi.com

EHRs and the Stark Law

In order to foster the dissemination of the EHR, there needs to be definitional clarity and regulatory relief from Stark Law concerns.

[John E. Steiner Jr., Esq., The Cleveland Clinic Health System]

The electronic health record (EHR) recently has become one of the most widely discussed, analyzed and promising developments in healthcare. For those who focus on the legal and regulatory aspects of the EHR, there is substantial discussion about how to make the EHR work in our highly regulated healthcare environment.

Most observers agree that federal direction and commitment are needed to establish and promote EHR standards across the country. Those standards, once established, should allow for rapid adoption of EHR and its benefits. At a high level, those benefits include improving the quality of patient care practices by, among other things, improving the accuracy and timeliness of the medical record and providing rapid access to patient information as well as clinical decision support software.

If a national standards setting effort is required to permit a new technology to take hold (as has been shown many times before), then federal government leadership is essential. EHR projects currently under way or in development by hospitals and large health systems are intended to expand beyond the physicians employed in those systems and reach community-based physicians. How this expansion occurs and at what cost to the parties are still somewhat open-ended questions. There are practical legal issues associated with EHR expansion. For example, in its 2005 report on Medicare Payment Policy to Congress, the Medicare Payment Advisory Commission stated: "Legal issues and uncertainties over legal restrictions may hamper efforts to create local health information exchange networks ... and should be re-examined."

One such restriction is the "Stark Law." This law is designed to address the perceived irreconcilable conflict of interest between the power of a physician to refer and to profit from those referrals. The Stark Law is an exceptions law. That means that broad prohibitions are stated at the beginning of the statute and then numerous exceptions to those prohibitions are provided.

The two Stark prohibitions are:

1. **Referral Prohibition:** Physicians may not refer to an entity with which the physician (or immediate family member) has a financial relationship and when the referral is for one or more designated health services, unless an exception applies (see Figure 1); and
2. **Claims Submission Prohibition:** Neither the physician who makes a prohibited referral nor the entity that provides the designated health services for which the referral was made, may submit a claim to Medicare or Medicaid (see Figure 2).

Each prohibition is broadly worded. A violation of either prohibition does not require a showing of intent to violate the law. Instead the law is "self-executing," and failure to know and follow the law can result in the improper receipt of federal health program funds by a physician or the entity from a prohibited referral or claim submission. The critical link in the Stark Law is between the physician (a referral source) and the entity where the referral is made for designated health services (a list of about 20 categories of healthcare items and services). That link is called a financial relationship and may be either an ownership or investment interest or a compensation arrangement. For purposes of the EHR discussion, if a hospital or health system provides EHR capability to a referring physician's office and there is a financial relationship with the physician, the Stark Law probably is implicated. Such support may be hardware, software, personnel training, upgrades, clinical decision support, etc. In most EHR projects, if a financial relationship exists between a physician and a hospital or health system, it probably will be a compensation arrangement, as opposed to an ownership or investment interest.

John E. Steiner Jr., Esq., is the chief compliance officer and privacy official of The Cleveland Clinic Health System and is actively involved, both internally and externally, in many of the current legal and regulatory issues presented by the EHR.

For example, a physician may receive compensation from a hospital to serve as a medical director. That physician, who refers patients to the hospital for designated health services, also might receive EHR support from the hospital. If the hospital provides something of value to the referring physician, that value is referred to as remuneration. The crux of the current discussion of Stark and EHR is what remuneration may be provided by an entity to a referring physician in terms of EHR support, where the entity has a financial relationship with the referring physician. Unfortunately the current Stark statute is very broad and a regulatory exception to Stark to adequately address EHR dissemination currently does not exist. Further, definitional ambiguity exists with terms associated with the EHR, such as standards and interoperability. Thus it is difficult to craft a Stark exception in this area that works both for the private sector and for government oversight agencies. Nonetheless both groups are working hard to determine the Stark uncertainties associated with the EHR.

Definitional Challenges

Just as the definition of remuneration under the Stark Law presents regulatory obstacles, it also is a challenge to craft an acceptable definition of EHR or, more broadly, patient care support systems, that works for many different purposes, including a Stark exception. In particular, the medical and legal field is struggling with how to define the EHR. Responses to litigation discovery requests for "medical records that are maintained electronically" is one example of definitional ambiguity. State laws are, of course, a key resource for addressing this issue. For example, the Ohio Revised Code refers to the medical record as data in any form that pertains to a patient's medical history, diagnosis, prognosis, or medical condition and that is generated and maintained by a healthcare provider in the process of the patient's healthcare treatment.

Another source is the Medicare Conditions of Participation that specifies that the medical record must contain information to justify the admission and continued hospitalization, support the diagnosis, and describe the patient's progress and response to medications and services. Generally recognized and accepted principles for describing the EHR should relate to characteristics or capabilities of the software that supports EHR, including:

- Contains the patient's medical history and is an authoritative document that describes the healthcare services provided to patients;
- Provides a method for coordinated communication of patient treatment plans between physicians and health care facilities;
- Provides a source for documentation that supports healthcare service claims;
- Serves as a source or record of data for health outcomes research and related public health purposes;
- Serves as a repository for health data for research and education;
- Serves as a tool for clinical decision making and may have application for evidence-based medicine;
- Provides readily available data for planning and related business decision making.

These attributes of an EHR reflect how flexible and useful the EHR can be, if implemented across many provider sites. These same attributes illustrate the need for definitional clarity and regulatory relief from Stark Law concerns in order to foster the dissemination of the EHR. ■

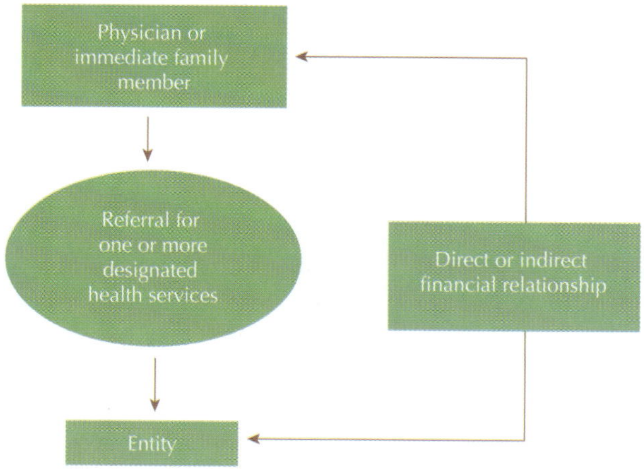

1. Designated health services are tied to common procedural terminology codes.
2. "Ownership or Investment interest" or "Compensation arrangements," or both.

Figure 1 Referral Prohibition

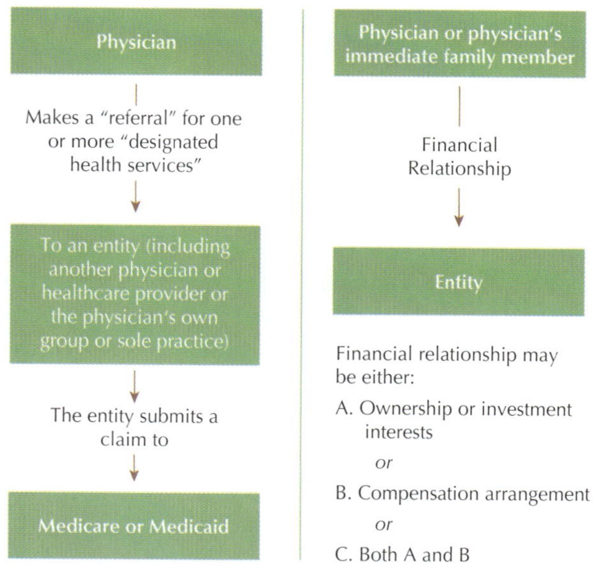

Figure 2 Claims Submission Prohibition

Building the Future

Turner Construction Company is the nation's leading builder of healthcare facilities. Each year, we deliver more than 100 healthcare projects with an annual volume of over $1.3 billion. Founded in 1902, Turner is the only builder that offers clients a nationwide network of offices in 44 markets throughout the U.S. Each office has the knowledge of the local environment in order to provide the best service to our clients, as well as the skills and resources for providing all types of construction services for all facility types including acute care, tertiary care, cancer treatment, research, heart facilities, ambulatory surgery and senior housing.

Turner created a specific market segment group to bring a more focused understanding of the healthcare industry to its local offices. Turner Healthcare sees that healthcare projects obtain the correct resources in order to achieve the goal of building a facility that is flexible, attracts patients and physicians and will take the hospital years into the future.

Turner offers a broad range of services to clients planning new facilities or additions and renovations to existing facilities. These are just some of the areas in which we have expertise.

- Pre-construction consulting;
- Construction management;
- General construction;
- Design-build;
- Medical equipment planning and procurement; and
- Commissioning.

Turner delivers its services in a number of different ways, each dependent upon the needs and expertise of its clients. Regardless of the type of service provided, clients can be sure of the quality and professionalism of our staff. Turner is very much at ease providing pre-construction consulting to a client with extensive in-house resources or assuming the total responsibility of design (as part of a team), construction and maintenance of a client's facility.

Over 70 percent of Turner's Healthcare contracts are "repeat" business from clients, a very good indication of the company's ability to render the type of service most desired by customers. Our reputation for quality and integrity are often cited as major factors in winning client confidence and avoiding project delays, unrealistic cost estimates and budget overruns. Turner's clients are assured of cost-effective, quality-driven construction services.

Our reputation for quality and integrity are often cited as major factors in winning client confidence and avoiding project delays, unrealistic cost estimates and budget overruns.

Turner's healthcare clients include many well-recognized tertiary and academic facilities including Harvard Medical School, Yale-New Haven Hospital, Vanderbilt University Medical Center, UCLA Medical Center, New York University School of Medicine and University of Chicago Hospitals. Research clients include Emory University, Johns Hopkins University, Memorial Sloan-Kettering, and Fred Hutchinson Cancer Research Center.

Turner's national presence and financial strength allows us to offer many value-added benefits to clients.

- Our historical cost database of over 1,000 projects, when escalated annually and adjusted geographically, provides an unmatched tool for controlling costs and potential value analysis of systems.
- Turner brings all of the advantages of national exposure to trends and systems, but with a unique geographical diversification through its local offices. Today's trends of flexibility (through the use of modular bay sizes, universal utilities and redundant systems) as well as digital medical delivery systems enables facilities to maintain state-of-the-art programs.
- Turner is the national sponsor for The Center for Health Design offering programs to help educate both healthcare providers and architects that the "built environment can enhance patient outcomes." The program covers evidence-based design research, research examples and putting the evidence into practice.
- Turner sponsors an educational program presented by Siemens, "The Digital, Integrated Healthcare Enterprise," which outlines transforming healthcare delivery through the innovative use of technology.
- The Turner Knowledge Network (TKN) is an interactive, Web-based training and information resource available to owners, architects and Turner employees, as well as selected work partners, especially subcontractors and their managers and supervisory employees. Subcontractors can access important information and training needed to meet today's construction challenges. As projects have become more complex and risks increase, it has become more important than ever to be highly selective in choosing the most qualified subcontractor to work with on complex projects.
- Turner Logistics provides purchasing opportunities that enable clients to take advantage of "direct from the factory" purchases of major construction equipment such as chillers, air handlers, boilers, etc., as well as medical

and lab equipment. Logistics is able to leverage the purchasing power of Turner's annual construction volume, which reached over $6 billion in 2004, by setting preferred pricing structures according to our aggregate volume, providing clients with the best value for their time and money.

- The Turner Logistics Medical & Research Products Group (MRPG) offers the only fully integrated solution to planning, purchasing, installing and integrating medical equipment, delivering a new level of service by providing stakeholders in the process a single point of contact and responsibility throughout the entire project. Services include budget development, pre-procurement, procurement, installation management, relocation management and turnover and close-out.
- Subguard provides coverage against losses directly and indirectly caused by the default of a subcontractor and/or supplier under the terms and conditions of the subcontract/purchase agreement. Being able to select the subcontractors who work on our projects and select the remedy to a default, immediately, are significant advantages.
- CCIP (Contractor Controlled Insurance Program) is a consolidated insurance program covering Turner and its subcontractors of all tiers. It covers all work performed at jobsites, provides workers' compensation and general and excess liability insurance. The advantages of CCIP are projected savings at the start of the project, no deductible requirements, savings that cannot be eroded by losses and no administrative burden to the owner.

Turner's founder, Henry C. Turner, stated, "We are awarded most of our work based on reputation. Preservation of our reputation demands a commitment to quality, service and operating within approved budgets and schedules. This commitment is the foundation of our company."

Turner believes that if you create and maintain a positive image, the word gets around. This leads not only to repeat clients, but also to new clients who know your reputation. It's all about building relationships. People are as important as bricks and mortar; without the people, you don't get the job. Throughout its history, the company has been associated with the highest standards of service, quality, integrity and personal attention to clients as emphasized by its founder who consistently referred to clients as "respected friends." This philosophy of mutual respect continues to this day. ■

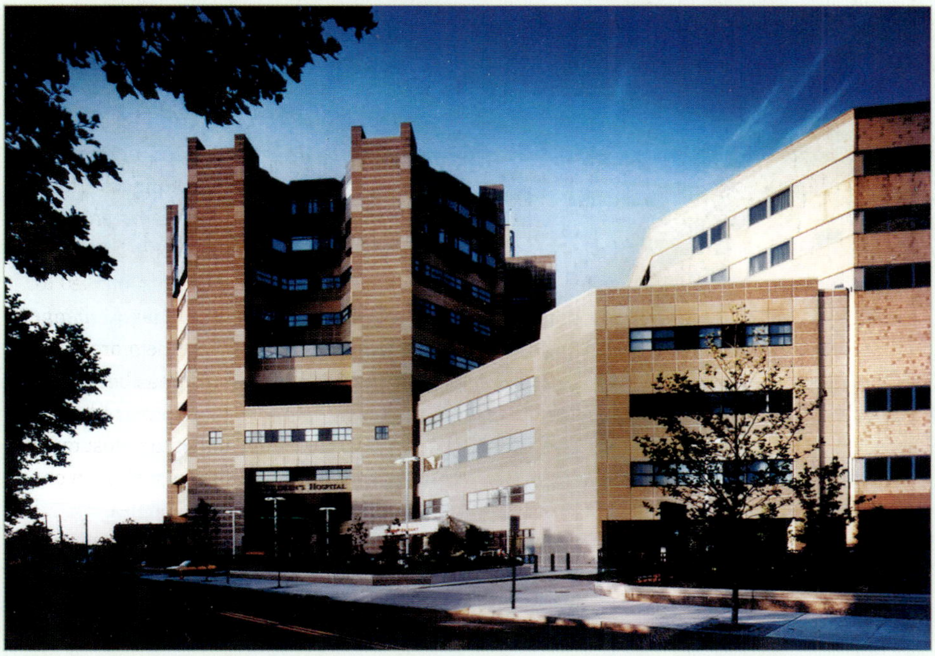

Figure 1 Yale-New Haven Hospital

Turner ≡ Healthcare

Turner Construction Company is the nation's leading healthcare builder providing general contracting and construction management services for all types of facilities.

Thomas C. Leppert
Chairman and
Chief Executive Officer

Peter J. Davoren
President and
Chief Operating Officer

Rodney J. Michalka
Executive Vice President
of New Business Initiatives

Donald G. Sleeman
Executive Vice President and
Chief Financial Officer

The Turner Corporation
901 Main St.
Dallas, TX 75202

Turner Construction Company
375 Hudson St.
New York, NY 10014
Phone 212.229.6000
www.turnerconstruction.com/healthcare

Business Contact
Robert D. Levine
Vice President &
General Manager
Turner Healthcare
5300 Virginia Way, Suite 200
Brentwood, TN 37027
Phone 615.324.3881
Fax 615.324.3899
rlevine@tcco.com

Meeting the Financial Challenge Of the 21st-Century Hospital

When building an integrated digital hospital, it is important to have a team that works in concert to assure that downstream savings accrues from good upstream planning.

[Robert D. Levine, Turner Construction Company]

It's pretty hard to travel anywhere in the United States without passing a hospital campus that doesn't have a crane sitting on the property. We are experiencing a surge in hospital construction that is unprecedented with numbers approaching $16 billion annually.

On average, it takes four to five years to plan and construct a new hospital. To be competitive, hospitals need to be built by 21st-century standards and be integrated digital hospitals. Major tailwinds are creating a once-in-a-lifetime opportunity to redefine our healthcare delivery system and how we develop the buildings that house them. Those tailwinds include:

- **Obsolescence.** Many if not most of the existing medical campuses were built in the 1950s. Although many additions and renovations have been done, one fact that can't be denied is that the core structure is over a half-century old. No other industry is attempting to use 21st century technology in a 20th-century building.
- **Demand.** We've all read about how the 83 million baby boomer generation will be affecting Social Security and Medicare when they retire. Most of these boomers are in their 50s right now and are already beginning to influence hospital usage. It has been indicated that if we build one 100-bed hospital per week for the next 10 years (50,000 beds), it would only just begin to address the upcoming demand – some think as many as 500,000 beds are needed.
- **Technology.** New generation equipment is creating utility (such as fiber optic) and space demands as most systems in the hospital are now digital as well as more versatile. Current space configurations, as well as inflexibility, are causing renovations to be costly, time-consuming and patient-unfriendly.
- **Demographic shift.** As the baby boomers have aged, their geographic preference for housing has shifted to the suburbs. Hospital campuses are still located in urban centers or suburban areas that are no longer areas of population growth. As a result, as hospital consolidation has taken place, instead of additions and renovations on existing campuses, hospitals have opted to build a new replacement hospital in new areas of population growth.
- **Favorable financing and reimbursement.** Notwithstanding the constant pressures of reimbursement, the overall climate for capital markets is greatly enhanced by the relative low level of interest rates.

As we begin the major overhauling of our healthcare system, many trends in the development of the 21st-century hospital become apparent: trends such as built-in flexibility (universal patient and exam rooms, modular bay sizes, universal utilities), an environment conducive to healing (larger patient and operating rooms, positive distractions such as water features and aromatherapy, natural light such as skylights, interventional rooms, digital way finding, decentralized nursing stations) and, perhaps the most important trend of all, the integration of the digital systems.

The integrated digital hospital takes in much content, such as Web-based medicine, pharmacology, patient registration, invoicing and payments, after-hours medical information, supply chain management, telecommunications and health records. Just on the telecommunications side, we are integrating CATV/MATV/Education TV distribution systems, structured cabling (voice, data, video) systems, telemedicine and teleconferencing; intercom, nurse call/code blue systems, infant abduction systems, public address systems, security/CCTV systems, telephone and voice mail systems, LAN/WAN, network transmission facilities, data center facility design, emergency power (UPS, generator), physiological monitoring and audio/video presentation systems.

Robert D. Levine heads Turner's Healthcare group, providing the company's 45 local offices with specialized resources on the unique aspects of healthcare construction. He has over 40 years of experience in the construction industry and has been involved in the completion of nearly $3 billion of healthcare projects across the country, including Mt. Sinai Hospital in New York.

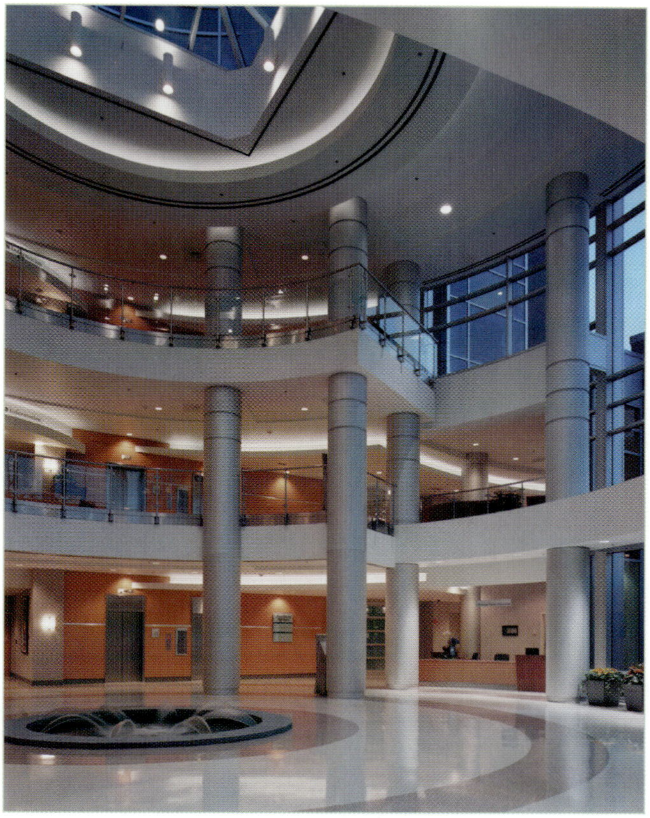

Figure 1 Inova Heart and Vascular Institute in Fairfax, Va.

When you take a step back, however, all of these trends put upward pressure both on the size of the building as well as the cost of construction. For example, patient rooms that used to be 250 square feet 10 years ago are now 300 to 350 square feet to allow for added space to accommodate parental and spousal rooming, computer workstations both for patients and visitors, and inboard toilet rooms to better facilitate proximity to the bedside. Operating rooms are approaching 50 percent space premiums to allow for the added integration of interventional medicine (imaging and surgery occupying the same space). Single-patient rooms versus a ratio of 75 percent single/25 percent semi-private can increase costs by over 10 percent.

Additionally, the added cost per square foot to develop natural light such as skylights, healing gardens, universal patient and exam rooms, universal utilities (which allow for just-in-time delivery of medical equipment), redundant mechanical systems as well as dual utility sources all increase the cost per square foot. And lastly, hospitals, as massive users of energy and water, are trying to be good corporate citizens by addressing Green Buildings with all of the opportunities that go with LEED certification.

LEED certification provides a framework for assessing building performance and meeting sustainability goals and promotes expertise in Green Building through a comprehensive system offering project certification, professional accreditation, training and practical resources. By addressing the major LEED categories, which are sustainable sites, water efficiency, energy and atmosphere, material and resources and indoor environmental quality during design and construction, a hospital can significantly improve its environmental impact, but not without some degree of added initial cost.

This added challenge of cost can and must be overcome in order to take advantage of this current opportunity to make a difference. And the principal way to do this is by combining the analysis of the capital budget with the operating budget. Notwithstanding that these funds come from different sources, it will be virtually impossible to fund these projects without taking into account the savings downstream during the operation of these new facilities. If, in fact, the built environment can affect patient outcomes, then we must include in the financial analysis the fact that single-patient rooms, although costly up front, will decrease patient length of stay, increase infection control, minimize staff turnover by increasing nursing efficiencies and ultimately improve patient outcomes.

There are two dramatic areas where these two interrelated budgets can come together; one is clinical and one is mechanical. The work of the Center for Health Design, a nonprofit advocacy group headquartered in Northern California, includes an emerging science called "evidence-based design," which is the tracking of information through their Pebble Projects. The idea behind the Pebble Projects is to quantify the clinical and financial advantages of designing a building that addresses the concept that a building that embraces an environment of healing will improve patient outcomes, reduce staff turnover, improve community relations and therefore increase contributions. Thus a business case can be made for designing and building better buildings. The Center for Health Design has presented in their regional conferences the following three examples:

- **Bronson Methodist Hospital, Kalamazoo, Mich.** The design features included access to nature (indoor garden, natural light, landscape views); control (intuitive way finding, private rooms, information access); positive distractions (artwork, music, nature); and environmental features (daylight, water sounds).

Using these design features, the areas of measurement were employee turnover, patient outcomes, length of stay, cost per

weblink

Read about how hospitals are leveraging technology to create value in "The Business Case for EHR" in this book and on the Web at www.hctproject.com.

unit of service, waiting times, patient satisfaction levels, organizational behavior and staff productivity.

The following selected results occurred: 11 percent decrease in nosocomial infections; savings due to fewer patient transfers; market share increase; nurse turnover rates decreased to 6.5 percent; increased employee satisfaction; and patient satisfaction increased to 95.7 percent. Overall, there was a positive correlation between the design and key measures of higher quality of care.

- **Methodist Hospital, Indianapolis.** The design features were similar to those for Bronson Methodist Hospital and included natural light, single rooms, healing gardens, digital services and access to nature.

The areas of measurement were clinical outcomes, satisfaction, education and personal growth, and cost and efficiency.

The following selected results occurred: 75 percent fewer patient falls; 90 percent reduction in unit-to-unit transfers; patient dissatisfaction dropped from 6.7 percent to 2 percent; improved medication error index; and reduced caregiver workload index.

- **Karmanos Cancer Institute, Detroit.** The design features were social support (rooming in, computers outside every room); and performance efficiency (enclosed area for unit clerk, clutter-free hallways).

The areas of measurement were employee turnover, length of stay, patient satisfaction levels and pain control.

The following selected results occurred: 16.8 percent increase in patient satisfaction; 3.8 percent nurse attrition rate; 30 percent reduction in medical errors; 6 percent reduction in patient falls; 16.4 percent decrease in patient use of narcotics; and average variable costs decreased $1,000 per patient.

All of these Pebble Projects entailed increased costs and put added pressure on the capital budget. By including in the analysis what the operating savings would be downstream, the combined analysis created a win for those hospitals.

In addition to the clinical advantages, another major area of opportunity to combine first cost and operating cost is in the mechanical systems. On average, almost 50 percent of the cost of new construction can be attributed to the mechanical, electrical, plumbing and fire protection systems. Mostly these systems are designed with the first costs in mind. Occasionally, a life cycle analysis will be performed to determine which system will use the least amount of energy. Also important, and through what is called "commissioning," an analysis of which system will benefit the operational efficiencies over the lifetime of the building can be developed. Interestingly, by concentrating on first costs only, we are looking at only the first two years of a 40-year life cycle. By looking at the 40-year life cycle, we can gain the following benefits:

- Increased system efficiency means reduced energy consumption;
- Smoother building turnover;
- Reduced warranty callbacks;
- Reduced occupant interruptions;
- Reduced troubleshooting efforts;
- Improved air quality;
- Focus on proactive and preventive maintenance;
- Increased operation and management of the systems; and
- Improved building documentation.

Occasionally, a life cycle analysis will be performed to determine which system will use the least amount of energy. Also important, and through what is called "commissioning," an analysis of which system will benefit the operational efficiencies over the lifetime of the building can be developed.

According to Siemens, Lakeside Hospital in Omaha, Neb., decreased its plant management personnel from four to one using Siemens' digital tracking system for maintenance and operation after its new hospital opened.

The proper way to combine the analysis of these two interrelated financial resources is by putting together an integrated team up front comprised of planners, financial consultants, architects, engineers and construction managers all working in concert to assure that downstream savings (operational budget) can accrue from good upstream planning (capital budget). These team members all bring their own specific expertise of development, and having them on board together from the very early stages allows for the conceptual analysis of activities, something that can't be done if they are brought on board one by one as the project moves downstream. ■

Meeting Evolving Healthcare Demands for Secure and Reliable Wireless Solutions

Quick and reliable access to patient records, improved *point-of-patient care*, and uncompromising security safeguards protecting patient information are some of the requirements driving the adoption of technology in the healthcare industry. To be successful, however, these systems must be reliable, secure and able to scale to the unique demands of a hospital environment.

Since 1999, Bluesocket®, Inc. has been a leading provider of open and secure wireless solutions for healthcare organizations looking to extend patient information resources and medical information systems to the patient bedside. The company provides a complete and integrated series of products that can be easily deployed to set up and manage a secure and scalable wireless local area network (WLAN).

Bluesocket's BlueSecure™ Controllers provide reliable wireless access and offer strong management features that allow hospital administrators to control users, conserve bandwidth and develop multilevel procedures and policies that protect sensitive patient information to comply with HIPAA regulations.

BlueSecure Controllers are used today by leading hospitals not only to provide rapid and secure access to patient information, but also to enhance the relationship between patients and the healthcare staff. Wireless networks are used at the front office to gather initial information from patients and conduct triage operations, while emergency room doctors and nurses rely on wireless mobile systems to scour remote medical databases and collect information on patient allergies and prior illnesses. In the operating room, BlueSecure Controllers are used as the hub of 802.11-based voice-over-IP systems, allowing doctors to reach out to colleagues for on-the-spot consultations.

Mount Carmel Health, one of the largest healthcare systems in Ohio, for example, is using BlueSecure 5000 Controllers to provide secure connections to wireless "computers-on-wheels" and to allow bedside access to patient and pharmacy records. More than 1,200 doctors and 1,000 volunteers rely on the wireless network to record patient information on the spot and to provide immediate updates to the medical staff, preventing costly errors.

The security shield offered by BlueSecure Controllers can be enhanced with the addition of the BlueSecure™ Intrusion Protection System (IPS), a radio frequency intrusion detection and protection tool that includes independent purpose-built sensors designed to protect a wireless network from all types of "rogue" devices, including unauthorized access points and neighboring WLANs.

More than 1,200 doctors and 1,000 volunteers rely on the wireless network to record patient information on the spot and to provide immediate updates to the medical staff, preventing costly errors.

Bluesocket's BlueView™ Management System provides centralized management of single or multiple WLANs, as well as real-time discovery of all APs within your wireless networks, scheduled and automated maintenance functions and a trusted and simple way to enforce policy management and procedures as it works with the BlueSecure™ Controllers and BlueSecure™ Access Points securing your WLANs.

Bluesocket's BlueSecure Controllers and solutions are also well-positioned to be the wireless hub and "last mile" connection to remote patient monitoring systems, and are vital technology tools in channeling content to students in teaching hospitals and medical facilities that are preparing future doctors and nurses for the challenges of tomorrow. ■

Bluesocket is the leader in open wireless security and management solutions that simplify the complexities of mobile enterprises.

Ralph Calistri
President and CEO

Dave Danielson
Vice President Worldwide Marketing

Alex Kim
Vice President Business Development

Bluesocket, Inc.
10 North Ave.
Burlington, MA 01803
Phone 781.328.0888
Fax 781.328.0899

Business Contact
Julie Paradiso
Corporate Communications Manager
Phone 781.494.1004
jparadiso@bluesocket.com

On the Road to the EHR

As its first step, a hospital should begin EHR implementation in the health information management department with an on-demand electronic document management system.

[Richard Cohen, ChartOne] [Roberto Mameli, ChartOne]

When it comes to embarking on the journey toward an EHR (electronic health record), many organizations first focus on automating the patient floors – as these areas have been the target of hot-button issues such as patient safety through the collection, sharing and analysis of electronic information. High-profile failures with the patient-floor approach – such as Los Angeles' Cedars-Sinai Medical Center, which scrapped its $34 million computerized physician order entry (CPOE) system after physicians revolted – are leading organizations to wonder whether their journeys might begin in a potentially more valuable setting.

A critical step in creating an EHR is to have a single electronic record of a patient's entire history, indexed for easy and simultaneous retrieval across functional areas. As its first step, a hospital should begin EHR implementation in the health information management (HIM) department with an on-demand electronic document management system (EDMS).

EDMS: A Vital Component of the EHR

Although an EDMS is often described as an application for the HIM department, this is only partially true. In the broadest sense, an EDMS automates the workflow of the HIM department, providing HIPAA-compliant access to an electronic version of the patient chart. The American Health Information Management Association (AHIMA) divides EDMS capabilities into six categories: automated forms processing; electronic signature, document annotation and edit; document capture (both from paper and electronic sources); document indexing, bar coding, character and form recognition and forms redesign; document retrieval, viewing and distribution; and document management. Thus, although an EDMS primarily supports the HIM department, its effects are felt throughout the hospital and, with browser-based access, extend to the hospital's associates, such as payers, regulatory agencies, physician clinics and service providers.

According to the AHIMA, HIM computer systems historically have not been included in enterprisewide IT strategies. This has often resulted in two untenable situations: insufficient HIM automation or the housing of a separate information system within the HIM department, one that is not integrated with the rest of the hospital's IT systems. In both instances, access to the longitudinal patient record is dependent on HIM staff, and the benefits of automation fail to be leveraged from department to department. In addition, most HIM departments are still making paper their primary delivery vehicle for patient information, and even the most efficient, well-staffed hospitals that rely heavily on paper cannot grant simultaneous multi-user access to the patient record.

This is why the EDMS is increasingly being recognized as a critical component of the EHR, the piece that ensures the simultaneous availability of historical patient information to the numerous constituents whose functions depend on this access.

Leveraging the Web for On-Demand Medical Records

Compared with clinical document technologies, which often demand radical workflow changes, a hosted EDMS is relatively low-impact yet has a high return. Although workflow in the HIM department does require change, HIM staff members are able to customize the EDMS to meet the operational realities of their specific hospital.

With a hosted EDMS, the IT resources needed for implementation are minimal, and with almost 75 percent of the typical hospi-

Richard Cohen is CIO at ChartOne where he spearheads information technology, information business systems and all application service provider operations. Before joining ChartOne, Mr. Cohen was CIO at Zentropy Partners and held a variety of other business and technology leadership positions. **Roberto Mameli** is vice president of engineering at ChartOne, where he guides technology and product development. For over 15 years, he has helped leading technology companies such as Oracle and Macromedia innovate and grow through the use of Internet technologies and the development of standard-setting enterprise products.

tal's documents created electronically (even though they are still predominantly printed and stored on paper), the majority of the effort required to supply documents to an EDMS is already done; these existing electronic documents require only interfaces to move them into a single electronic repository of patient information. Therefore implementation is relatively simple and quick (six months, on average). In addition, using Internet technologies based on industrywide standards, organizations are able to achieve higher levels of interoperability with other systems, a critical success factor when it comes to information sharing.

Financially, a hosted EDMS also makes a lot of sense. Hospitals do not need to make large capital outlays to get started with a hosted EDMS. The service is an operational expense, with break-evens normally occurring anywhere from six months to 1.5 years after implementation and significant net savings accruing in year two and beyond. In addition, hospitals benefit from a heightened level of technological robustness, security, availability and scalability that they might otherwise be unable to afford.

Stakeholders across the hospital are motivated to participate in the successful implementation and acceptance of electronic patient chart technology because they gain access to records via their Internet browser; employing this familiar tool minimizes training needs and makes getting started with the EDMS very fast and easy. The browser-based approach is particularly helpful for physicians, who can use their Internet browser to view and complete charts without ever coming to the hospital. This seemingly minor triumph is more powerful than one might imagine, as it begins to engender physician support of and participation in point-of-care technology usage.

Any discomfort in changing entrenched paper-based work habits is more than offset by the hosted EDMS' numerous benefits. Simultaneous electronic access to patient charts means that the chart tug-of-wars that pit, for example, physicians against coders, ER staff against utilization management staff, finally cease. The administrative and clinical efficiencies that result from having more complete patient information accessible at the touch of a computer key, no matter what the time of day and how many others might also be using the information, yield a number of benefits, including the ability to:

- Enhance the revenue cycle by allowing HIM functions to be performed faster, billing to more accurately reflect the services the hospital provides and fewer claims to be denied for insufficient documentation – all along the way ensuring regulatory compliance;
- Cast a wider recruiting net for difficult-to-staff positions like coding, as such functions can be performed remotely – also a prime staff retention factor;
- Improve the satisfaction of physicians and other caregivers by lending greater immediacy, convenience and flexibility to their interactions with the patient record – for example, physicians can sign off on charts from wherever they have Web access;
- Provide better service to patients by giving them a greater sense of being "known" by the hospital – for example, if they visit the emergency room shortly after a hospital stay and records are at a new physician's fingertips – and being able to both guarantee greater medical record security and share more complete information about who has seen what portion of the record at what time, and what action (e.g., viewed, printed) they took; and
- Reallocate precious hospital space from chart storage to revenue-generating activities and HIM staffing resources to more valuable tasks than simple "paper wrangling."

In fact, these benefits can be gained so quickly, with so little up-front capital investment, that hard-dollar savings can be used to fund additional EHR components or other needed hospital projects.

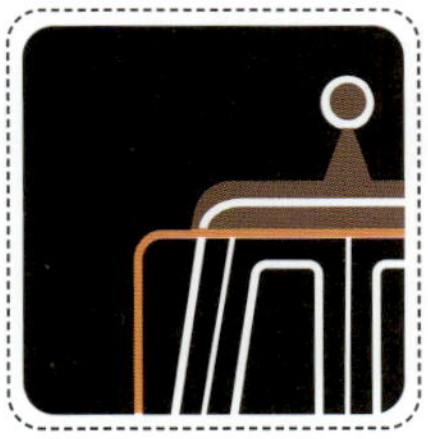

Simultaneous electronic access to patient charts means that the chart tug-of-wars that pit, for example, physicians against coders, ER staff against utilization management staff, finally cease.

Ensuring Security, Availability, Scalability and Speed

The first concern on most people's minds when the topic arises of using the Internet to share patient information is security. Ensuring the security of patient information on the Internet is a far easier task than ensuring the security of paper records, which can be lost, misfiled, left out in the open and otherwise exposed to inappropriate viewing. The right safeguards are essential, however, and include, at a minimum, hardened data centers, isolation of the data layer from any external access, two-factor authentication, data encryption, access logging, role-based security, automatic log-offs and access control.

For a small organization, providing this level of security may be exceedingly difficult because of the law of diminishing returns: Once a certain level of security is attained, it takes increasingly larger investments to make even minor improvements. These investments are not out of reach for a hosted application provider, as they can be leveraged across a wide swath of clients.

In a hospital environment, the stakes are just as high for guaranteeing the availability of patient information via the Internet. The inability to gain access to electronic patient information when it is required could interfere with the revenue cycle, even jeopardize patient care. Here again, organizations can benefit from a service provider's ability to invest more heavily in redundant systems and fault-tolerant infrastructure. The ability to cache information within the hospital's infrastructure also ensures that information remains accessible even when the Internet is not.

> Web-based applications ... take advantage of Internet standards that support the delivery of vast quantities of information efficiently and rapidly. Where applications have been designed ... for the Internet, response time is quick ...

Scalability is also an important consideration when implementing an EDMS. Few facilities design their IT infrastructures to gracefully accommodate exponential growth. Hosted applications built on high-performance Web architectures are designed with exactly this in mind. Their basic design includes horizontal cloning, resource pooling, load balancing, "hot" expansion and use of co-location facilities on the Web backbone.

Hand in hand with the question of scalability is the issue of processing speed. Won't a high volume of users utilizing a data-laden tool over the Internet result in a slow, frustrating system? Web-enabled applications can be slow, as they are front-ending legacy systems. Web-based applications, on the other hand, take advantage of Internet standards that support the delivery of vast quantities of information efficiently and rapidly. Where applications have been designed from the ground up for the Internet, response time is quick, even during high-volume periods.

As a final point, because of the speed of technological advancements themselves, a hospital going at it alone will discover that the quest to be leading edge is an endless and costly one. Partnering with a service provider can give organizations access to the "latest and greatest" without the associated risks, as the success of these companies is largely dependent on their ability to stay ahead of the technology curve.

Interoperability With Other Systems

To arrive at a complete EHR, organizations need to take a component-by-component approach because of the sheer size of the project. Each component needs to work with the next component, which means that the components should be built on industry standards such as XML, HTML, Health Level 7 and others. Nonetheless interfaces to these systems can and should be created to maximize the efficiency and usefulness of the added components.

Service providers often have an advantage here, as they interface with multiple legacy applications. Their experience in creating functional interfaces can be applied to the implementation process and ensures quick results. Hospitals are advised to start with a connection to their admission, discharge and transfer systems; updates here should automatically be reflected in the hosted EDMS to help maintain a cohesive record. Optimal next targets are transcription, laboratory, pharmacy, the emergency department, computerized physician order entry and radiology. Hospitals can then move on to capture, via interface, any document that was created in electronic form.

Extending Beyond the HIM Department

The final reason to start EHR implementations with a hosted EDMS is the number of external organizations the HIM department touches that will also benefit from electronic information access. Remote workers, outsourced service providers, auditors, government agencies and others with a rightful need to view the patient record can gain access under tightly regulated conditions. Data bridges, in turn, help hospitals build stronger, more efficient and profitable relationships with these business partners. A hosted EDMS allows only secure, authorized and auditable access to medical record information, so a hospital does not have to balance the risk of exposing its technology infrastructure to outsiders against the advantages of broadening access.

In addition, organizations should consider that a hosted EDMS' utility can extend beyond the HIM department and its functions – for example, to "de-paper" the business office, to support clinical research and facilitate the development of evidence-based clinical guidelines, and even to replace the majority of filing cabinets in the facility devoted to duplication or long-term storage of medical record information.

Into the foreseeable future, paper will be generated in the patient care process that will need to be managed, records will still require authentication and completion, payers will require documents to support claims, records will be subpoenaed and delivered into jurisprudence and, perhaps most importantly, historical data that did not originate electronically will be required in the patient care process. That these functions may need to be performed simultaneously means that the hosted EDMS is now and will continue to be an essential component of the EHR. ■

Maximizing Hospital Capacity By Automating the Patient Flow Process

On-Demand Medical Records

ChartOne provides Web-based electronic medical record products and services that provide the necessary foundation on the way to an EHR. ChartOne develops, markets, implements and manages customer-driven, people- and technology-based solutions that provide affordable, secure and timely access to patient chart information throughout the healthcare delivery chain. ChartOne has over 20 years' experience providing services in health information management departments, with over 1,000 customers and 1,500 employees.

Our Products

ChartOne's technology and service solutions enable efficient management of the patient chart both inside and outside the medical facility. ChartOne offers a scalable suite of enterprise level document management and workflow applications as well as a broad range of services highlighted below.

eWebHealth Suite

eWebView™: Provides secure, long-term electronic chart viewing and storage for clinicians, billers and others. Multiple users can access a single record simultaneously while reducing the costs associated with storage and maintenance of paper charts.

eWebED™: Gives quick, easy access to patient records in the ED for optimal clinical care. eWebED also gives referring physicians access to medical records from their offices and expedites physician billing.

eWebCoding™: Allows coders to work from any remote location – even from home. The world's first Web-based clinical coding solution, eWebCoding, allows organizations to attract and retain quality coders, increase coder productivity, reduce DNFB and decrease costs.

eWebSignature™: Allows physicians to sign off on charts remotely and electronically for faster chart completion and billing.

eWebCompletion™: Streamlines the chart completion process by routing incomplete charts to physicians via the Internet, reducing chart deficiencies by up to 50 percent.

eWebRelease™: Provides scanning and online access to records, requests and authorizations. Reduces turnaround time and labor costs for the release of information function.

Professional Services

Release of Information Services: All or some release-of-information functions for patient records can be outsourced. ChartOne's Release of Information Services can help improve requester satisfaction, reduce turnaround time and save on equipment, storage and staffing costs.

Disclosure Reporting Services: Capture, track, maintain and report on all requests to view any portion of patients' protected health information – meeting HIPAA disclosure requirements.

Storage Services: Optimize storage of medical records to free up space for revenue-generating activities.

Coding Services: Eliminate coding backlog and reduce DNFB and accounts receivable days with ChartOne's end-to-end coding services that include hardware, software, clerks and coders.

Chart Management Services: Use ChartOne for permanent or temporary file room staffing and management for a variety of services, from purges to conversions and special projects.

Value

Depending on the mix of ChartOne products and services opted for, the customer can experience:

- Improved revenue cycle management;
- Faster coding of charts and responding to denied bills;
- Operational savings and/or efficiencies;
- Improved productivity; and
- New opportunities to leverage hospital space for revenue-generating activities – all without large up-front capital outlays.

ChartOne ensures that each step of the patient chart process is implemented quickly and managed professionally, while meeting all HIPAA and other regulatory requirements. ChartOne's solutions are designed to ensure they require only minimal internal IT support. ■

CHARTONE™
chart management solutions

ChartOne's on-demand medical record solutions combine innovative, Web-based document management technology with superior professional services to automate health information and revenue cycle management.

Brian Cahill
Chief Executive Officer

George Abatjoglou
Chief Financial Officer

Peter Henderson
VP Product Operations

Scott Seero
SVP Sales

ChartOne, Inc.
3 New England Executive Park
Suite 200
Burlington, MA 01803
Toll-Free 800.733.2679
info@ChartOne.com
www.ChartOne.com

Business Contact
Sally Fleishman
info@ChartOne.com

Making the ThinkPad® X41 Tablet Work For You and Your Healthcare Organization

We listened when our customers, business partners and sales specialists told us we needed to develop a tablet. They wanted a tablet to help improve the ease with which healthcare workers could capture critical data and help them improve patient care with easy access to secure patient information. They asked for a tablet that was smaller and lighter than the average tablet notebook that didn't compromise on security, performance, battery life or expansion capabilities. In other words, they asked for a tablet that was a ThinkPad PC.

The ThinkPad X41 Tablet offers a new trifecta in tablet innovation: writable slate, full-size keyboard and light weight.[1] Starting at 3.5 pounds and 1.14 inches thin, the ThinkPad X41 Tablet is 18 percent lighter than the next-lightest convertible tablet among leading vendors and delivers the longest standard battery life of any 12-inch convertible tablet (applies to select X41 Tablet models with 8-cell battery).[2, 3, 4]

The form factor and functionality of the ThinkPad X41 Tablet is ideally suited to be utilized as a primary technology device in the healthcare environment. It's a device that can help healthcare organizations meet some of their most important organizational demands: efficiency, accuracy and security. The ThinkPad X41 Tablet enables healthcare workers to input customer data into the network system in real time either via handwritten notes or via standardization form data; utilizing either the digital handwriting recognition functionality or by typing the data in via the full-size keyboard.[5] The ThinkPad X41 Tablet can also help healthcare organizations protect their patient data through the Client Security Solution and integrated Fingerprint Reader (select models), which combine to create the most secure tablet available.[6] The Client Security Solution includes an integrated security chip and Client Security Software, helping to protect and encrypt vital proprietary information and security passwords, encryption keys and electronic credentials. No other manufacturer offers stronger security as a standard feature.

In their drive to improve all aspects of patient healthcare, professionals at the University of Virginia Health System consider the deployment of tablet PCs to be an important next step. For example, tablet PCs provide immediate access to extensive patient information at the point of care, including past history, medical tests, treatment, diagnosis and education material. In addition, mobile tablets in a complete network solution can help eliminate the need to re-enter patient data on a stationary terminal, helping to drive down administrative costs, potentially reduce errors in patient data and help liberate physicians to spend more time in patient care.[7] "We expect tablets to become an integral component of our healthcare process," said Corb Ardrey, information systems manager for the University of Virginia Health System, which is evaluating the ThinkPad X41 Tablet for possible use in more than 100 clinics in Charlottesville and throughout the state. "Equipped with state-of-the-art wireless, security and the full power and functionally of a traditional notebook PC, tablets will help enable our healthcare professionals to be productive in ways that better serve our patients."

A convertible tablet PC based on Microsoft© XP Tablet PC Edition 2005 offers mobile and healthcare professionals the choice of working in two ways: as a tablet with digital pen or as a traditional notebook PC. Equipped with the ThinkPad signature full-size keyboard, the ThinkPad X41 Tablet provides 170-degree viewing, an optional integrated fingerprint reader for unsurpassed security, the latest ThinkVantage™ Technologies for reliability and convenient wireless connectivity and flexible one-step expandability through the optional new ThinkPad X4 Dock. The X41 Tablet also offers standard anti-reflective and anti-glare coatings to maximize indoor viewability. For mobile workers who demand anytime and anywhere access, users can combine the ThinkPad X41 Tablet's unique battery options to deliver all-day computing, offering up to 8.5 hours of battery life with the optional 8-cell system battery and separate extended-life battery.[8]

Tablet Scenarios …

- Current collection and entry of patient information is time-consuming and has a high possibility of transcription errors.
- Physicians are not able to see as many patients per day as desired.
- Paper based medical records are less secure, can be easily lost or stolen, and are not instantly accessible to all.
- Traditional notebook-based solutions don't provide a way to electronically capture signatures of physicians or patients.
- Password-based security can be cumbersome and often requires expensive calls to the helpdesk for password resets.

… With a ThinkPad X41 Solution

The ThinkPad X41 Tablet and X40 series extended-life battery are an ideal solution because:

- The inking capability allows doctors to do away with clipboards; notes and signatures can be captured digitally.
- The lighter form factor and longer battery life than some tablets allow physicians to carry the X41 Tablet for up to 6.8 hours, with the 8-cell battery and extended-life battery options, without having to recharge.
- In tablet mode, the standard anti-glare and anti-reflective screen enables a doctor and his colleagues to review records together.
- Built in wireless provides a secure link to the hospital patient databases.[13]
- The available integrated fingerprint reader, with Client Security Solution, can help keep patient records secure while allowing multiple profiles to be registered.

The ThinkPad X41 Tablet relies on ThinkVantage™ Technologies to make the difference for today's mobile and healthcare workers. These include the Active Protection System, an integrated motion sensor that can detect certain types of sudden changes in movement and temporarily park the hard drive to help protect data from some falls

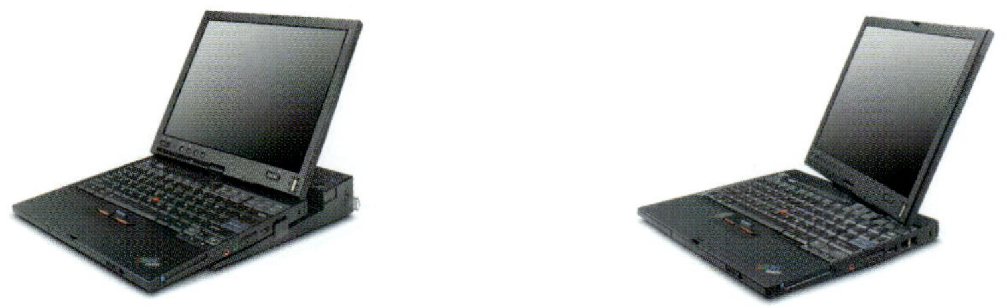

or drops. Also, Rescue and Recovery is a one-button solution that includes self-recovery tools to help users diagnose, get help and recover from a software crash, even if the primary operating system will not boot.

To see innovative healthcare solutions designed around our ThinkPad X41 Tablet, visit our Lenovo Innovation Center Web page at www.thinkpad.com/innovation. The Innovation Centers, located in Research Triangle Park, N.C., and Beijing were developed to provide a venue for solving real customer issues with innovative technology solutions, leveraging customer and partner collaboration.

About ThinkVantage Technologies

ThinkVantage Technologies are available on ThinkPad notebooks and ThinkCentre desktops and help make PCs less dependent on IT staff or user intervention for basic tasks such as deployment, backup, maintenance and security. They free up users and IT staff to focus on competitive advantages in their business. According to industry analysts, costs associated with deployment, support and disposal account for approximately 80 percent of the entire PC life cycle cost. More information is available at www.lenovo.com/thinkvantage. ■

Endnotes

1. *Full-size keyboard: As defined by ISO/IEC 15412.*
2. *Travel weight: Includes battery: weight may vary due to vendor components, manufacturing process and options.*
3. *Thinness: May vary at certain points on the system.*
4. *Leading vendors: Based on manufacturer's published figures or CNET.com results for Top 5 convertible tablet vendors in first quarter 2005 notebook sales as reported by IDC.*
5. *See number 2.*
6. *See number 1.*
7. *Complete Network solution: Other equipment purchased from other vendors is required for a complete network solution.*
8. *Anytime, anywhere access: Wireless network access is required and not included. Subscription may be required and fees may apply.*

lenovo

Lenovo is an innovative, international technology company formed as a result of the acquisition by the Lenovo Group of the IBM Personal Computing Division. Lenovo's executive headquarters are in Purchase, N.Y., with principal operations in Beijing, and Raleigh, N.C., and an enterprise sales organization worldwide. The company employs more than 27,000 people around the world.

As a global leader in the PC market, we develop, manufacture and market cutting-edge, reliable, high-quality PC products and value-added professional services that provide customers around the world with smarter ways to be productive and competitive.

We base our success on our customers achieving their goals: productivity in business and enhancement of personal life.

Business Contact
Carole Smith
WW Sector Sales Champion
Lenovo International
caroles1@us.lenovo.com
Phone 914.701.2865
www.lenovo.com/us

Lenovo Innovation Centers
www.thinkpad.com/innovation

The French Perspective

To address increasing demand due to demographic changes and to improve the affordability of healthcare in France, the time has come to modernize healthcare information systems.

[Sylvie Ouziel, Accenture France and inVita]

Healthcare in France Today

The French government provides diverse and comprehensive healthcare coverage for all citizens. For more than 96 percent of the population, medical care is either entirely free or is reimbursed 100 percent. French people can also choose among healthcare providers, regardless of income level.

French health insurance is a branch of the social security system and is funded by workers' salaries, indirect taxes on alcohol and tobacco, and by direct contributions proportional to income. Currently 85 percent of health expenditures are paid by the national social security program. The rest is paid by private health insurers.

More than 80 percent of French people have supplemental insurance, often provided by employers. Additionally, treatment costs for those who suffer from long-term illnesses are completely reimbursed.

Organization of the Healthcare System

The state exercises control over the healthcare system through central, regional and departmental services. Two large organizations work under the Ministry of Health: General Health Management, and Hospital and Healthcare Management. Numerous healthcare facilities function under the direction of these two large organizations.

The healthcare establishment is composed of three types of institutions: public hospitals, private clinics and not-for-profit healthcare.

In all hospitals, doctors, biologists and dentists are paid as "hospital practitioners." Public hospitals are financed primarily by endowment funding that is paid for by health insurance funds.

Private clinics were originated by surgeons and obstetricians and eventually evolved into private hospitals. A 1991 law requires all doctors in private clinics to share medical files with colleagues and to create a medical care commission to formulate evaluation procedures.

Another sector of the French healthcare system, nonprofit private hospitals, was originally denominational and currently makes up 14 percent of inpatient services among French medical care institutions. Like public hospitals, they are financed through endowments but have the right to privacy like private clinics.

The cooperation between the public and private sector is a positive feature that allows citizens to avoid the waiting lists for surgeries often associated with socialized medicine. The unique combination of government-financed medical care and private medical services produces a healthcare system that is open to all and provides the latest in medical technology and treatment.

Setting the Stage for E-Health in France

Since 1990, France has been working on several e-health initiatives to improve the quality of care and increase efficiency. In March 2002, a law was enacted which granted French citizens access to their medical files. The problem, however, is that coordination along the continuum of the French healthcare system lacks structure. Any one patient can have medical records residing in different hospitals, with different physicians, creating a fragmented health record separated by geography. In this way, collaborative care cannot occur in a uniform or efficient way.

The DMP – France's Answer to the EHR

France took a step toward implementing e-health when a law was passed in August 2004 stating that every French citizen should have a personal electronic medical record – dossier

Sylvie Ouziel is a partner in charge of Accenture's Health & Life Sciences practice for France, Belgium and the Netherlands. She is a member of the Strategy practice and specializes in post-merger integration, organization design and international outsourcing experiences.

médical personnel or DMP – by July 2007, and that care reimbursement could be reduced if a citizen fails to present a DMP to a physician.

The national DMP initiative is pushing healthcare providers to invest in new technologies or upgrade internal clinical information systems to:

- Deliver faster, safer diagnoses, based on a better understanding of patient history and current health status;
- Reduce redundant clinical testing and imaging;
- Avoid patient complications due to drug interactions;
- Create medical statistics for epidemiology and to serve as a basis for health investments; and
- Introduce transparency to make it easier to set protocols, create policy and structure how care is delivered.

The DMP is expected to improve health "value for money" by reducing the costs of poor quality, which the Health Quality Agency estimates to run at least 15 to 20 percent of France's total health budget.

A combination of France's social security system and private insurers will underwrite the cost of the DMP initiative. These funds will be managed by a public interest group.

How the DMP Will Work

DMP systems will collect and centralize information from automated sources such as imaging facilities and laboratories, as well as data keyed in by office-based and hospital physicians.

The DMP system, with a Web interface, will be accessible via the Internet to the patient and to providers with a health professional card (an electronic card supplied to healthcare professionals). Only practitioners to whom the patient will have granted access will be able to view the file.

The new version of France's health card, when introduced in 2006-2007, will serve as a patient identification tool and fit into the DMP system. The new card will include several features it doesn't include now, including a photo, PIN number and a patient ID to verify identity.

The national DMP system will rely on "hosters," meaning private companies who will be paid to host the national electronic health record on behalf of payers, providers and patients. The hosters will be validated by the state according to quality and commitment, and will be employed by service contracts. Services will be sold on a transactional basis and paid by social security funds through a public interest group.

Hosters will also be responsible for managing the physician-to-patient relationship, while ensuring continual availability of service 24/7 in a redundant and safe technical environment. Hosters will need to submit a robust disaster recovery plan and will need to meet the native scalability challenge their applications will face in terms of storage. Hosters must also ensure data integrity, confidentiality and access traceability.

A dialogue body will be established to communicate between DMP hosters and public powers on topics such as service levels, norms and interoperability, pricing and deployment.

DMP hosters will also have to "translate" proprietary formats (such as imaging or biology) into easily readable formats, such as a PDF file that can be read by any Internet browser. These translations will have to occur as software versions evolve to ensure information remains readable for the lifetime of the medical records.

All access to the DMP will be highly authenticated through appropriate encryption and electronic signature processes. Hosters will also employ time-stamping for each and every document to certify who posted what and at what time.

The DMP Initiative – Current State

The DMP is the largest national e-health initiative today in France and follows the launch of electronic reimbursement several years ago. Another precursor to the DMP was the introduction of France's health cards four years ago. These steps have paved the way to adding clinical content, which is the main focus of the DMP initiative.

Accenture has been supporting France's evolving health network since the end of the 1990s, gathering firsthand knowledge of the issues around medical information sharing and collaboration. In 2003 Accenture helped create a dedicated subsidiary to work on the DMP project, called inVita. inVita, a leading group of services and technology firms, works together to address the necessary dimensions of the DMP. It includes representatives from La Poste, 9 Telecom, IntraCallCenter, Sun, EMC-Documentum, SeeBeyond, BEA and Accenture. Working with several, nonprofit health insurers, inVita developed a prototype of the DMP.

French payers and providers show different levels of readiness to connect to the DMP. The DMP project is already triggering clinical IS (information systems) projects in hospitals and hospital groups, but these are occurring locally.

Hospitals are probably further along in connecting to the DMP than other groups. For example, current law already dictates that all patients leaving a hospital receive a copy of their hospital documents showing any care received. These records will be routed to the DMP, where they will be stored and tagged, ready to be linked to patient records as the DMP is built. inVita's target hospital networks.

Physicians surveyed by Accenture are largely in favor of the national DMP; however, over 50 percent have PCs and laptops

weblink

Read about healthcare challenges in the United States in "The Impact on Healthcare Costs for American Companies" in this book and on the Web at www.hctproject.com.

that are older than five years and will not handle the high-speed Internet connections needed to log on and access patient records on the initial DMP platform.

In terms of patient records, inVita's goal is to add 500,000 patient records by the end of 2005, 4 million records by 2006 and 40 million records by July 2007.

Several live pilots have been established in Lels, Rouen and Paris prior to national deployment this year. All testing and results from these projects have been favorable.

system is to learn by doing. Getting started helps to actively solicit buy-in from providers by showcasing early project wins and by encouraging reluctant players to get in the game.

Next Steps

Deployment of the DMP is imminent. Unfortunately significant infrastructure items will not be in place before September 2005, including high-speed connections, physician authentication cards in hospitals, modems and full support for legacy systems.

It's best to build patient records from bits and pieces of information, with the understanding that some information is better than none.

Privacy Concerns

Data confidentiality within the DMP framework is a complex issue. Although it seems appealing to encourage patients to share as much information as possible, patients who are eager to maintain their privacy might not want all caregivers to see their full records. A compromise must be achieved that does not sacrifice quality of care in the name of patient rights.

DMP project coordinators have suggested that patients should be able to "hide" a medical event from certain caregivers. This means, of course, that a huge responsibility is placed on physicians to educate patients about the risks involved in withholding information.

It is important to note that some emergency data (such as allergies) will be placed in an easily accessible part of the DMP, perhaps with an automated voice synthesizer to deliver information to a physician calling in an emergency. For these data, patients must accept less confidentiality (meaning lighter protection of data) because the information may be needed to save a life.

Lessons Learned

Bringing players up to speed and hearing all concerns about the DMP project has been a tremendous job for inVita. Reaching out to patient advocacy groups, physician unions, hospitals and original health organizations has already required a great deal of time, and all players need to be kept in the loop as the DMP system is launched. This step is especially important in a decentralized environment like the French healthcare system, as it is easy for physicians and hospitals to act independently and develop solutions that are incompatible with the evolving DMP.

The main lesson of the DMP initiative is that e-health pioneers must take a pragmatic approach toward implementation and must find the right compromise between theory and action. Tying together countless IS systems is a daunting task; the best way to test the

The risk is greater, however, in waiting for these steps to be taken rather than proceeding. If project participants wait for the ideal moment when all people, processes and technology are in place, the initiative will stall and fail. It's best to build patient records from bits and pieces of information, with the understanding that some information is better than none.

The solution is to engage a durable approach that will adapt over time during what promises to be a multiyear venture. Participants know they will soon prove some initial assumptions wrong, requiring redesign and reconfiguration; however, the DMP will be stronger as a result and lessons learned can be applied to the next phase. The best tactic is to start with physicians and hospitals that are already wired, then gradually add providers as technology permits.

Summary

In 2000, the World Health Organization stated that France provides the best overall healthcare in the world. Recent initiatives to introduce e-health mechanisms are bound to help France maintain this ranking by improving diagnoses, reducing redundancies and providing more information to providers for better-quality care. France's primary e-health initiative, the DMP, will go live in September 2005. It promises to improve coordination among caregivers by outsourcing the management of the system to third-party DMP hosters. The challenge will be keeping a project of this magnitude moving forward. The project faces significant challenges including complex privacy issues and players at different stages of technology readiness. The biggest risk, however, is allowing the project to get sidetracked by technical issues. The strategy being employed by inVita and all project participants is to get started now to gain momentum while resolving technical and process issues as they appear. By staying focused and systematically adding providers to the system, the DMP will gain critical mass and deliver its promise of improved healthcare for all. ■

2

Achieving Interoperability & Collaboration

Interoperability permits the automatic exchange of clinical data from one computer to another while maintaining the integrity of the information. It is essential for improving the quality of care and for creating a platform that allows the healthcare system to evolve. Accelerating the adoption of standards is required for facilitating collaboration and for implementing an interconnected electronic health information infrastructure nationwide.

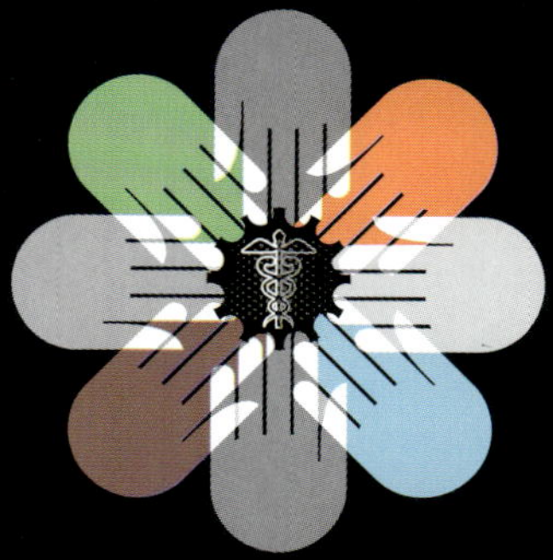

Interoperability

Computers need to interoperate so they can store and act on data from other computers in a reliable and beneficial way without human intervention and translation.

[Marshall Ruffin, M.D., M.P.H., M.B.A., F.A.C.P.E., Accenture]

What does interoperability mean? Imagine you have traveled to London from the United States and arrive in the morning after an overnight flight; you fall asleep in your hotel to overcome jet lag and awake in the mid-afternoon somewhat revived and eager to clean up and get something to eat. You shower and prepare to use your corded electric razor only to discover that the electrical outlet in England does not receive the electrical plug of your American razor. You suffer from a failure of mechanical interoperability – the plug doesn't match the wall jack. So you ring up the front desk and you ask for an adapter. A member of the hotel staff brings the adapter quickly and you plug it into the wall socket. Now your razor can interoperate with the electrical system in England, right? Not necessarily. When you turn on the razor nothing happens. The electrical standards in England, the voltage and amperage, are different than they are in electrical systems in the U.S. So while you have mechanical interoperability with the converter given to you, you do not have electrical interoperability. For your electric razor designed for the U.S. to work in England, you need both an adapter for mechanical interoperability (plug-to-jack interoperability) and a transformer for electrical interoperability, which changes the voltage and amperage to what your razor requires. At this point either you ask the hotel staff if they have a transformer, or you ask the hotel staff to sell you a manual razor and shaving cream. The electrical appliance you brought from the United States does not interoperate with the electrical system in the U.K. on two levels because mechanical standards and electrical standards do not match.

Similarly, imagine that after you shave with the manual razor you dress and leave your hotel hoping to find an appealing restaurant. Looking about you do not see one, so you approach the nearest person to ask directions. That person happens to be a visitor from Germany who speaks little English and does not know the city at all, having just arrived the day before from Berlin. Here again you face a failure of interoperability. That person does not speak your language well enough to converse with you. You turn to another person walking by dressed in a tweed jacket and kilts and ask him about restaurants in the neighborhood and he replies in exemplary English that he is a visitor to London from Inverness, Scotland, and cannot recommend any restaurant. You have interoperated in language but not in content knowledge. The third person walking by is Asian and smiles agreeably so you ask your question with little hope of interoperating. To your surprise and delight she answers in a British accent with a "cheers" and a question about what type of restaurant you would like. She is second-generation English and her parents are on the faculty of University College London. With her you can interoperate with language and content.

Now think of interoperability as it relates to computers. The computers must connect together in some way, over some network, in order to interoperate – meaning they must physically connect to the network in the same way with the same sort of plugs, such as ethernet plugs. They also need to share operating systems and network protocols in order to connect one to another, so one computer recognizes the other computer on the network. Anyone who has tried to add a computer to a network knows the bewildering complexity of protocols, switches, IP addresses, authentication and identification, and other facts needed to achieve interconnectivity between PC and network. Interconnecting a PC to a network is the first step, but not the only step, to interoperability. Once the PC, whether wired or wireless, connects to the network it will not give its user access

Marshall Ruffin, M.D., M.P.H., M.B.A., F.A.C.P.E., is a partner of Strategy and Business Architecture for the Health & Life Sciences practice of Accenture. He recently served as the initial clinical director of the National Care Records Service for the National Health Service in the United Kingdom. Dr. Ruffin currently is the executive director of the Interoperability Consortium (Accenture, Cisco, CSC, HP, IBM, Intel, Microsoft, Oracle) that is developing the technical reference architecture for the regional health information organizations in California.

to an application, such as an electronic medical record (EMR), without proper authentication by ID, password, retinal scan, voice print or other means of reliably identifying the user and determining that he or she may access the contents of the EMR application.

Once the PC has connected to the network and the user has been given access to the EMR application, the user may be able to access the content of patients' records. A human can interpret the language on the screen and make sense of it, provided the coded numbers for diagnoses and laboratory results and pharmaceuticals and procedures are accompanied by their translations in English. A computer cannot do these things. A computer needs codes it expects, otherwise it will not understand the content of a message it receives from another computer. A human who understands English can see an ICD-9CM code and, if the English translation accompanies the code, understand the meaning of the code. A human can do the same with a SNOMED-CT code; that is, understand it, as long as the English translation of the code accompanies the code. A computer cannot understand, so to speak, an ICD-9CM code if it is expecting a SNOMED-CT code, and vice versa.

Interoperability requires standardized language (terminologies, data, information models and document structures) and messages so the integrity of the content of the information exchanged is preserved. Without interoperability, there can be no useful exchange of information.

Without interoperability of clinical content between computers, one must print paper records from one computer, a human must interpret the information content on the paper and then that human must type into the second computer the information in a format the second computer will store reliably. This happens in the hospital pharmacy when a fancy physician order entry system used by doctors on the inpatient care units is not integrated with the pharmacy information system, so the fancy CPOE system, unbeknownst to all those hospital employees and doctors proud of the new CPOE system, prints its orders in the pharmacy on paper and a pharmacist types the order into the pharmacy information system. In most exchanges of healthcare information between providers, between providers and payers, between doctors and pharmacies and durable medical equipment vendors and between physicians and hospitals, the translation function takes place by people interpreting paper records printed from one computer before entering by hand the content into the second computer.

A scanned document, unless formatted carefully and passed through an optical character reader software application, is an image in the recipient information system, available for viewing but not for extraction of data for entry into a database.

Computers are not as facile with English and data as we humans. To store, communicate and act on information they need data carefully formatted, with codes they expect, properly formatted and in messages in the right order. To interoperate, computers need a carefully defined structure of messages, using standards such as Health Level 7 (HL7); and information, using a reference information model (RIM) such as HL7 RIM, and documents; using common document formats such as HL7 clinical document architecture (CDA). Without these standards, computers cannot reliably exchange the information content of laboratory results, operative reports, radiology interpretations, diagnosis codes, discharge summaries, prescriptions and lists of allergies without human intervention and translation. Without these standards, the computers cannot interoperate – though they may be on the same network.

So why is interoperability important? It permits the automatic exchange of clinical data from one computer to another while maintaining the integrity of the information content, so diagnosis codes sent from one computer are interpreted and stored as diagnosis codes by the recipient computer, and allergy data sent by one computer are received by another computer as allergy data. The network is essential but not sufficient for interoperability.

Think of all the claims that pass from doctors' offices to insurers on paper, having been created in the doctors' office computers and printed to paper for mailing to the insurers, and the legions of clerks who take the paper records and type their contents into the insurers' claims processing systems. Think of all the paper prescriptions hand written or computer generated by physicians and typed into pharmacy information systems by pharmacists or clerks. Think of all the paper reports from consulting physicians and reference laboratories and diagnostic radiology groups received by doctors' offices and either scanned or typed into those physicians' office practice electronic medical records.
A scanned document, unless formatted carefully and passed through an optical character reader software application, is an image in the recipient information system, available for viewing but not for extraction of data for entry into a database. Scanned documents generally do not contribute content to databases. Interoperability of content with standardized terms and messages,

and data and information models permits computers to exchange coded data and to interact on the data exchanged, so that an electronic medical record can alert a physician when it receives an abnormal laboratory result from a laboratory system, such as from a blood gas measurement in an intensive care unit that can trigger changes in oxygen concentration, or ventilator rate per minute or tidal volume of the ventilator oxygenating a patient. Computers need to interoperate so they can store and act on data from other computers in a reliable and beneficial way without human intervention and translation. The velocity of actions speeds up and treatment decisions can occur more quickly than they can with human intervention for translation.

The economic benefits of interoperability are enormous. Imagine you had to speak with an operator every time you wanted to make a cellular telephone connection because the various cellular networks did not interoperate. You use Sprint. Your friend uses AT&T. You would need to call a Sprint operator, who would call an AT&T operator, who would dial your friend's telephone number before establishing a circuit for you and your friend to speak before both operators can hang up. For this model to work, almost the entire population of the U.S. would have to become operators in order to facilitate the number of telephone calls we Americans take for granted every day. All the telephone companies in the U.S. have adopted interoperable standards for dialing and connecting telephone calls so that computers can switch calls and set up connections without expensive and slow intervention by human operators. The cellular and landline telephone networks interoperate, and so our society enjoys enormous productivity benefits.

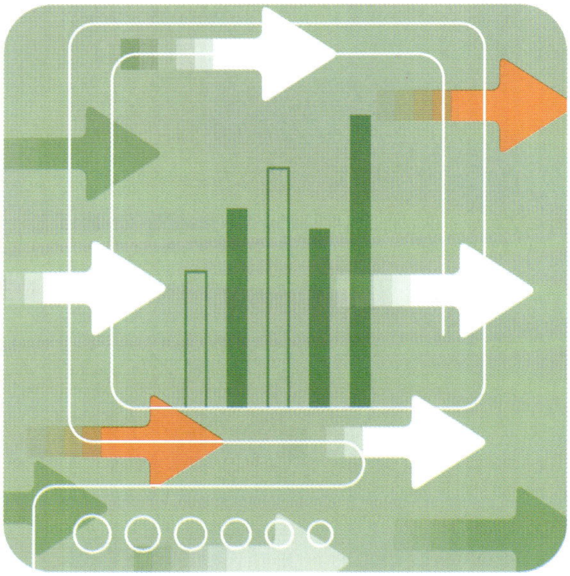

So too with the Internet and the World Wide Web – the standards permit interoperability insofar as Web pages on a server attached to the Internet anywhere can be viewed by computers with Web browsers anywhere. Through a Web browser you can schedule a hotel room or a rental car or reserve an airline ticket, all because your Web browser formats data in the way that the computer systems of the hotel and rental car company and airline expect the data to be formatted. With this same technology for interoperability, you can check the weather, the value of your stocks or your medical record without another person having to translate your request into the format of another computer.

The economic and political benefits of interoperability derive from the automatic exchange of information between computers. Interoperability reduces labor costs and increases the velocity of information exchange; it expedites and lowers the costs of commerce. Interoperability allows computers to exchange information without human interference, assuring doctors that laboratory their patients' results will be available in their patients' electronic medical records as soon as the computerized laboratory equipment have calculated the results; it means a doctors' staff can instantly send claims for a day's work to the patients' various payers, and the doctors' practice management system will receive from the payers' computers, just as quickly, results of claims adjudication and remittance advice for those claims found acceptable by the payer. Delays with paper processing that may be on the order of days and weeks in the interoperable digital world shrink to seconds and minutes. Cash flow improves and clerical staff work declines – provided the physician's computer system has been set up to interoperate with the computer systems of the payers used by his patients.

There are costs to interoperability in hardware, software and network access, and in standardization of data and information in clinical and financial transaction systems that exchange data. However, once the standards have been implemented and the computers can interoperate, the velocity of commerce increases, the friction of interaction between businesses and their customers declines and the costs of commerce decline. In the short run, adoption of digital communications and standardization of information exchange hurts and costs money. It hurts because it requires change in the ways business happens. It costs money because hardware and software and network access cost money, and because the language of work must change from free text to coded information interpretable and storable by computers. In the long run, the standardization reduces the costs of commerce and reduces the costs of both producers and consumers, especially for activities that require searching many sources of information, or updating sources of information remotely.

Think of the friction of finding sources of information in paper form on obscure topics, the publications of a little-known author or the medications used to treat an unusual tropical disease. Visits to libraries and searches through card files and stacks of journals often take days or weeks. Now with a Web browser and the English language, you can perform those searches in seconds with PubMed or Google. How can a large multispecialty group practice using paper medical records alert its patients taking Vioxx that the medication has been recalled by the manufacturer and they should contact their physicians to discuss other treatments? It will have to alert all of its patients by mail, since it has no simple way to scan paper charts for those patients who have received prescriptions for Vioxx, and no way of knowing if those patients who responded to the letter represented all of the patients taking Vioxx. On the other hand, with an EMR and software for e-prescribing, the group practice can identify and contact only those patients who have received prescriptions for Vioxx and make certain it reaches each and every one of them directly, increasing the velocity and accuracy of care and reducing the friction of information management.

What steps can a healthcare community of doctors, hospitals, pharmacies, nursing homes, home health agencies, durable medical equipment vendors and dentists (to name a few of the providers of care in a community) take to establish interoperable digital health records which they can share? For providers, payers and patients to share the myriad of standards for messaging and content of medical records, they must share a complete technical reference architecture for defining the documents and content to be exchanged between participants on the network. A community will have as much a political as a technical challenge to establish such a reference architecture. When any two people or organizations want to share data, they need only agree on standards among themselves. When a company wants to exchange data in standard format with all its customers or all its suppliers it faces a one-to-many challenge, and needs to establish the standards for communication and convey them to all those with which it wishes to communicate electronically. However, in healthcare, a patient may have many providers of care and a provider will have many patients, with many forms of insurance and many pharmacies of choice. A community sharing medical records electronically produces a many-to-many challenge that requires some third party to define the standards for the community – either the government or the community itself in the form of a shared organization. The community needs a trusted broker to establish the shared standards for all participants in the exchange of EMRs. In the paper world, the analog are the carriers of paper – the U.S. Postal Service, FedEx and UPS. In the digital world, for interoperability, every computer needs to connect to a shared network and share messaging and format and content standards in order to exchange medical information reliably. No aggregation of individual point-to-point exchanges will serve the purpose, at least not economically.

How do interoperable EMRs form in communities? In some countries with centralized healthcare systems, such as in England, the government defines the interoperability standards. The National Health Service (NHS) has defined the data and messaging standards for a summary EMR for every person in England, and calls that summary record the "National Spine." Right now the computer systems used by all the providers of healthcare in England, including dentists, home health nurses, nursing homes, diagnostic centers, pharmacies, general practitioners, hospitals and consultants are receiving new EMR software that will communicate with the National Spine. England has one source of organization and funding for this gargantuan effort, the NHS, which is planning to spend more than $20 billion over 10 years on the effort.

England has one source of organization and funding for this gargantuan effort, the NHS, which is planning to spend more than $20 billion over 10 years on the effort.

In the U.S., with our pluralistic and fragmented industry and dislike of big national government programs, we are moving toward a model for interoperable EMRs that promotes standards for interoperability and gives providers of care and payers for care economic incentives to modify their information systems to send and receive patients' data according to those standards. The standards will be defined by consortia of private sector organizations such as the Interoperability Consortium (started by Accenture, Cisco, Computer Sciences Corporation, Hewlett-Packard, IBM, Intel, Microsoft and Oracle) and endorsed by the federal government through the Office of the National Coordinator for Health Information Technology.

HHS and other payers now are expressing their strong interest in the widespread adoption of interoperable EHRs and are formulating the government grants and contracts to initiate development of regional health information organizations (RHIOs) that will establish communication-based interoperability, data security and privacy standards for all providers and payers and others who would exchange healthcare data in digital form. Because the costs of interoperable electronic health and medical records will be lower than those costs for maintaining and communicating paper records, the federal government believes that after catalyzing the conversion from paper to EMRs in some communities – with grants – the business case for EMRs will become obvious to most medical communities, and regional health information organizations (RHIOs) will appear spontaneously, adopting the interoperability standards that the first government-funded RHIOs will adopt, based largely on the Federal Health Architecture that already exists. ■

Verity: Greater Visibility Into Your Processes, Business and Content

What would you see if you had greater visibility into your company's content and processes? With enterprise search solutions from Verity, you see customers and competitors in context. Where your market is going, not where it's been. Faster, cheaper ways of doing things. Challenges before they become crises. You see a business where ...

business for processing. Accountants must understand changing tax regulations, how your business is evolving, and then use that knowledge to minimize liabilities and mitigate risks. Everyone in your company – from the receptionists and call center representatives who answer your customers' questions, to the people designing, making and selling your products – needs to be able to discover, analyze and process real-time information. That's what visibility into your content and processes is all about, and that's the type of visibility that only Verity can provide.

Information Is Everywhere

Information is spread across your business in thousands of applications, databases and servers. It is stored in hundreds of document, presentation, spreadsheet and other file formats, and on paper and electronic forms. Some of that information is accessible to everyone, while some of it is restricted to just a few. And all of it

Germany he can't find the specifications documents he needs to do his job – getting your factory up and running. Verity gives him and every other employee in your company the visibility they need to do their jobs, whatever their roles are and wherever they're located.

Everything Happens in Real Time

What makes information valuable is not how much it costs to produce, but how much and how quickly it gets reused or processed. Take the reports written by engineering teams throughout a project, information you collect from customers when they initiate a support request or the competitive content you purchase from industry analysts and media. The information in each of these decreases in value the longer it sits untouched. That loss of value can be seen in project teams recreating existing work, decreased customer satisfaction and intelligence, and missed opportunities that you paid analysts good money to tell you about.

Verity gives every employee in your company the visibility they need to do their jobs, whatever their roles are and wherever they're located.

Everyone Is a 'Knowledge Worker'

An assembly-line worker in a manufacturing plant. A claims adjuster assessing and recording the damage to a car after an accident. An accountant reviewing R&D programs to find projects eligible for tax credits.

Which of these are knowledge workers? They all are. And they all need better visibility into your intellectual capital. Employees on a factory floor must know and follow increasingly complex manufacturing procedures. Claims adjusters must know a wide variety of insurance products, gather content from customers making claims and send that information back into the

increases in value when you understand how one document relates to another document, to the people who use it and to the processes it drives. All together, these make up your intellectual capital: your information, your people, your processes and the relationships between them.

In order for people to find and take action on a single document amongst all that information, they need secure visibility across all of it. That means you must make it all behave like a single set of content that can be managed, viewed and accessed with a common set of tools. Because if a mechanic retooling a factory in Michigan can't see into a content management system on a server in Munich,

Products are designed, manufactured and sold in real time. Customers use products, experience problems and require support in real time. The race with your competition is in real time. Your employees, customers and partners need Verity's real-time visibility into your content at every stage of its capture, processing and storage.

Visibility Into Your Business

In order to have greater visibility into your business, you need greater visibility into your content and your processes. Only Verity's solutions combine:

- Enterprise Search Solutions – Integrated search, classification, recommenda-

tion and monitoring/alerting – that provide visibility into your content.
- Content capture and business process management applications that enable visibility into your processes.

This integrated approach creates solutions that meet your unique requirements better than point solutions are capable of, while delivering lower total cost of ownership and shorter implementation cycles.

Visibility Into Your Content

Verity is the recognized market leader in intelligent content services (ICS):
- Search;
- Classification & Taxonomies;
- Recommendation;
- Monitoring & Evaluation;
- Question & Answer Interfaces; and
- Federated Solutions.

With the broadest and deepest line of integrated enterprise search products available, Verity is uniquely able to deliver solutions that give you broader and deeper visibility into the content spread across your business. This ranges from departmental search of file and Web servers, to evaluation of content in diverse applications in order to meet specific business objectives such as HIPAA and Sarbanes-Oxley compliance, email monitoring and mining, and tax credit analysis.

Visibility Into Your Processes

Verity's integrated content capture and business process management solutions make manual processes more efficient and give you visibility into the content driving your business processes. This increases your control over your business by making in-process content actionable in real time through:
- Paper-to-electronic Content Capture;
- Web-based Content Capture;
- Electronic Forms; and
- Process Workflow.

Extended Visibility

Sir Isaac Newton once said, "If I have seen further, it is by standing upon the shoulders of giants." Verity provides our customers with shoulders to stand on in the form of top-tier partners and our world-class professional services organization.

Partners

Verity is committed to building strong partnerships that allow our customers to benefit from the most complete set of solutions possible. Our partners provide specialized solutions that manage information across legacy applications, as well as solutions customized to the unique current and future needs of vertical industries and horizontal applications. We also partner with companies that allow us to enhance the value we deliver through specialized consulting services, taxonomies and content and technology integration. However, our most valuable partners are our customers, who give us the insight and understanding into their needs that we need to develop products that solve the business problems they face in the real world.

Professional Services

The Verity Professional Services organization exists solely to optimize the visibility our solutions provide to our customers. Instead of outsourcing our consulting, training and technical support, we view these services as strategic assets. As a result, our customers benefit from the direct links between the programmers who develop our software and the Verity consultants on client sites, the educators in our classrooms and the technical support representatives solving problems by telephone, email and online via our dedicated customer support website. ■

Verity®

Verity provides enterprise search software that enables organizations to discover, analyze and process all the information within their enterprises. Verity's solutions include integrated search, classification, recommendation, monitoring and analytics and business process management and content capture solutions that deliver the true real-time process control and forward-looking visibility required by complex businesses.

Anthony J. Bettencourt
President and
Chief Executive Officer

Steven R. Springsteel
Senior VP of Finance and
Administration and
Chief Financial Officer

Nicole Eagan
Senior VP and
Chief Marketing Officer

Michael D. Mooney
Senior VP, North American Sales
& Business Development

Verity
894 Ross Drive
Sunnyvale, CA 94089
Phone 408.541.1500
Fax 408.541.1600
www.verity.com

For more information
Verity Business Development
Phone 408.541.1500
info@verity.com

Getting to Action From Your EHR Data

Business intelligence software helps healthcare organizations to integrate clinical data from multiple sources and allows that information to be easily viewed, shared and analyzed.

[Bob Gressens, Business Objects] [David Manchester, Business Objects]

What Exactly Is an Electronic Health Record?

The National Health Information Infrastructure initiative targets that every American should have an electronic health record (EHR) within 10 years. But what an EHR actually is, and what that means for healthcare organizations, remains unclear. Most commonly an EHR is thought of as an electronic tool used by physicians and clinicians to record their notes, order tests and drugs and store their patients' information. Most modern EHR applications do all those things and much more, but the use of computing tools by the clinician while the patient is in the exam room is only part of the whole EHR picture.

It's actually more accurate to say that patients don't have one record, they have several. These records comprise a mix of physical (paper notes, X-ray film) and electronic files (images, digital wave outputs, text notes). There are varying amounts of administrative, financial and clinical data specific to each patient on each of these records and, of course, these data sets are created by many different healthcare organizations and the patients themselves. These organizations are far from being on the same page as to how they share that information. There is universal agreement, from Newt Gingrich to Sen. Hillary Clinton, that getting all that data into an EHR accessible by physicians and patients will have two major benefits.

Two Big Benefits for an EHR

The first rationale for the EHR is to improve the quality and efficiency of the care process as patients experience it. The focus has been on getting tools and applications into the clinicians' hands at the point of care. These tools are intended to deliver the patients' medical history, medications, lab results and other pertinent information to the clinician, while at the same time being able to record the clinicians' notes, take their orders for lab tests, diagnostic imaging, prescriptions and referrals to other clinicians. In addition the tools are often designed to suggest care protocols to the clinician while warning against potential hazards such as medication errors. Clinician use of the EHR should make the patient's experience safer, more efficient and more effective.

The second reason for an EHR is to analyze overall patterns of care within a population, using the data recorded in the data repository that is the foundation of an EHR. Those interested in the population level include health plan and hospital medical directors checking whether their patients are being treated with the most appropriate care guidelines, private and government payers looking at high-cost "outliers" or the cost-effectiveness of treatments and clinical researchers assessing post-approval drug safety. As more clinical data is captured electronically and analyzed, more innovation will occur in how it's used.

So Why Care About Business Intelligence?

Two trends are intersecting that increase the potential for this analysis while healthcare organizations struggle to reduce costs and improve performance. The first is that even though clinician adoption of the EHR is only increasing slowly, more and more clinical information is being transmitted and captured electronically. That information includes not only basic but useful diagnosis and procedure information on claims, but also lab results, radiology reports, medication histories and clinical notes transcribed into XML or other searchable formats. The second is that the tools with which significant value can be extracted from this data are becoming more powerful and easier to use. In fact it doesn't really matter whether a clinician is using an EHR at the point of care; there is now enough data available for medical directors, researchers and clinicians to make meaningful interventions in

Bob Gressens is the director of business development of Business Objects. His experience includes two decades in the sales and business development of enterprise software, with prior experience at Siebel Systems and Oracle. **David Manchester** is responsible for healthcare marketing at Business Objects, helping organizations understand the strategic value of business intelligence.

the overall management of the care process, including in the care of individual patients, without having to wait for days or weeks for special IT reports. What they need is the ability to easily collate and manipulate this data from multiple sources: This is the lair of an emerging application called business intelligence (BI).

Business Intelligence Using the EHR

There are many potential uses of BI using clinical data, often created using the EHR and stored in clinical data repositories. Below are some brief examples of how the use of BI has changed clinical care processes, and has improved patient care as well as financial performance.

Inpatient care: Hospital profit margins are extremely sensitive to variations in inpatient care such as patient length of stay, staff and equipment use. Yet a recent study published in *Health Affairs* showed significant variation in resource use in the care of similar patients even between prestigious academic medical centers[1]. The information collected in EHRs can be used to determine the resources used in patient care. Using a data mart storing information from both the EHR and various departmental clinical and financial systems, BI systems allow the assessment of the use of supplies, staff and procedures, and equate that back to decisions made by individual clinicians. The analysis can drill down to individual patients, such as types of supplies used in surgery or imaging, and cross-match that with length of stay, frequency of re-admissions, outcomes and overall costs – all of which might have significant impact on overall profit margins per admission, as well as being a key to improving patient outcomes. That information can then be communicated back to clinicians.

Population care management: Gathering information from many divergent clinical and financial databases, health plan medical directors have been attempting to profile the overall care delivered by contracted physicians to their populations for over a decade. But the effectiveness has been limited in part because the data used has been out of date and difficult to analyze and communicate. Despite these limitations, looking at macro-level claims data has enabled the discovery of outliers that may have serious consequences for payers, providers and patients. For example, two physicians were responsible for a dramatic increase in cardiac procedures in Redding, Calif., in the late 1990s – clearly visible in the Dartmouth Health Atlas analysis of surgery rates. This had severe consequences for the hospital's parent, Tenet Healthcare. But that information was hard to find. BI promises to deliver this type of analysis much closer to real time, and make it far more available to analysts within hospitals, health plans and government agencies responsible for looking at physician practice patterns, population health or even fraud.

BI is also useful for direct care management. For example, Active Health Management (recently acquired by Aetna) has been using close to real-time analysis of medical, pharmaceutical and lab claims to directly contact doctors and patients if their system flags a potentially adverse event. Similarly, BCBS of Kansas City has been using BI to determine whether their members with diabetes or heart conditions are seeing their doctors on a regular basis, receiving recommended tests or filling the correct prescriptions. In these cases, contacting the doctors and patients concerned allows for better and less expensive care.

As more clinical data is collected via EHRs and various other clinical and financial databases, the use of BI for this analysis and consequent intervention in care management will become more common and more effective. Kaiser Permanente is making a huge investment in its HealthConnect EHR and associated data warehouse and BI tools. John Mattison, CMIO of Kaiser Permanente of Southern California, described the goal of the BI function as giving the ability to perform analysis to anyone, given their role and appropriate security level, in order to come up with more creative ways to answer problems. "The goal is to have best practices where they are known and create a good model to discover best practices where they are not yet known," and then to feed that clinical content to clinicians at the point of care. Mattison believes that within five to seven years provider organizations that don't find a way to combine the EHR with this BI and overall process improvement function will be unable to compete, as Kaiser will be able to demonstrably provide better value at a lower cost. As more end payers start to "pay for performance," these competitive pressures will increase.

BCBS of Kansas City has been using BI to determine whether their members with diabetes or heart conditions are seeing their doctors on a regular basis, receiving recommended tests or filling the correct prescriptions.

weblink

Read how modernizing legacy systems enables organizations to strengthen the connections between patient systems and payer claims systems in "Claims Management and Legacy Integration."

Public health and bioterrorism: As information is collected in the EHR in public health clinics and emergency rooms, clinicians and public health officials are beginning to use BI to track potential disease outbreaks. For example, physician group Emergency Medical Associates uses BI in conjunction with its encounter records to track disease outbreaks, such as TB, or possible bioterrorism attacks. Based on key words used by patients in articulating their symptoms, patients are placed into disease groupings, and the number of patients in each grouping is then compared with statistical norms. Unusual levels or trends of symptoms could indicate the early stages of an outbreak.

Patient safety. Patient safety, particularly around medication administration errors, has become a critical issue for healthcare providers. Intermountain Healthcare in Utah has been perhaps the leading proponent of collecting and analyzing data on medication use and associated adverse drug events. Using the connection between BI and their EHR systems, Intermountain has created a robust and complete error reporting system, and after feeding that back to clinicians, it has seen reductions in error rates that significantly exceed comparable provider systems. This has a direct impact on patient safety, patient outcomes and lives saved.

The overall implication is that the management of healthcare organizations including hospitals, large physician organizations, and private and government payers will be able to examine their clinical and business processes much more closely.

The Technology Behind Business Intelligence

These examples of BI use the data that's collected as part of the wider EHR in the patient's journey around the healthcare system. Even without direct clinician use of an EHR, a significant amount of clinical data is available already in electronic format, albeit in different silos. The goal of BI is to access information, regardless of where it resides, giving all the relevant decision makers a single view of the true data. A good BI application performs several related tasks:

Data integration – BI applications extract, transfer and load from multiple transaction database types into special databases called data marts.

Data integrity – Sophisticated BI applications have internal controls to check that the data integrated is correct and conforms to proper business rules.

Prebuilt datamarts and reports – Modern BI applications provide prebuilt data marts and "canned" analysis, often presented in a "dashboard." This gives immediate value to users, without requiring a learning curve or dedicated IT resources.

The Impact of Business Intelligence In the EHR World

As EHRs help create much more clinical, financial and administrative information about patients, BI will change how healthcare organizations use their data. While some effects are obvious, other innovations are as yet unknowable. But they will share common threads.

The first will be increased speed of reporting. Frequently the data in transaction systems can only be reported on after several days or weeks, requiring extensive intervention from IT staff. BI allows that data to become actionable information within days or hours.

The second is "democratization" of critical information within organizations, achieved by the much wider distribution of BI tools and data, and consequently a greater ability for different teams to analyze key business and clinical processes. This data can also be shared securely online between different stakeholders such as hospitals and affiliated physicians, health plans and even patients. Overall the increased use of this information will enable more sophisticated cross-stakeholder collaboration for processes like disease management.

The third thread is the increased ability for critical decisions to be made by operational and strategic executives, without needing special IT or analysis skills. BI applications will increasingly appear on the executive information system dashboard. For healthcare organizations this will allow greater oversight of financial, clinical and operational issues.

The overall implication is that the management of healthcare organizations including hospitals, large physician organizations and private and government payers will be able to examine their clinical and business processes much more closely and see changes in those processes much more quickly. BI will enable organizations to view the types of activity and innovation that are valuable from both a clinical and cost-effective perspective in the complex process of delivering patient care. ■

Endnote

1. *Fisher, et al.; "Variations In The Longitudinal Efficiency Of Academic Medical Centers," Health Affairs Web exclusive, October 2004. http://content.healthaffairs.org/cgi/content/abstract/hlthaff.var.19v1.*

Improving Performance in Healthcare

Business Objects

Business Objects is the world's leading business intelligence (BI) software company. With more than 30,000 customers worldwide, including over 80 percent of the Fortune 500, Business Objects helps organizations gain better insight into their business, improve decision making and optimize enterprise performance.

Business Objects has both broad and deep experience in helping healthcare organizations improve performance and provide higher-quality customer care. Many leading healthcare organizations – including Emergency Medical Associates, various Blue Cross Blue Shield plans, Renal Care Group, HCA, Kaiser Permanente and Intermountain Healthcare – use Business Objects business intelligence solutions to understand and manage their critical performance indicators.

Companywide information access and analysis enables healthcare businesses to monitor clinical treatments for quality, safety and cost control. It also empowers healthcare companies to identify efficient service and workflow practices.

Business Objects business intelligence solutions enable healthcare companies to:

- **Increase workflow efficiencies** by analyzing consolidated data from clinical, administrative and financial areas;
- **Improve patient care and optimize resource management** by tracking and predicting healthcare service utilization;
- **Meet government legislative controls** by delivering measured and accountable patient-centric care metrics;
- **Monitor and analyze patient diagnosis and condition** to facilitate timely and effective clinical decisions;
- **Control costs, improve contracting decisions and eliminate waste** by closely managing inventory and provider performances; and
- **Increase efficiency and detect fraud** by analyzing historical information, and tracking and closely monitoring current claims data.

Dana-Farber Cancer Institute, a teaching affiliate of Harvard Medical School and a leading U.S. cancer research and care center, relies on Business Objects to deliver reports packed with the latest information about patient flow, staff schedules, service volumes and clinical trials.

With Business Objects, Dana-Farber monitors the number of patients scheduled into each clinic on a daily basis. Reports alert workers when the volume is at capacity, so schedulers know to move appointments to different days and times. This evens out patient flow, which leads to improved safety, shorter wait times and higher staff satisfaction. Other reports track and analyze the type of services provided to patients and show whether those services have increased over time, helping Dana-Farber management predict future staff, equipment and space needs.

Dana-Farber also uses Business Objects to support a wide variety of clinical research activities and helps researchers recruit research participants, manage study operations, monitor data quality and generate research papers.

Business Objects' market-leading business intelligence platform, BusinessObjects™ XI, offers the BI industry's most complete and trusted platform for reporting, query and analysis, performance management and data integration. BusinessObjects XI includes Crystal Reports®, the industry standard for enterprise reporting. Business Objects has also built the industry's strongest and most diverse partner community, with more than 3,500 partners worldwide. In addition, the company offers consulting and education services to help customers effectively deploy their business intelligence projects.

Business Objects has dual headquarters in San Jose, Calif., and Paris, France. The company's stock is traded both on the Nasdaq (BOBJ) and Euronext Paris (ISIN: FR0004026250 - BOB) stock exchanges. More information about Business Objects can be found at www.businessobjects.com. ■

Business Objects, the makers of BusinessObjects XI and Crystal Reports, is the world's leading business intelligence (BI) software company.

Bernard Liautaud
CEO and Chairman of the Board

Hervé Couturier
Senior Vice President, Products

Greg Wolfe
Senior Vice President and General Manager, Americas Operations

David Galloway
Group Vice President
Worldwide Customer Support

Business Objects
3030 Orchard Pkwy.
San Jose, CA 95134
Toll-free 866.681.3435
Phone 604.681.3435
Fax 604.681.2934

Business Contact
Carrie Hout
Accenture Partner
Development Manager
Phone 415.357.7742
carrie.hout@businessobjects.com

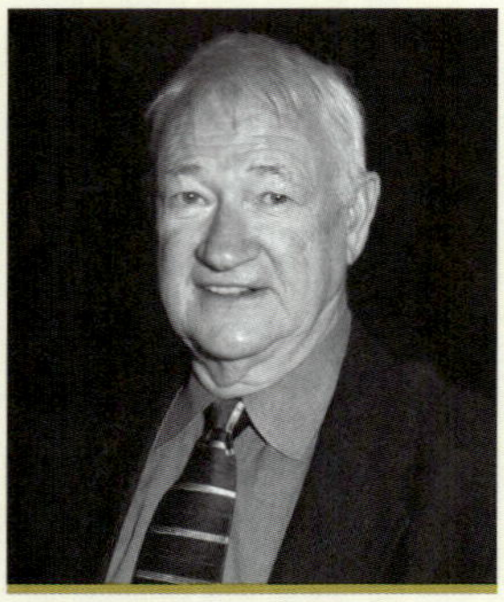

Ed Hammond
Professor Emeritus
Duke University

W. Ed Hammond, M.D., is professor emeritus of community and family medicine and professor emeritus, biomedical engineering at Duke University. He is an adjunct professor in the Health Sectors Management Division of the Fuqua School of Business. He has extensive experience in the design and implementation of electronic patient records. He is a co-developer of The Medical Record, a clinical and billing record system.

Q&A With Dr. Ed Hammond

Professor Emeritus at Duke University explains the historical evolution of technical standards.

HCT: *From a technology standpoint, what's required for EHR implementation?*

Ed Hammond: I think it's important to discuss, briefly, what an EHR (electronic health record) is. It seems to me that historically, almost every organization that starts to do something with the EHR attempts to define what an EHR is. And, invariably, that is always an open issue. There is no universal definition of that term. Clearly an EHR serves multiple roles. Its major role is documenting the care of the patient. In addition to that, increasingly in the future if not so much in the past, it's been the source of information for research and analysis. It certainly performs a legal service in the sense of documenting what happened to the patient. It's the source of decisions related to reimbursement. So there's a multiplicity of purposes.

The EHR also is used in many different sites; most specifically the difference between the EHR used in the inpatient environment may be very different from the EHR in the outpatient environment. In the inpatient environment, largely it is a process of dealing with an acute event. The data that's collected is stored in the EHR and has a more immediate value. You do a test, analyze the data and do a treatment. So you're trying to solve an acute care problem where your changes are rather rapid. And the long-term value of that, I think, is much more limited than it is in the outpatient world. In the outpatient world, the data tends to change more slowly. Much of that data is focused on either chronic problems or in screening problems and trying to determine the health status of an individual, preventative care and that type of thing, and thus changes occur at a slower rate and therefore the data has more persistent value than it does in the inpatient care setting. I think those are two distinctions that need to be combined in the EHR. Another factor that impacts the EHR is that most patients go to more than one site for care.

A recent study suggested that patients see from three to five different providers in different sites of care. To get a complete picture of the patient, we need to be able to bring all of that data together in a single EHR to understand what's really going on with the patient. So the combination of data from a primary care setting, a secondary care setting, a specialist's setting and an inpatient setting is necessary to provide a complete view of the patient. Women, for example, typically will have a primary care physician as well as a gynecologist; at a minimum that scenario gives you two sources of data that need to be combined into a single record. So when we talk about EHR implementation, I think that's the kind of thing that we're talking about. There is another perspective of the EHR that will impact implementation as well. That perspective is the different views of the EHR. I think the first view is the one that I've really been talking about, and that's the view that I call the provider view.

This view is an institutional view, either inpatient or outpatient, and is the documentation of events occurring in the organization delivering the care. It's used for credentialing of physicians; it's used for the reimbursement process; it's used for accreditation; it's used for patient care; it's used for auditing quality and patient safety; it's used for research; and it's used for education. Two other views of the EHR are being developed; one is a population view that may be identical to the summary record at which there is an aggregation of data about a patient from multiple sites of care. The population view also serves for health surveillance, where you're looking for outbreaks of disease or analyzing similar episodes of care in a regional area or in a particular population group. In most cases, that population data functions as the public health documentation and involves multiple sites of care. And more recently, there is increased sophistication and awareness of individuals – consumers, if you will, of healthcare – into their own healthcare, so they're a much more knowledgeable group and much more interested in being involved in the decisions made about their healthcare. They want to be informed sufficiently so that they can make decisions and trade-offs between risks of death and quality of life. And again, much of that results from an EHR.

So a personal health record is another view of the EHR that most groups believe is important for involving the patient in his or her healthcare. I think part of this is that the changing model of healthcare has raised questions about who the individual is , an identifiable person, which accepts the responsibility for an individual's care. Who worries to make sure that the chronic disease, whether it's hypertension or diabetes or asthma, is under control? Who worries about whether the patient does all the right things to make that happen? Who worries about whether the levels of the medication are adequate to control the disease and things of that nature? Increasingly the model doesn't seem to identify that individual. The role of a primary care provider as the gatekeeper seems to have disappeared, and again that responsibility appears to be falling back to the patient, to the citizen, to the consumer. And to do that effectively requires that data. So I think that again is a requirement.

Now in terms of the implementation, that's an open-ended question. To some it would involve defining what the architectural structure of the EHR is, whether this is a series of data points stored in a relational database or, perhaps, in others' view, it's a series of documents that are stored, and some of those documents constitute the EHR. And some of the standards work that's being done supports that view. So there's not a single agreed-upon answer to the question of what an implementation is, and I don't think that we will see a single answer to that question. Certainly in the next 10 years, I think you'll see a variety of things.

The role of a primary care provider as the gatekeeper seems to have disappeared, and again that responsibility appears to be falling back to the patient, to the citizen, to the consumer. And to do that effectively requires that data.

HCT: *What's the historical evolution of technical standards?*

EH: My assumption is that we're talking about health data standards, rather than healthcare standards. And to my knowledge, there were probably three or four different groups that approached the standards that would be used, health data standards, for different purposes.

ANSI created a standards group called ASC X12 for the purpose of creating transaction standards. In other words, this group created the standards that were responsible for carrying the transaction data that is used for the reimbursement process. The HIPAA legislation in 1996 identified the X12 standards as the transaction standards that would be used for reimbursement purposes. Another group, the National Council of Prescription Drug Programs (NCPDP), started because of the need for pharmacy-based systems for PBMs to reimburse for prescription drugs. The NCPDP created its first transactions standard for the reimbursement of clinical drugs back in the late '80s and early '90s, and this is the dominant standard for that purpose.

DICOM came originally from the American College of Radiology and the National Electronics Manufacturers Association, which jointly created a standard that was used in PACS systems. Basically these are the imaging standards that are used primarily for radiology and are now expanded to almost any images involved in healthcare.

HL7 (Health Level 7) got its start when a group of people were trying to create a hospital information system from what's called the best of breed. In other words, you look at the best ADT system, you look at the best laboratory order entry system, you look at the best materials management system, you look at the best pharmacy system and things of that nature and you need to put those together.

HL7 began as a clinical messaging standard that was used, initially, primarily in single settings, namely hospitals, to carry the data from one department to the other to create a consolidated look at the patient. Initially HL7 focused largely on that inpatient environment, and most of the electronic systems were in the inpatient world because that's where most of the money was. But over time, that change began to move into the outpatient world. So HL7 continued to support clinical data in both the inpatient and the outpatient arena.

Q&A With Ed Hammond

As the needs of what we were doing required more standards, HL7 changed its scope to cover some of those needs. Now HL7 is really addressing the broad set of standards that are required for EHR. Implementation of that includes definitions of EHR functionality; it includes the clinical data architecture; it includes clinical statements, clinical templates, data types, a reference information model and so forth. So HL7 now covers a very broad horizontal scope of the things that are associated with the implementation of the EHR and the movement of data from various sites to be able to consolidate that.

The RSNA, HIMSS, and DICOM, in beginning to try to connect PACs systems and radiology information systems with the rest of hospital information systems, began to broaden its scope a little bit. This was later in the world of standards, so it recognized the existence of standards and started looking beyond standards for specific and single purposes and at the broader aspects of putting standards together. So the IHE (the integration of the healthcare enterprise) activity started, and the kinds of things that are required to make an enterprise system that uses standards came out of that.

There are two other groups that I would talk about in terms of evolution of standards. One of these is the ASTM E31 Committee. Dr. Clem McDonald led the effort; I was a major part of that. The first kind of standards that we created in ASTM were similar to the standards that HL7 created, and those first standards were focused on moving laboratory data, primarily from the commercial clinical laboratories to provider institutions. ASTM has had typically smaller groups working on topics, but they've been fairly broad and included such things as dealing with the EHR in terms of content, in dealing with transcriptions, in dealing with standards related to security, privacy and things of that nature.

Most recently the ASTM's major contribution is the continuity of care document standard that's been used to move electronic data from one place to the other. MedBiquitous is a very recent ANSI-approved standard organization that is trying to create standards that would support distance learning and education and patient simulation and activities of that nature. The American Dental Association has had standards focused entirely on the dental community for a number of years. Veterinarians have created standards – more in other groups than independent efforts – but they have been identifiable as veterinary standards.

So basically in this country we've ended up with six or seven groups that have been creating standards that, when they first started, had a clear-cut and understandable difference in purpose and being, but in pursuit of those standards and in meeting the needs – the broad needs of the people that use those standards – have begun to increase their scope to the point where almost all the standards activities have overlaps in redundancy with other standards efforts. And a specific example that recently occurred is that the NCPDP standard for capturing and reporting prescription drug data was used in an overwhelming percentage of transactions involving prescription drugs, and as such, these databases, whose contents have been acquired through the process of reimbursement, are the most complete record of all the prescription drugs the patients are taking.

As e-prescribing has come into vogue, the Medicare Modernization Act is going to require electronic prescribing of drugs over the next three years. The NCPDP standards appear to be the ones most likely used for this, taking advantage of that database. But the problem is when you begin to look at the broader requirements of e-prescribing, you begin to need clinical data. At a minimum, you need some physical parameters such as the height or the weight of an individual to be able to calculate the correct dosages; you need to have something about the diseases a person may have that would impact the metabolism of the drugs; you begin to need some social kind of information, the ability of the patients to take complex drugs. So that variation has now expanded the requirements beyond just the drugs and how they were administered.

The NCPDP, for example, is working on a medical data standard that will increase that capture. So you begin to see the overlap between ASTM and the CCR, HL7 and its messaging standards, the NCPDP, and through claims attachment you begin to see the overlap among the standards groups. In fact, the IHE effort in moving clinical documents begins to overlap with this as well. So you've got all of these groups, including the ADA, that has a little bit of everything that had this overall redundancy. So it will be interesting to see how we solve that problem, because probably worse than no standards is too many standards There's not a clear-cut way of finding which standard you want to invest your money in using, and consequently you don't use any standards. So that's sort of where we are and how we got there. ■

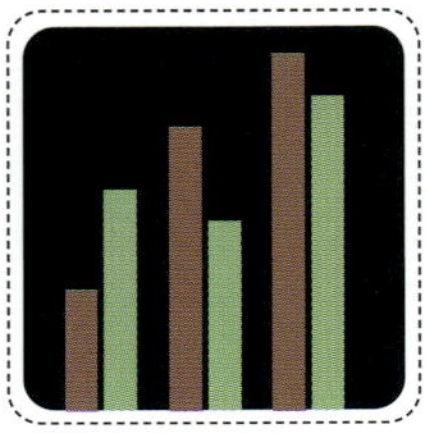

So HL7 now covers a very broad horizontal scope of the things that are associated with the implementation of the EHR and the movement of data from various sites to be able to consolidate that.

Panasonic Toughbooks®: Powerful Wireless Computing Solutions for Healthcare

Throughout the healthcare industry, the demand for mobile computing and wireless solutions grows every day, driven by a combination of market, regulatory and technical trends.

The amount of data generated by the U.S. healthcare industry is growing faster than in perhaps any other industry in the world. Advances in the generation, transmission, storage, display and implementation of digital information offer the promise of better, more cost-effective healthcare. However, in order to mitigate risks, the industry is drafting new technical and procedural standards that protect patients' rights to privacy while enabling greater choice. These standards will force data producers and consumers to adopt secure mobile and wireless technologies to manage digital patient records.

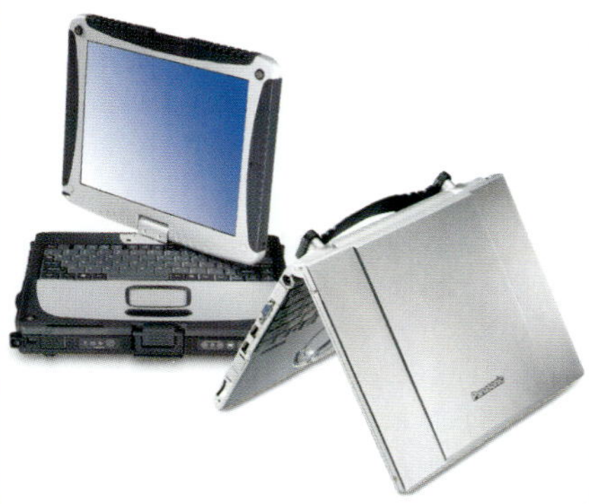

In addition, because miscommunication in prescription deliveries contributes to more than 10,000 deaths per year in the United States, the Food and Drug Administration has begun rolling out standard data format, structure and input methods. Using bar codes and other automatic data capture technologies, the FDA aims to reduce medical errors in hospitals and doctors' offices. Also in development are standards for delivering this information – securely and in real time – with a number of integrated next-generation WLAN and WWAN technologies, including 802.11, the IEEE wireless networking standard and CDMA and GPRS.

And of course, the healthcare industry has a need for computers that are portable, powerful, reliable and rugged – able to withstand the bangs, spills and mishaps that occur in any busy healthcare workplace.

That's where Panasonic's Toughbook line comes in.

For over 15 years, **Panasonic Computer Solutions Company** has manufactured the industry's most reliable mobile PCs – wireless and durable **Panasonic Toughbooks®**. Portable and lightweight, Toughbooks are healthcare's ultimate mobile computing partners. They're built to withstand the daily rigors faced on the job, feature extra-long battery life and are equipped to run sophisticated, healthcare-specific applications.

Consider the powerful Toughbook T2, a lightweight yet remarkably durable mobile PC. Ideal for on-the-go healthcare professionals, it includes a hand strap for easy bedside use. Like many Toughbooks, the T2 is available with a pressure-sensitive touchscreen display – perfect for use when wearing latex gloves. And because it's powered by Intel® Centrino™ Mobile Technology for maximum unwired freedom, medical workers will always be connected.

Or consider the versatile Toughbook 18 – the first-of-its-kind rugged mobile PC. Ideal for healthcare applications, it boasts long-lasting battery life, an outdoor-readable LCD and converts from a powerful notebook PC to a tablet PC with one quick swivel. Powered by Intel® Centrino™ Mobile Technology, the Toughbook 18 is sealed and sanitizable. Because it's a Toughbook, it moves easily from room to room and can withstand the bumps, drops and spills that can occur in a healthcare environment. Plus it keeps healthcare professionals in constant, real-time communication with integrated wireless WAN options, including CDMA1xEVDO/1xRTT and EDGE/GPRS/GSM. Best of all, in tablet form the Toughbook 18 allows medical workers to easily update patient records by hand, take notes and convert those handwritten notes into text.

Contact us for more information about how the Toughbook line can work in your environment. ■

Panasonic produces the industry's most reliable mobile PCs – legendary Panasonic Toughbooks®. Rugged and wireless, Toughbooks are total computing solutions for today's mobile healthcare workforces.

Rance Poehler
President

Panasonic Computer Solutions Company
Three Panasonic Way
Secaucus, NJ 07094
Phone 800.662.3537, Option 8
Fax 201.271.3480
panasonic.com/toughbook/healthcare

For more information
Phone 800.662.3537, Option 8
toughbookhealthcare@us.panasonic.com

EHR Messaging and Data Standards In the United States

The evolving needs of the healthcare industry – especially for EHR implementation – demand uniform messaging standards and consistent use of those standards.

[John Quinn, Accenture]

Connectivity is important both to patient safety and cost-effectiveness in healthcare. Keeping costs down through compatibility of new IT systems – workstations, CT scanners, MR imagers, film digitizers, shared archives, laser printers and host computers and mainframes made by multiple vendors and located at one site or many sites – can be greatly enhanced through a single clinical messaging standard.

When clinical information can be exchanged among various IT systems – within a hospital and among external health providers, public health entities and even insurance plans – the corresponding medical information, diagnoses and images are captured and communicated sooner, physicians reach diagnoses sooner and treatment decisions can be made more quickly. In the future, even individual patients may be able to request, receive and manage their own personal health information via the Internet using secure messaging standards. In a restricted way, this is already happening today.

The goal is clear: a fully integrated healthcare system that allows secure transfer of personal health information within the United States or abroad. The U.K., Canada, Australia, Finland and other countries are well on their way to implementing their own set of EHR applications and data integration standards. Surely this country should also be a leader in healthcare information technology.

While the federal government has recognized the need for messaging standards to enable improved levels of interoperability and data comparability, progress toward widespread use remains difficult. One of the U.S. government's goals is to accelerate adoption of EHR standards such as Health Level 7 (HL7), that will facilitate implementation of an interconnected electronic health information infrastructure nationwide.

Collecting and Moving Clinical Data In the Organization

Collecting patients' clinical and demographic information starts the moment they first schedule an appointment, which is where the challenge of working with various messaging standards becomes evident. Figure 1 is a summary of the types of information that can come together at a patient's physician office via other physicians, payers, reference labs, diagnostic centers and hospital records – every one in a differing format. It illustrates the complexity of getting to a compatible EHR.

This is a partial listing of possible IT system types that identifies some of the different information sources – all with mostly incompatible message standards or differing implementations of those messaging standards for each information source. In short, the data and the supportive process must "match" at both the source and destination computer systems.

Outside of healthcare, automating a process – such as ordering an airline ticket over the Internet – is based on an industry-standard, intuitive information sequence familiar to anyone with a PC. However, little true standardization is actually deployed on any level within the fragmented healthcare industry. Placing a prescription order, receiving lab test results, billing for a patient visit or referral to a specialist – communications become an exercise in risk management. Especially alarming is that a typical hospital runs dozens of different computer systems. Large academic institutions may have more than 100 online systems.

Because almost every provider organization relies on off-the-shelf software solutions, an open and profitable market for third-party vendors of healthcare applications has resulted in the U.S. and most other countries. This market consists of a number of relatively small vendors that are mostly unique to the healthcare

John Quinn is chief technology officer in Accenture's Provider, Health & Life Sciences practice focusing on emerging healthcare information systems technologies. He has over 29 and 32 years' experience in the healthcare and computer industries respectively. He has participated on the HL7 board of directors since its inception 18 years ago and has served as the chair of its technical steering committee for the last 14 years.

Process / Function	Physician office	Hospital
Scheduling	Practice management	Scheduling
Admitting / registration	Practice management	ADT / clinic registration
Medical chart	EHR	EHR
Patient billing	Practice management	Billing
Pathology / lab	Reference laboratory	In-house / reference lab
EHR	EHR	EHR
Radiology	Radiology diagnostic center	Radiology system

Figure 1 Different Formats of Clinical Information

market and a few recognizable "big brands," such as Siemens and General Electric. By and large, these software solutions are extremely configurable to the wide variety of processes that exist across the industry. Similarly all interfaces are also configured to match the exact data and process being supported for every computer interconnection in every organization.

Going Beyond the Organization

Until now we have limited our considerations to a single organization. However, there are two different theaters for messaging standards: 1) moving data inside an organization (inter-organizational), and 2) moving data back and forth among separate locations and organizations. The seemingly simple process of transferring diagnosis or allergy information from a hospital to a specialist can quickly expose the weakness of the system.

Once EHRs are transferred to other facilities or organizations – or even other countries – the technical challenges become more complex. True plug-and-play standards are far more important, as there is neither the time nor the resources to both match data and the process across organizational boundaries.

HIPAA – This 1996 federal set of regulations that is still being deployed covers communications between providers and payers as well as federal laws protecting the privacy of health information and the security measures necessary to ensure that privacy. HIPAA also includes provisions that require the Health and Human Services (HHS) department to identify and adopt national standards for electronic healthcare transactions, while integrating crucial protocols to protect individual privacy. These standards include the Accredited Standards Committee X12 standard, the National Council for Prescription Drug Program standard and the HL7 standard.

Electronic Prescribing and EHR – The Medicare Modernization Act of 2003 (MMA) requires the Secretary of HHS to promote and secure the adoption of electronic prescribing by 2010 as defined in the act. Unlike HIPAA, MMA is very specific in its definition of the relatively technical concept of electronic prescribing. MMA requires that electronic prescribing systems contain a subset of what we expect in an EHR or electronic medical record (EMR) system. In short, MMA requires what we might call a "light" version of EHR by 2010 – significantly earlier than the president's goal of 2014.

Modes of Messaging

There are several variations in the style and content of messaging standards. Some of these differences result from the needs of different business and clinical purposes. Others result from a growing awareness of user requirements, improvements in modeling methods and increasingly rigorous efforts to define the implementation issues.

Variations in standards specifications are inevitable; however, implementation guides with a common style of documentation and more consistent content can ease understanding and implementation of messaging standards.

Because they deal with arbitrary processes and a seemingly unlimited amount of data, messaging standards applications are very complex. Variations in standards specifications are inevitable; however, implementation guides with a common style of documentation and more consistent content can ease understanding and implementation of messaging standards.

There are two general ways that healthcare information is typically communicated between computer systems:

- **Unsolicited Update** – Unsolicited updates are messages that are "pushed" from a source computer system as the result of a pre-specified event. This type of event-driven messaging is what is most typically used between computer systems inside of provider organizations.

- **Query Response** – Similar to accessing your financial records over an ATM, a query response is initiated by the user. Query response messages are a coupling of two messages. The first message makes a request of data specified in a query. The second message is a coupled response to the query that contains the request information or possibly an explanation of why the data can't be sent.

Role of the NCVHS in Recommending Standards

The National Committee on Vital and Health Statistics (NCVHS) is the public advisory body to the secretary of HHS and was directed by the HIPAA law to make recommendations of specific national standards for electronic clinical messaging formats.

In a letter to the secretary of HHS, the subcommittee stated that "standards for EHR are important because they will facilitate significant improvements in the quality of patient care, promote patient safety, control rising healthcare costs, enhance the productivity of clinical research and strengthen the nation's ability to identify and respond to healthcare emergencies. They are critical for a National Health Information Infrastructure."

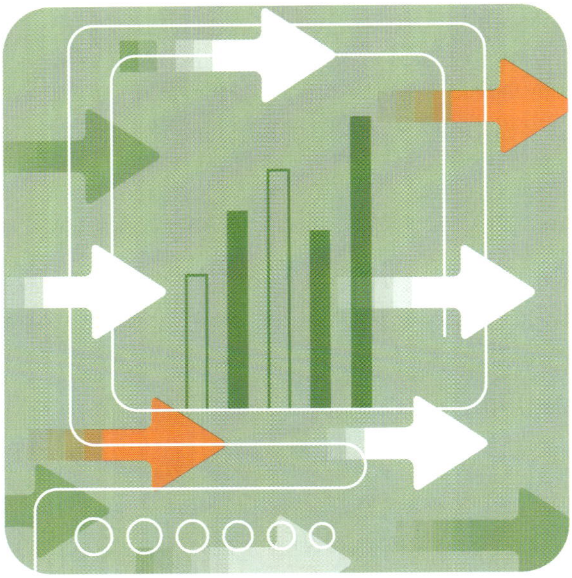

The subcommittee recently recommended that HHS make the standards voluntary by outlining industry use of standards rather than creating new regulations. It also suggested HHS use its leading healthcare market position to accelerate the development, adoption and coordination of EHR standards.

Because HHS has been so slow in promoting the implementation of further standards, committee members believe that making clinical standards voluntary – but using HHS and other government agencies as early adopters – may result in widespread adoption faster than mandates, contrary to the national mandate for standardized electronic transactions authorized under HIPAA.

HHS has enormous influence in the healthcare industry. With control over Medicare, Indian Health Service and other health programs, and joint authority with states over Medicaid, HHS is by far the largest healthcare payer in the nation. Other federal agencies, especially the Departments of Defense and Veterans Affairs, are among the largest providers of healthcare in the nation.

To harmonize the various EHR message format standards, the NCVHS Subcommittee recommends that standards developing organizations (SDOs) share data elements and definitions with the U.S. Health Information Knowledgebase, a data registry. The subcommittee's proposal also gives a glimpse of its future work to standardize clinical data: "NCVHS has limited its EHR recommendations to message format standards. The committee plans to further investigate medical terminologies and code sets and will also consider EHR standards for clinical documents and the content and structure of patient records."

Messaging and Data Standards – The current list of SDOs and different messaging standards proposals are summarized below. In addition, there are various data vocabulary standards, such as LOINC (Logical Observation Identifiers, Names and Codes) – codes used as universal identifiers for laboratory and other clinical transactions that facilitate the exchange and pooling of results, such as blood hemoglobin, serum potassium or vital signs, for clinical care, outcomes management and research. The different terminologies also add to the complexity of standards, such as the American College of Pathologists' SNOMED Clinical Terms (SNOMED CT). This terminology provides a common language to enable a consistent way of capturing, sharing and aggregating health data across specialties and sites of care. Some applications for SNOMED CT include EMR, ICU monitoring, clinical decision support, medical research studies, clinical trials, computerized physician order entry, disease surveillance, image indexing and consumer health information services.

EHR/EMR – For purposes of discussion in this article, an EHR contains information about a patient's health and is used to communicate a patient's health status to a physician or other caregiver. EHR Systems (or EHRS) is developing into a formal standard definition by HL7's EHR Technical Committee and its published normative EHR standard. EHRS support the creation and communication of an EHR. EMR is a similar (and overlapping) term used to describe a more formal definition of an electronic collection of patient information and the processes surrounding the collection and use of that data. It can also extend to a specific (state-by-state defined) legal definition. In general, EMR (like EHR) systems are computer systems that both hold the EMR and are used by a physician to document and retrieve information about the patient in the normal course of providing care. At this point in time, the terms EHR and EMR are sometimes difficult to distinguish and many users of the terms do not really distinguish a distinct different meaning to the terms.

Electronic Prescribing – Already noted earlier, electronic prescribing, as set forth by the MMA, requires electronic prescribing systems to feature items such as a patient's medication history, allergies and other information, such as diagnosis, problem lists and laboratory results.

Major Standards Organizations

There are several SDOs accredited by the American National Standards Institute (ANSI) that operate in the U.S. healthcare arena, and in some cases, in other countries as well. SDOs produce standards (also called specifications or protocols) for specific healthcare areas such as pharmacy, medical devices, imaging or insurance (claims processing) transactions.

Following is an overview of the major SDOs in use in the U.S.:

Health Level Seven (HL7) – Provides standards for management and integration of data supporting clinical patient care and healthcare services. HL7 endeavors "specifically, to create flexible, cost-effective approaches, standards, guidelines, methodologies, and related services for interoperability between healthcare information systems." It is unique in encompassing "the interface requirements of the entire health care organization" rather than focusing on the messaging requirements of a single department.

- **Version 2** – This messaging standard (Application Protocol for Electronic Data Exchange in Healthcare Environments) from HL7 is the most widely implemented standard for healthcare information in the world and seen as the "workhorse" of data exchange in healthcare. Later versions (such as the current 2.5) have evolved and feature enhanced functionalities over earlier versions as well as support for newer syntax coding technologies such as XML.
- **Version 3** – Similar to V2.x in functionality, V3 is a standard for exchanging messages among information systems that implement healthcare applications. However, V3 is a more robust standard based on a formal development methodology that includes the use of modeling both for data (a reference information model) and processes (use case scenarios). It uses rigorous analytic and message-building techniques and incorporates more trigger events and message formats while also greatly reducing options. Unlike V2, the Version 3 standard is definite and testable, and provides the ability to certify vendors' conformance. Version 3 uses an object-oriented development methodology and a Reference Information Model to create messages.
  - **Reference Information Model (RIM)** – This cornerstone of V3 is a large model language and pictorial representation of the clinical data (domains), and identifies the life cycle of events that a message or groups of related messages will carry. Shared between the domains, the RIM is the model for all domains to create their messages.
  - **HL7 Methodology** – The HL7 Development Framework is the methodology for the development of HL7 Version 3 and its messages.
  - **Vocabulary Standards** – The vocabulary standards vary by the data item in a message. Standards are chosen by HL7 and the NCVHS. They make use of established standards when they exist for the data item (e.g., ICD for a diagnosis); when possible, non-health specific data are coded from standards established by organizations such as the UN's ISO (e.g., race and religion).

The CDA standard makes documents both machine-readable and human-readable to enable easy retrieval and readability for users while at the same time managing the integrity and attestability of the specific collection of data contained in the document.

Clinical Document Architecture (CDA) – Previously known as the patient record architecture, CDA provides an exchange model for clinical documents (such as discharge summaries and progress notes), and is an important step toward implementation of EHRs. The CDA standard makes documents both machine-readable and human-readable to enable easy retrieval and readability for users while at the same time managing the integrity and attestability of the specific collection of data contained in the document.

Digital Imaging and Communications in Medicine (DICOM) – A standards committee of the American College of Radiology and the National Electrical Manufacturers Association (ACR/NEMA) that supports DICOM, an industry standard for the transmission of a wide range of medical images (in radiology, cardiology, pathology and dentistry). DICOM enables digital communication between diagnostic and therapeutic equipment and systems from various manufacturers.

National Council of Prescription Drug Programs (NCPDP) – Has defined a standard for sending drug prescription information from pharmacies to payers for prescription management service and for receiving approval and payment information – all at close to real time. The council is currently working on standards for adverse drug reactions and utilization review and mapping of their prescription "script" standards to HL7s in-hospital pharmacy order messages.

Clinical Data Interchange Standards Consortium (CDISC) – Leads development of standard data models that improve process efficiency while supporting the scientific nature of clinical research, particularly the end-to-end data flow of clinical trials, from the source(s) into an operational database, through analysis to regulatory submission. The relevant data sources vary among patient records (e.g., case-report-form data), clinical laboratory data, data from contract research organizations, shared data between companies with corporate mergers or development partners, and other sources.

X12N – A transaction standard of the ANSI-accredited Standards Committee X12's insurance subgroup (N) that is also part of the Transactions and Code Sets Rule specified by HIPAA. The X12N standards include transactions for claims/encounters, attachments, enrollment, disenrollment, eligibility, payment/remittance advice, premium payments, first report of injury, claim status, referral certification/authorization and coordination of benefits.

American Society for Testing and Materials (ASTM) – One of the largest voluntary standards development organizations in the world, ASTM develops technical standards for materials, products, systems and services. The ASTM Committee E31 on Healthcare Informatics develops standards related to the architecture, content, storage, security, confidentiality, functionality and communication of information used within healthcare and healthcare decision making, including patient-specific information and knowledge. Specific to EHR, ASTM has been developing the continuity of care record to ensure the portability of patients' clinical data between settings of care.

American Dental Association (ADA) – Provides the HIPAA standards similar to X12 but specifically related to the dental industry and payers of dental services.

American National Standards Institute (ANSI) – Active in both national and international standardization, ANSI itself does not develop standards, but provides the framework of rules and accreditation of standards that SDOs develop. The Institute ensures that access to the standards process, including an appeals mechanism, is made available to anyone directly or materially affected by a standard under development. ANSI's involvement in EHR is through the standards organizations that are accredited by ANSI. ANSI also sponsors the Health Information Standards Board to provide a forum for coordinating the activities of the multiple ANSI-accredited healthcare standards groups.

Integrating the Healthcare Enterprise (IHE) – An initiative by healthcare professionals and industry to improve the way computer systems in healthcare share information. IHE promotes the coordinated use of established standards such as DICOM and HL7 to address specific clinical needs in support of optimal patient care. Systems developed in accordance with IHE standards-based implementation guides communicate with one another better, are easier to implement and enable healthcare providers to use information more effectively.

Electronic Health Record Vendor Association (EHRVA) – A trade association of EHR vendors that supports and promotes national efforts to create interoperable EHRs in hospital and ambulatory care settings. Its chief objective is to promote a rapid adoption of EHR to help improve the quality of patient care and the productivity of the healthcare system.

Healthcare Information and Management Systems Society (HIMSS) – The healthcare industry's membership organization; it advances healthcare public policy and industry practices through its advocacy, educational and professional development initiatives. These promote information and management system contributions that help improve patient care. HIMSS supports EHRVA by providing staff to assist with meetings and conference calls, as well as to provide guidance relative to trade association operations.

Summary

EHR messaging standards are key to enabling efficiency gains and improved service across the U.S. healthcare industry. However, the complexity of reliably moving data and processes among IT systems continues to resist a useful solution. The NCVHS, the main advisor to HHS, sees voluntary adoption of EHR standards as more efficient than new regulations. This includes a call to the major SDOs to share data elements (such as messaging and EHRS standards, and electronic prescribing) to accelerate and enhance the development of an integrated healthcare system that allows secure transfer of personal health information.

As an independent and trusted advisor to many healthcare institutions and SDOs, Accenture is an experienced facilitator of IT solutions for the healthcare industry. We see the increased involvement of the U.S. government – through the NCVHS – as a necessary prerequisite for the development and adoption of a messaging standard. ■

How Secure Are Your Electronic Communications?

Simple question, right? But is there a simple answer?

The reality is that electronic communications are rapidly replacing hard-copy communications in the healthcare industry, posing real issues for all of its constituents.

The critical issues for medical insurers are lowest-cost processing and auditable paper trails that can verify the authenticity of documents.

Regulators demand compliance with more effective anti-fraud programs.

At the same time, many doctors and physicians' practices are moving toward the paperless office, creating concerns about the safety and integrity of patient data.

And patients deserve real-time electronic access to their doctors, too, with all the reassurances of privacy of health records.

Virtually all of the pieces to this puzzle involve some form of electronic communications – whether a fax, an email, a PDF file, a Web form or a Word document. Any one of these electronic communications is subject to tampering and can be changed, either maliciously or accidentally. Even unintended errors or omissions can cause significant problems with billing or compliance.

Take a simple example – the faxed order. A leading national medical products company specializing in mail-order diabetic supplies receives a staggering number of faxes every month from physicians issuing doctors orders that support the medical need for issuance of supplies and services reimbursed under Medicare. But, all too often, busy physicians neglect to date the forms, or do so illegibly. This forces the suppliers to have to go back to the doctors to properly date the orders in order to be eligible for Medicare reimbursement – an inconvenience, but also an unnecessary cost element and a compliance risk owing to potential untimely billing.

Incorporating the United States Postal Service® Electronic Postmark® Service, AuthentiDate has crafted a HIPAA-compliant solution that provides trusted third-party proof of the date of the document and remedies the problem. The result: lower administrative costs, fewer lost orders and improved days sales outstanding (DSO). At the same time, tampering of faxes is automatically detected and flagged, an important benefit in an industry sector that receives heavy anti-fraud audit scrutiny from regulatory agencies such as Medicare's CMS and the OIG.

A second area is the authentication of documentation for billing-support purposes. Working with leading home care providers like Apria, Lincare, American Home Patient and Rotech, AuthentiDate's CareCert™ solution increases the certainty and speed of reimbursement for durable medical equipment usage from federal and state healthcare programs.

Because erroneous and illegal claims submission are key elements in healthcare fraud and abuse, companies seeking reimbursement from federal and state agencies have to clearly document the medical need to support their claims, often going through three process cycles with physicians to obtain the appropriate justification. Use of CareCert, which electronically processes CMNs and written confirmation of verbal orders, can cut that down to one cycle, bringing DSO down from as much as 90 days to as little as 30 days.

Many vendors claim to meet these needs, but a successful IT-enabled solutions approach must integrate the following elements:

- Ease and flexibility of use – Simple and dynamic user interfaces that support multiple data formats like faxes, Word documents, email and Web-based forms;
- Strength of technology – Extensible architectures built on industry standards; and
- Trusted third-party authentication and verification capability built into the system to reduce compliance risk and audit cost.

Yes, there's more work to do before the healthcare community's need for secure electronic communications is fully satisfied. But does technology exist today to address that need while improving ROI as well as regulatory compliance and risk mitigation? Absolutely! ■

AuthentiDate™

AuthentiDate is a leading provider of content-authentication solutions that address the healthcare community's unique needs for secure electronic communications.

Suren Pai
President and
Chief Executive Officer

John Waters
Executive Vice President and
Chief Administrative Officer

O'Connell (Ben) Benjamin
Vice President Products
& Technology

Jakes Srinivasan
Vice President Corporate
Development

AuthentiDate
225 Liberty St.
Two World Financial Center
43rd Floor
New York, NY 10281

Business Contact
Jakes Srinivasan
Vice President Corporate
Development
Phone 212.329.1100
jsrinivasan@authentidate.com

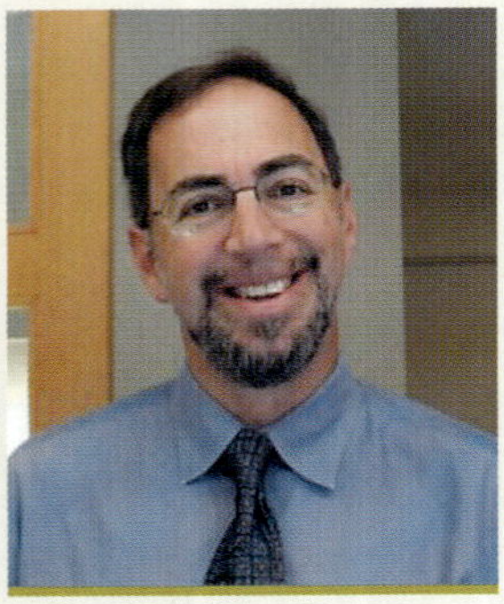

David Lansky
Executive Director
Markle Foundation

David Lansky, Ph.D., is the senior director of the Health Program and executive director of the Personal Health Technology Initiative at the Markle Foundation. Dr. Lansky has 20 years' experience with healthcare policy issues and is focusing on the adoption of interoperable health information technology throughout U.S. healthcare, with an emphasis on patient and consumer representation.

Q&A With David Lansky

The executive director of the Markle Foundation explains why interoperability is essential for improving the quality of care and for creating a platform that enables innovation.

Healthcare Technology: *Can you tell us a little bit about the Markle Foundation and your role there?*

David Lansky: The Markle Foundation is a philanthropic organization, a 501C3 charity. Our interest has always been in how information, communications and technology can better serve society. For example, we were one of the first funders of the Children's Television Workshop which produced Sesame Street. So we've had a lot of interest in how media communications can be used to benefit the public interest. The last four years we've been interested in how electronic health records (EHRs) and the interoperability of health records can best be applied to improve the healthcare system. In particular, we have an interest in how patients and consumers can themselves be part of that process, and can be better involved in managing their own care and managing their own information. In terms of my role, I am director of the Health Program, and my particular interest is the question of how consumers and patients become more involved in their healthcare. We have come to believe that creating an interoperable health information environment is an important first step before we can do all the things we'd like to do to have patients more involved.

HCT: *Why is interoperability so important?*

DL: I think there are two primary challenges. One is to improve the quality of care that's delivered now, and the second is to create a platform that would allow the healthcare system to innovate and evolve.

The first challenge I mentioned, improving safety and quality, is driven by the many well-documented cases of medication errors and inadequate quality of care today – much of which could be addressed by having information when it's needed, where it's needed, in the right person's hands. An interoperable health information environment would allow professionals and patients to move information from where it is now to where it's needed in a more timely and reliable way.

We need to recognize that people move around a lot, they change doctors, they change plans, they move between communities, they have many different doctors at once. Many people may believe that because they primarily see only one doctor their information is in one person's hands, and of course it isn't; it's scattered all over the place. So it's very important to create an environment in which that information can be accessed appropriately. I don't think it's as obvious to the public as it is to the people working inside the system. As a result of this fragmentation, it is very hard to develop new ways of organizing care itself; it's very hard for healthcare innovators to succeed.

We see that the healthcare system has been relatively inflexible in the way it's organized, partly because information is locked inside the "silos" of a very fragmented and disjointed system. So by having a platform in which information can move more freely, we think that will create an environment where there can be more creative solutions to how to deliver healthcare as well.

HCT: *What are some of the requirements and challenges?*

DL: Undoubtedly, one of the requirements is that end users – doctors, hospitals, pharmacies, clinics – need to have some level of EHR installed as a starting point. And we're certainly not very far along in that. But

Markle's work has not focused primarily on how to get end users to adopt EHRs. We want to make sure that once they do, whatever they've adopted can communicate and exchange information appropriately with other components of the healthcare system.

We see three challenges to creating a more interoperable health information environment. The first group of issues that surrounds the need to define commonly accepted standards and see them widely and uniformly adopted. If all the different healthcare organizations are out there today, buying whatever they want, building whatever they want, there's no particular requirement or even guidance that would ensure that what each organization or each doctor or each hospital installs is capable of communicating information in a standardized way with every other organization. Until all of the parties in the system recognize and use the same standards, it'll be very hard to achieve interoperability – very expensive, very difficult.

Once the standards have been identified, how do we then encourage their adoption? It seems unlikely that we will see the government or major payers mandating that all providers and suppliers adopt uniform standards. So how will we, in a voluntary system, get many different organizations all to agree to use the same standards? We must not only have agreement to use the common standards, but we also will need providers to adopt uniform profiles or implementation guides. In order to solve a particular problem, even a simple problem like moving a prescription from a doctor's office to a pharmacy electronically, or retrieving a lab result from a laboratory to a doctor's electronic health record, there are a number of different standards that come into play. It's not just identifying standards, it's bundling those standards into a particular solution, and doing that in such a formal way that everybody who implements those standards in their own systems will do it in the same way. Today there are few commonly accepted implementation guides – bundles of standards applied to a common task. Right now the standards organizations do a great job of identifying standards for each part of the process, but nobody has the job of assembling all the parts together into a complete and uniformly applied solution.

The last standards-related need is certification. Once we have standards, once we know what the implementation guides look like, how do we know that anybody who claims to be selling a system that supports interoperability can actually do it, that the system will actually talk to other systems, other networks. There's a lot of interest now in having some independent entity certify which products are complying with the standards and which are not.

The second set of challenges emerges from the need to assure the privacy and security of personal health information. Regardless of how elegant and brilliant and efficient the technical process is, what really matters most is that the public trusts this system to be private and to treat their information respectfully, and to allow them to control where their information goes and when. And obviously, given the privacy spills of the Internet in the last few months, there's a very high public concern about having their health information online. We think that it's an absolute priority to design this system to permit interoperability, and at the same time to do everything possible to assure the security and privacy of information. That really means two things. One is preventing anything from being spilled when it shouldn't be, and the second is to make sure that if something bad happens, the consequences are universal and severe.

The public has to know that anybody who breaks any of the rules around privacy is going to face a severe sanction. So getting the privacy and security program to be uniform across the country – again without new mandates or laws that will address these things – is a second really big challenge. Underlying that is that the states do things differently, so you have 50 different jurisdictions, and you have to somehow achieve some uniformity despite the fact that the states certainly have the right to do their own thing.

Finally, if you know you need universal standards, and you know you need policies for privacy and security, and you want these things to be relatively uniform so that a person in Orlando has as much confidence in the system as a person in Seattle, who is going to establish these nationwide policies and standards? The question, in a nutshell, is who decides what the rules are going to be? And again we have no national institution or entity with the authority to decide how this system will work. However well-intentioned all the different hospitals and doctors and providers in the country might be, right now they have no one to turn to get these questions answered.

HCT: ***Do you think we'll have widespread adoption in five years?***

DL: I would be surprised. I would not be optimistic that we can make a five-year time line. The steps I mentioned before – setting standards, seeing them adopted, defining implementation guides, establishing common privacy policies – all of that will take time and a shared commitment across the industry. But perhaps most critical – the public has to insist upon it; the public has to say "we demand a safer, more reliable, more efficient system." For example, just personally, I will virtually never go to a doctor who doesn't use electronic medical records, I don't think it's safe. So I think it's important for a lot of Americans to begin to feel that way and to say to their doctor: "Are you using an EMR to manage my information?" ■

SAS® Gives Healthcare Organizations *The Power to Know®*

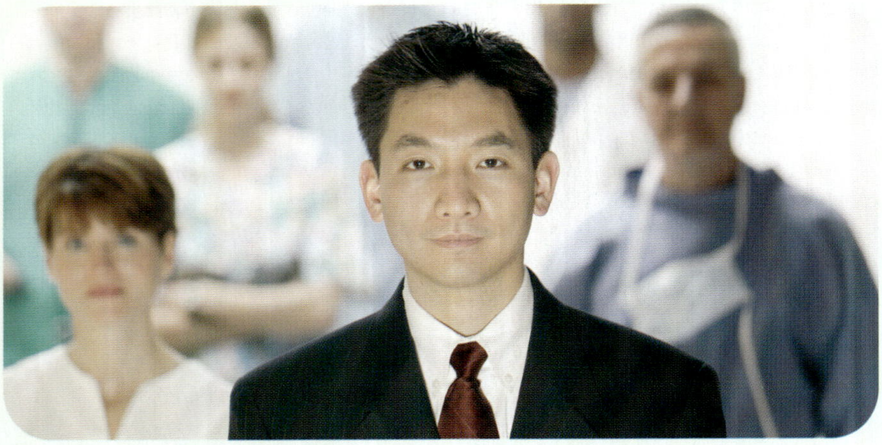

Managing healthcare organizations is much like managing healthcare: Sound decisions require accurate knowledge of complex, interdependent variables. That's exactly what SAS solutions do for healthcare leaders – turn complex data into the business intelligence needed to produce the most successful outcomes.

Healthcare Providers

Healthcare providers manage massive quantities of data. Because it is scattered across various business units, labs and diagnostic departments, this data is rarely integrated. Hospitals and health systems use SAS to collect data from many different source systems, access cleansed data and view key metrics using the Web. We help our customers improve clinical outcomes, bolster the quality and safety of patient care and make the transition to evidence-based practices.

We have tailored our SAS Performance Management for Healthcare solution to meet the specific business intelligence needs of healthcare providers. This solution enables executives to view performance at an aggregate level while allowing clinicians to compare their individual performance to accepted benchmarks.

Hospital and health system executives and clinicians use SAS to:

- Align strategic priorities with departmental goals, objectives and measures;
- Determine the cause-and-effect relationship between measures, such as between length of stay and patient satisfaction;
- Pinpoint quality and safety issues by unit, service line and provider;
- Achieve expense-reduction goals by arming clinicians with accurate and timely information;
- Forecast clinical service needs based on utilization rates and referral patterns; and
- Reduce length of stay without compromising care.

Health Insurance

Health plans must manage the risk that premiums will be overwhelmed by claims. Historically, health insurers analyzed membership, provider and claims data, but this analysis has been database-restricted, incapable of allowing more comprehensive analytics to cross these intelligence silos. Insurers need more if, for example, they are to control costs by predicting which individuals or providers will submit higher claims in the future. To engage in more forward-thinking analysis, our insurance customers use powerful predictive analytics to tackle a greater range of data: membership, enrollment, provider care delivery patterns and group demographics. We help health insurers create a unified platform to facilitate comprehensive forecasting, prediction and customer self-reporting.

With our assistance, SAS health plan customers:

- Determine which claims from healthcare providers are likely fraudulent;
- Draw correlations between treatments, diagnoses and provider practices to deliver more effective disease management;
- Improve consumer-directed healthcare analytics and quantify quality metrics;
- Enable pay-for-performance contract management for healthcare providers; and
- Perform outcomes analysis to support evidence-based medicine.

All SAS solutions for healthcare are built on the SAS Intelligence Platform, which provides a flexible foundation for delivering the information and intelligence your healthcare organization needs. As a gateway to all SAS functionality, this integrated architecture gives you quick access to consistent, high-quality information that supports improved processes and better decisions.

Why SAS?

SAS has served health and life sciences organizations for more than 29 years. In response to significant growth in this sector, SAS created its Health and Life Sciences Organization in 2003, dedicating substantial resources to serve these interconnected industries in a comprehensive manner – from sales and product development to consulting and customer service. We are a strategic partner to these organizations, supporting them in the important work they do to improve the health and lives of the people they serve.

SAS has recruited seasoned personnel from industry organizations – from both private and public sectors – to join its Health and Life Sciences Organization. This is a major reason for our success: Our people have worked in the field and know the current state of affairs in health and life sciences, as well as how the industry is evolving. Meet two of SAS' most senior strategists whose prior experience as healthcare executives benefits the Health and Life Sciences Organization every day.

The Power to Know.

Melissa A. Fitzpatrick, R.N., M.S.N., F.A.A.N., Principal Healthcare Strategist (Provider)

At the 2005 HIMSS Annual Conference, Melissa Fitzpatrick presented "Creating an Evidence-Based Practice Culture with Business Intelligence."

Fitzpatrick joined SAS in November 2001. With 27 years of healthcare experience, she has held a variety of leadership roles: nurse manager, cardiovascular clinical nurse specialist, director of nursing, adjunct professor and health system vice president at Dartmouth Hitchcock Medical Center. From 1997 to 1999, Fitzpatrick served as senior associate chief operating officer and the chief nurse executive at Duke University Hospital. She also served as the editor-in-chief of the *Journal of Nursing Management* from 2000 to 2003.

Fitzpatrick brings extensive clinical and operational healthcare expertise, scorecard design and implementation expertise, and clinical standards and compliance expertise to SAS and our customers. She has played an integral role in every healthcare provider sale at SAS, contributing to the wins at Brigham and Women's Hospital, Yale New Haven Health System, Maine Medical Center, Duke University Hospital, Atlantic Health System and Centra Health.

Fitzpatrick earned her bachelor's degree in nursing from Gwynedd-Mercy College and her master's in nursing from the University of Pennsylvania. She is a nationally and internationally recognized consultant, speaker and author on clinical and leadership issues in healthcare, with many peer-reviewed publications and book chapters to her credit. Fitzpatrick is a past president of the Foundation for Critical Care and the American Association of Critical-Care Nurses, the largest specialty nursing organization in the world. She was inducted as a fellow in the American Academy of Nursing in 1997, achieving the highest recognition in the profession of nursing. Fitzpatrick was selected as one of the Great 100 Nurses in North Carolina in 2002.

Richard B. Ingraham, Principal Healthcare Strategist (Insurance)

Richard Ingraham brings a unique understanding of the shared business and delivery issues, along with conflicting incentive structures, within the healthcare provider, payer and IT analytic industries. Ingraham has served in various executive capacities across both private and public entities within each of these three key driver industries of healthcare improvement. His insight into the opportunities for improved collaboration and coordination across the healthcare spectrum serves as a foundation for SAS' leadership within the health and life sciences arena. Ingraham represents SAS at major industry gatherings, including the Disease Management Association of America, America's Health Insurance Plans, National Health Care Anti-Fraud Association and the National Managed Health Care Congress. Ingraham currently serves on the National Anti-Fraud Project Executive Committee for the Office of the National Coordinator for Health Information Technology, administered through the American Health Information Management Association.

After serving in various health delivery program management capacities within the Florida Department of Health & Rehabilitative Services, Ingraham became business director for the Leon County Public Health Department in Tallahassee, Fla., in 1984 before moving to manage an investigative unit with the Bureau of Allied Lines, Florida Department of Insurance in 1986.

Over the next 11 years, as director and vice president of operations, controller and chief financial officer for Equicor, CIGNA and the Health Services Group, respectively, Ingraham has directed numerous managed care program design and development initiatives, as well as strategic acquisition projects. His knowledge of claims patterns and analysis for fraud detection was formed through his Florida Department of Insurance and Equicor posts. He presents expertise in risk stratification for disease and medical case management, medical utilization improvements, provider performance and quality benchmarking, process engineering and internal control projects.

Since joining SAS in 1998, Ingraham's efforts have focused on working with senior-level management teams in the healthcare sector to improve strategic decision-making processes and knowledge management, while aligning information technology capacities with business. ■

SAS® software is used for a variety of applications in more than 1,000 U.S. healthcare organizations, enabling healthcare leaders to turn complex data into the business intelligence needed to produce the most successful outcomes.

Dr. James (Jim) Goodnight
Chief Executive Officer

Jim Davis
Senior Vice President and Chief Marketing Officer

Kecia Serwin
General Manager, Health and Life Sciences Organization

SAS Institute Inc.
100 SAS Campus Dr.
Cary, NC 27513-2414
Toll-Free 866.791.3181
Fax 919.677.4444
www.sas.com

Business Contact
Kimberly MacClurg
Health and Life Sciences Specialist
Toll-Free 866.791.3181
Kimberly.MacClurg@sas.com

Selecting Technologies for an EHR

Evaluating technologies for an EHR is very different from choosing technologies for an individual organization.

[Joe Poats, Accenture]

The task of choosing technologies for an organization varies greatly from doing it for an electronic health record (EHR). The tasks themselves are similar, but the focus, priorities and evaluative criteria for selecting technologies are not. You need to define the community to be served by the EHR, understand existing assets to build upon, figure out how it would be funded and determine the interoperability requirements. Remember, for most technologies, the software is important, but not as important as the direction and commitment for continued development and how the solution gets implemented.

Define the Goal

Defining the goal is not always as simple as it may sounds. What problem needs to be solved? What community will be served? Consider the players who will benefit from the technologies being evaluated:

- A group of providers, payers and other interested parties in the community such as a regional health information organization (RHIO) to enable clinical and demographic data exchange and linkages;
- A physician group with an eye toward linking to consumers and other community players at the right time; and
- A hospital system (advanced clinical system including computerized physician order entry) considering linking to EHRs, consumers and other community players at the right time.

There are many other combinations and possibilities. The processes that can be automated and the data/standard requirements are vastly different depending on the defined goals and the players who stand to benefit.

Define Commitment

Who will pay for this? Who will benefit? The success of any technology initiative depends on the commitment of representative key players within an organization or community, so testing the readiness of constituents is a good idea. Early participation may also reduce resistance toward using technology once it is up and running. Physicians, nurses and other key clinicians must be heavily represented on the technology selection team. Also, involve key technical professionals to weigh in on the right mix of custom versus off-the-shelf solutions.

Understand the Vendor Landscape

If an organization is a fledgling RHIO, or a component of one, no off-the-shelf software package will work today. In fact, few vendors are even aligned with the concept of a shared EHR and lack the orientation toward developing community standards, sharing ideas and collaborating to achieve the necessary connectivity. The vendors are actually the integrators in today's market.

For physician-based organizations, there are a number of well- developed choices and some "up-and-comers" to evaluate. Likewise, hospital-based organizations also have a number of established software options. Many sources of market assessment data are available through KLAS, consulting firms and networking. It is absolutely critical to plan for the workflow and data flow required by the eventual EHR. Otherwise the end result will be mixed purposes and a zillion silos of data.

Also realize that no single vendor can solve all the clinical data exchange riddles. The requirements are immense (see Figure 1).

So do the homework before approaching vendors. Determine up front if the EHR will grow from the perspective of hospital-based systems, physician group-based systems, or payer-based systems.

Joe Poats is a partner with Accenture, responsible for provider technology services for North America. His role includes planning, designing and implementing process and technology solutions, and leading design and implementation projects for healthcare providers (hospital systems, academic medical centers, and large physician groups), involving complex process and technology change.

Evaluate Assets

What already exists and what standards are in place? What investments have already been made? Before doing outside research, understand and document current standards and architectures embraced within the community to be served. At this step, organizations must assess their own level of willingness to work with other groups. Because collaboration is so critical to the overall EHR initiative, it's important to determine up front whether the requisite information sharing can occur.

Address technical concerns, such as existing platforms and opportunities for interoperability. In addition, leverage HIPAA, e-prescribing and patient safety initiatives already in place to get closer to a connected EHR.

Existing health records can also be leveraged by populating the local EHR database with information from RHIOs or the National Health Information Network (NHIN). It should be noted however, that, although tapping into an existing RHIO facilitates the automation of clinical processes, it will still require new EHR functionality.

Determine EHR Workflow Requirements

Be sure to look at the supportive technologies through the lens of workflow and data requirements. Decide who will have access to information, what roles these players will have and how these roles affect workflow.

To get started, evaluate collaboration efforts such as regional and community-based health information organizations and networks. Players include large health plans, hospitals, physician groups, healthcare IT suppliers, public health organizations and the government. These groups come together to explore challenges and strategies related to healthcare IT and health information exchange. There are similar state and national initiatives, such as the NHIN.

Evaluating workflow requirements includes deciding who will maintain EHR data and what types of information will result, such as reference lab data, consultant notes, prescription records, immunization and allergy records, and hospital data (surgery notes, discharge notes, etc.).

Also determine how patients and consumers will be identified, such as by social security number, account number or other specialized ID. In addition, decide which clinical processes will be enabled by the EHR and at what point in time.

For legal purposes, the workflow plan must also incorporate a process for synchronizing to a legal record of care. Consumers must also be considered as part of the workflow. Work with collaboration partners to decide how a constituent's health status information will be updated and made available.

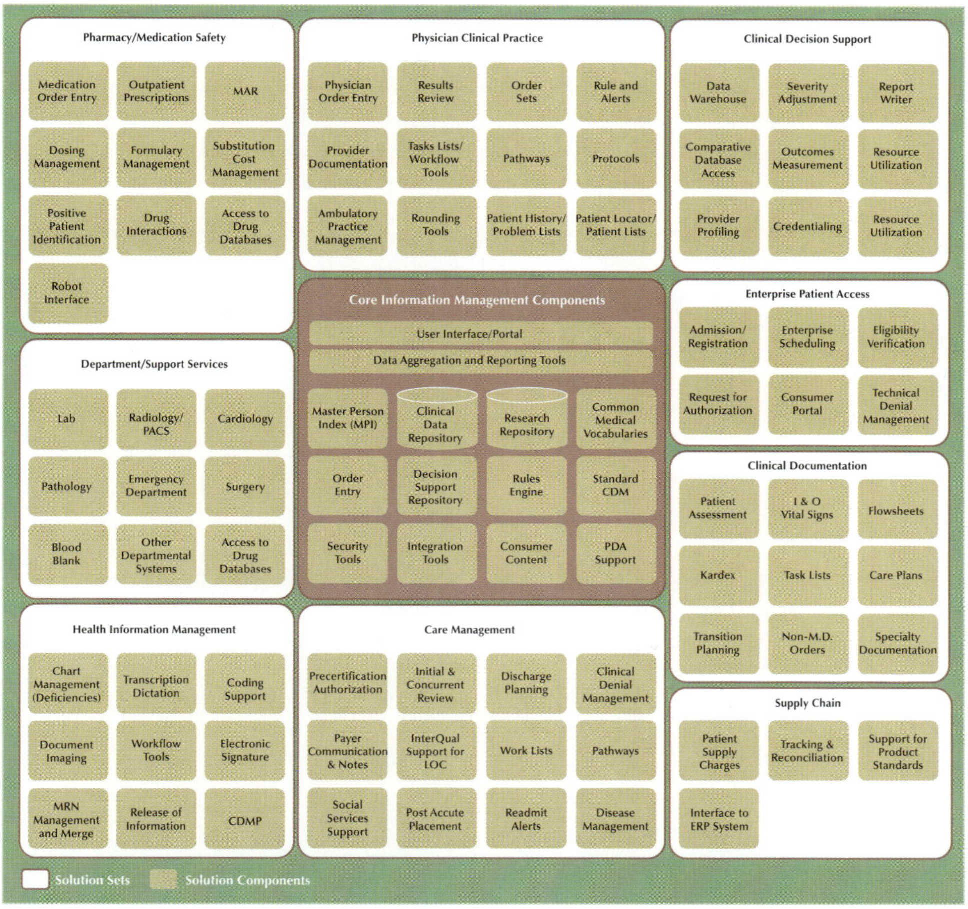

Figure 1 No single vendor supports all of the functionality required.

Determine EHR Technology Requirements

Next evaluate internal technology requirements. Consider the type of proposed infrastructure, including the network, portal opportunities, server utilities and who can access the system for security purposes.

Interconnectivity among different record-keeping systems must also be reconciled. For example, existing clinical data repositories, EHRs and computerized patient records must somehow coexist within the framework of the larger EHR initiative. E-prescribing systems and electronic payer processes must also fit into this scheme.

In addition, determine what type of user interface is appropriate for

Selecting Technologies for an EHR

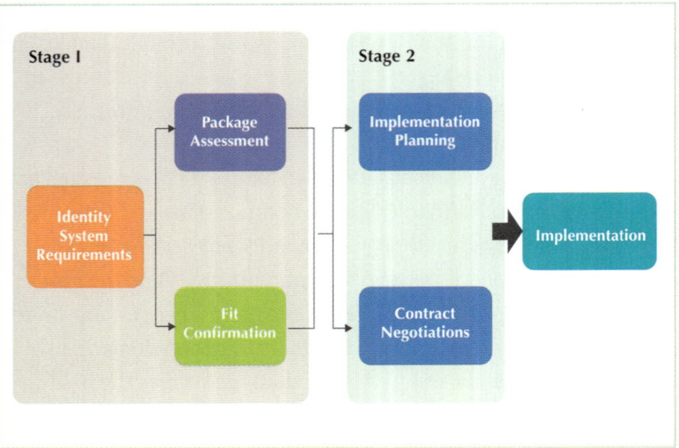

Figure 2 Model for Assessing Technology Choices

each constituent, depending upon individual needs and devices being used to access data. For example, a customer-facing portal varies greatly from a physician portal. It's also possible that Web screen access through the NHIN could allow authorized users to view data with little or no need to involve an EHR system vendor. This must be considered before talking to vendors.

Assess Solutions

Organizations and communities that have addressed the above concerns are ready to begin assessing technology choices. Figure 2 is a simple model for evaluating, assessing and confirming the correct choice.

The key questions in this process must include:

- Which work processes should be technology enabled?
- What are the critical business functions to support? Give prominence to these requirements in developing the request for information and request for proposal.
- Using the 80/20 rule, what are the key drivers of functionality? (Don't let requirements become littered with details).
- What risks must be addressed (e.g., financial stability, how new the vendor technology is and whether it is proven)? Ask for the vendor's history and product development track record and request a list of satisfied customers.
- How does the technology actually fit with outlined needs? A fit test provides an opportunity to really look at the technology in depth. Develop workflow-based scripts and conduct demonstration sessions to showcase the tools in action.
- What will this cost? Create an "apples to apples" view of the cost differences. Look at the total cost of ownership, not just up-front costs.
- How will this be accomplished? Create an action plan around project implementation.

First, break the project into different phases to create manageable sections. Also outline resource and key integration requirements during this planning stage. Importantly, compile and summarize a list of benefits to make the implementation compelling. Finally, draft a charter that addresses scope, governance and the multi-constituent roles and responsibilities.

The process approach for evaluating and selecting an EHR conceptually is in Figure 3.

Summary

The evaluation and selection process will depend on what players are trying to accomplish and where they are coming from. Focus on the functions and features of possible solutions, but first make sure there is an agreed-upon, balanced "scorecard" of criteria for selection. Use the evaluation process to achieve buy-in of those who will be affected, but avoid the proverbial "analysis paralysis." In most cases, how something gets implemented is more important than what gets implemented. ■

Can the core functionality in the vendor solution support our operational needs?	Can the core functionality in the vendor solution support our operational needs?	What are the technical considerations?
▪ Develop functional scenarios and demonstration scripts ▪ Vendor conducts demonstration ▪ End users and IS evaluate scripted demonstrations	▪ Develop a high-level workplan ▪ Identify internal and external resource requirements ▪ Identify conversion requirements ▪ Identify training efforts and expenditures	▪ Determine key standards ▪ Evaluate technical platform, reliability ▪ Review system scalability ▪ Evaluate integration options
What is the financial impact and total cost of ownership associated with the solution?	**What experiences and outcomes have other customers encountered?**	**What will be the future-state staffing model?**
▪ Get bids from vendors/integrators ▪ Evaluate total cost of ownership for current applications ▪ Identifiy impact on depreciation expenses for recently acquired systems	▪ Develop reference check criteria ▪ Interview customers with comparable size and complexity ▪ Interview customers with comparable migration experiences	▪ Identify current IS staffing and skill mix ▪ Determine support requirement for applications and infrastructure ▪ Develop future-state IS staffing

Figure 3 Sample EHR Evaluation Criteria

EHR Identity Management: A Proposal for the U.S.

In the United States, reliably matching EHRs with patients encompasses complex and far-ranging technical and social issues.

[John Quinn, Accenture]

With potentially over 300 million individuals and electronic health records (EHRs) accessible through a national health information network, the importance of "identity management" cannot be overstated. Identity management of an EHR involves a technology-assisted process that ensures a positive match between the elements of an electronic record that may be gathered from multiple source locations and the patient being treated. Correct identification is important with any computer-assisted process – from electronic banking to making a restaurant reservation – but with a patient's safety at stake, it takes on special importance.

If a physician or any caregiver receives the wrong health record content for a particular patient, the probability that significant harm may be done to that patient increases dramatically. For example, incorrect information about a patient's current medications and known allergies could lead to mistreatment resulting in a fatal drug-drug interaction or allergic reaction in the patient. This problem is compounded if the patient is unconscious at the time or otherwise unable to communicate.

Reducing the risk and occurrence of medication errors and adverse drug events, and thereby lowering the number of avoidable deaths, injuries and disabilities, is one of the key reasons for moving the U.S. toward an EHR system. Our approach to portable EHRs must strengthen this measure of safety, rather than add another risk.

Social and Political Factors

Before we evaluate the technical aspects of identity management, consider the current social and political factors that complicate patient identity management in the United States.

Attaching government identification or general numeric identifiers to individual citizens is politically sensitive. Though public resistance to creating a national person identifier may – in this case – be contradictory to its best interest, previous attempts have met strong resistance. For example, Congress swiftly, effectively repealed the HIPAA person identifier shortly after it was passed into law and publicity in the press brought it to the public's attention. Further, even though the Social Security number (SSN) – or a modification to the current SSN – could function as such an identifier, the laws that created the Social Security Act and various laws modifying the original act restrict its use for any but very narrowly defined uses. Even if restrictions were removed and funding was provided for a national database, studies have shown that the current SSN structure is inadequate for the job of a national healthcare identifier.

Another curious American phenomenon is the small subset of the population that – for various reasons such as personal desire, mental illness (e.g., paranoia), criminal records and illegal immigration status – consistently resists accurate identification. This opting out of the system becomes a serious problem when an individual deliberately ties his or her identity to another unsuspecting person (identity theft) and consequently intermixes two different medical records.

Issues at the IDN Level

In an integrated delivery network (IDN), the networkwide or enterprise patient identifier unites the patient's clinical and administrative information across the IDN (hospitals, primary care physician, specialists, ambulatory care centers, etc.) in a dynamic and ongoing exchange to provide information to the patient's caregivers and healthcare to the patient.

Correctly implementing identity management – identifying the patients and connecting them to their medical information – is a prerequisite to using the information in any medical record. This process is similar to accessing a bank account with the right account number, but is fraught with additional concerns about a

John Quinn is chief technology officer in Accenture's Provider, Health & Life Sciences practice focusing on emerging health care information systems technologies. He has over 29 and 32 years' experience in the healthcare and computer industries respectively. He has participated on the HL7 board of directors since its inception 18 years ago and has served as the chair of its technical steering committee for the last 14 years.

single medical identification number and a patient's history that may span many legacy identifiers when the information is sourced from multiple information systems that were established over a long period of time.

Managing the legacy identifiers in these multiple information systems is a key capability of any identity management system. Using an IDN enterprisewide identifier to manage multiple legacy identifiers is a key part of any IDN identity management program. Each individual may already have dozens of different legacy identifiers that may include: SSN, driver's license, individual hospital account and medical record numbers, lab system identifiers, pharmacy system identifiers, etc. – and the numbers keep growing. During the patient entry process (scheduling, registration, admission, etc.), a patient's identity is often confirmed with a selection of possible identifiers or key information (name, address, date of birth, etc.) that may or may not result in a unique match of identification.

Further challenges remain for the hospital's medical records department. Mismatched identifiers must be subsequently untangled by merging or unmerging records and by creating or deleting links among databases. In all these areas, there is little or no room for error, because incorrectly identifying patients could invite catastrophic outcomes.

Using EMPI to Manage Identity

The real challenge in identity management is integrating the numerous data sources – each one holding important patient information – and unifying disparate information silos into a single virtual record system through the dynamic and intelligent matching and linking of related patient records. This all needs to be done without overwhelming IT staff, users or hospital budgets.

In addition, the emergence of IDNs during the 1990s across the U.S. created a new set of technical challenges. Multiple hospitals were effectively merged into one network with their IT systems and medical records departments intact. These mergers usually happened without a specific IT plan (or funding) for enabling a conversion of the IT systems or a comprehensive merge of the medical records.

All this led to the creation of a new hierarchy to solve these problems: the enterprise master person index (EMPI). The EMPI evolved out of the previous hospital master patient index and represents the latest technology to manage medical records. An EMPI is the basis for a unique person identifier as a cross-reference across all systems, data records and applications throughout the healthcare information network. It plays a central role in the identification process from the moment of a patient's entry into the IDN, where a new enterprisewide ID – or a link to an existing identifier (or identifiers) – may be created. Integrating the EMPI in this phase is necessary to access and assimilate information from numerous data sources by managing new or legacy identifiers.

The EMPI can be a stand-alone system (unique to a hospital/caregiver's database) or part of a major clinical records system. How an EMPI is implemented by the IDN is usually determined by the system's architecture and its acquisition history within the organization. In any case, an overarching EMPI that embraces all systems is necessary to manage the multitude of patient identifiers within the environment.

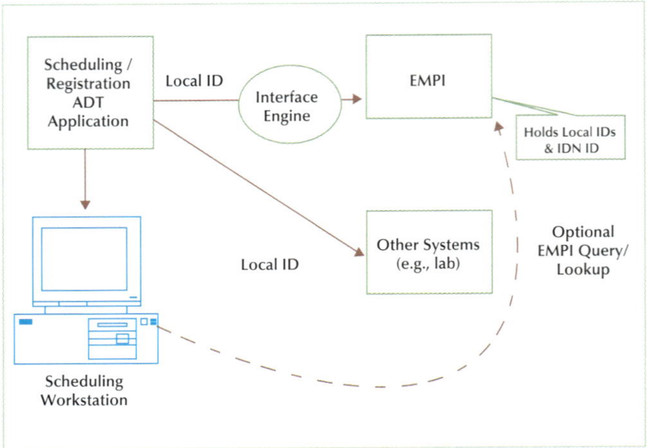

Figure 1 Passive EMPI Integration

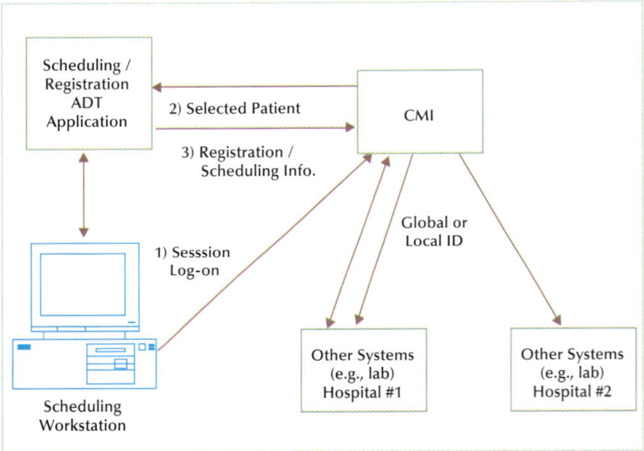

Figure 2 Active EMPI Integration

The operational real-time integration between systems is a less evident use of the EMPI. Here the EMPI ensures that a substitute legacy local identifier appropriate for the receiving system is used for messages sent to a system incapable of using the newer IDN identifier.

Most importantly, in addition to this internal IT management of identifiers between systems, patient identification starts during the patient's entry into the IDN – typically when a patient is scheduled or registers for a visit. Typically, there are two process approaches to establishing identity – passive and active:

- **Passive:** Look up, match and gather information relating a patient's identity to an existing ID – or create a new one –

after the initial encounter is completed; generally an automated process (see Figure 1).

- **Active:** Identity is matched immediately during the initial encounter; applies the EMPI rules and expertise while the patient is interacting with an IDN employee. However, this technical integration that gets information to the user right away by integrating the EMPI into the workflow is usually technically problematic (see Figure 2).

ID Is Key to Privacy

It's impossible to achieve positive and consistent patient identification without also considering the counterbalancing issues of privacy. As a medical record follows a patient, identity issues become synonymous with privacy issues.

For various (HIPAA-associated) reasons, privacy policies associated with the source clinical information systems may complicate or preclude distribution of medical records through a portable EHR.

For various (HIPAA-associated) reasons, privacy policies associated with the source clinical information systems may complicate or preclude distribution of medical records through a portable EHR.

In all cases, the medical records department has the final job of manually sorting out the known or suspected identification problems and "gray area" matches.

RxHub: An EMPI Example

An example of a large healthcare network across a very large population using EMPI numbers is the electronic prescription benefits exchange service, RxHub. Connecting physicians, patients, pharmacies and pharmacy benefit managers (PBMs)/payers, the RxHub exchange routes patient medication history and health benefit information between PBMs and physicians.

The exchange streamlines e-prescribing and smooths pharmacy claims adjudications for eventually up to 150 million covered members. In order to better manage this huge number of records, RxHub has implemented an EMPI based on Initiate System's Identity EMPI product.

However, RxHub's simplified EMPI application has an intrinsic simplification over the problem of matching medical records. If a patient does not have a benefit plan number that matches the information from the benefit plans, the request is simply rejected. This is an inconvenience, as it requires the patient spend time on the phone with the benefit plan to fix the problem.

At RxHub, errors do not in general create a patient safety problem, but are a payment inconvenience that can be straightened out later. The process does not support an immediate decision such as those faced by physicians in an emergency room. All of these problems are amplified at the regional and national level where it is not clear what service will exist that is similar to an IDN's medical records department.

This is an area where policy and legal change is probably necessary. Currently HIPAA allows state privacy rules that are more stringent to preempt national HIPAA requirements. At a minimum, mechanisms need to be created to coordinate a patient's specific privacy requirements and possible state requirements that might not normally apply where the EHR information is being used.

Summary

Improving patient safety – reducing medication errors and adverse drug events – is the key driver in a move to an EHR system with a reliable identity management capability. In addition to the formidable technical challenges of identity management, social and political factors in the U.S. (e.g., aversion to a national ID number system) complicate an identity management solution. The recent emergence of IDNs and the related technical complexity of maintaining identity management capabilities across numerous information systems led to the creation of the EMPI. Used as a stand-alone system or part of a participating IDN, the EMPI points the way to an EHR system featuring comprehensive identity management capabilities. With up to 150 million records, the RxHub electronic prescription exchange service is a good example of a very large healthcare network on the scale of at least one-half of a fully deployed national health information network that is using an EMPI today.

The obvious and most elegant solution to the identity management challenge in the U.S. would be a national identifier, similar to the one in use for almost 60 years in the U.K. However, because of the particular social and political factors in the U.S., we see an EMPI-based process as the most practical path. In addition, federal and state privacy policies should be coordinated to avoid further technical and practical hurdles for EHR implementation. ■

Current and Future Payer and Industry Needs Solved by Certification of EHRs

Organizations such as the Certifying Commission on Health Information Technology should be encouraged to make available a certification process for vendors seeking to deploy health IT solutions.

[Charles Kennedy, M.D., Wellpoint]

Providing Americans with high-quality, safe, affordable healthcare is behind the national push to use health information technology (HIT). In response to this increasing and ever more acute challenge, the Department of Health and Human Services established four goals as part of its framework for strategic action of 2004:

1. Inform clinical practice;
2. Interconnect clinicians;
3. Personalize care; and
4. Improve public health.

These goals have profound implications for our healthcare industry. It is anticipated that the deployment of the required technology to meet these goals will impact how physicians are paid and the type of information patients have access to, not to mention new hardware, software, intermediaries and other industry changes. However, all of the complexities and challenges of making these goals a reality distill into one significant underlying interaction: a patient and a physician seeking to improve health status. With this as our organizing principle and ultimate unit of measure, a clear set of actions emerges.

Steps Toward a National Health Information Network

Electronic health records (EHRs) are the central foundation for all subsequent systems, whether financial, clinical, research or administrative. EHRs are the anticipated technical foundation for the patient-physician interaction. Therefore, these systems must achieve the highest level of security, functionality, interoperability and data completeness. These systems face a tall order: maximizing the safety, health and effective care of patients while satisfying a very demanding and challenging end user – physicians. Creating such a system, however, is further complicated by our current environment of multiple, disparate systems with incomplete clinical and technical standards for deployment, poorly understood impact on workflow, user interface design challenges and multiple custom interfaces required for interoperability.

Definition and Role of Product Certification

Given the requirements of software development cycles, financial requirements and adoption periods, we must create a road map that spans several years. This road map must include objective criteria that grow in depth and breadth until the vision of a broadly deployed, value-adding EHR is realized. The road map's criteria must include a pass/fail metric as well as an objective, trusted party that can vouch for the accuracy of the certification results. Self-attestation by the vendor may be acceptable for select, obvious components of the software as well as certain steps in the recertification of products (such as a capability that was present and certified in the previous year for which no modifications to the standard or software have been made in the intervening time period). However, objective, testable criteria that are focused on real needs for real users must be the basis for the majority of the certifying process.

The certification of EHRs has a central role in the national effort to increase the availability, deployment, use and refinement of them. It is the most compelling strategy for realizing the vision and ensuring an objective measurement on the industry's or a vendor's progress in achieving this vision. A compelling certification provides an objective standard that all stakeholders in the healthcare value chain (hospitals, health plans, physicians and patients) can point to with confidence regarding the validity and accuracy of the anticipated system capabilities. This function will be required in order for health plans to play an effective role in this evolution of the healthcare industry.

Charles Kennedy, M.D., is vice president of Clinical Informatics at WellPoint, Inc. He has 20 years of healthcare experience, most recently as CEO of Care Assured, a technology start-up company. Prior to this, he served at BlueShield of California. Dr. Kennedy received his M.D. from UCLA and his M.B.A. from Stanford University.

Role of Health Plans in Driving Health IT Enabled Through Certification

Although there is still much uncertainty as to how HIT will be deployed, there are several potential points of leverage that a health plan can provide in driving HIT solutions. These include:

Accelerating Adoption Through Use of Plan-Based Clinical Data Sets

A substantial challenge in the deployment of HIT is the conversion from a paper to an electronic environment. Today physicians must operate in a mixed electronic-paper environment for prolonged periods of time or the health system must pay for substantial paper-to-electronic conversion projects. Health plans can play an important role in this conversion by offering the ability to prepopulate EHRs with a base set of clinical data derived from claims data sets available on broad sets of patients. These data sets can include ICD-9 codes for diagnosis, CPT codes for procedural information and NDC codes for prescribed drug information.

An EHR, certified for acceptable levels of security, will likely need to be present to access these value sets. A strong and industry-accepted certification process will enable this data delivery.

Some health plans have lab data sets developed through HEDIS measure generation. These data sets provide an opportunity to deliver value for both patients and physicians from the moment an EHR "goes live." However, health plans are unlikely to provide this data to environments where there is significant potential for inappropriate use, security or privacy breaches. Therefore, an EHR, certified for acceptable levels of security, will likely need to be present to access these value sets. A strong and industry-accepted certification process will enable this data delivery.

Accelerating Adoption Through Payment Incentives

Although HIT is expected to provide a positive return on investment, it requires substantial upfront capital and a meaningful product/network strategy to recoup these investments (both financial and clinical). Further, the current payment strategy provides challenges for hospitals and physicians that currently deploy systems to improve clinical performance. Fee-for-service medicine can potentially reward inefficiency and poor outcomes more than efficient, high-quality practices. This is because complications result in the need for more medical services which, in turn, result in greater payments to the physician. Pay for performance is a tool that can help resolve this issue by rewarding physicians for improved outcomes. Its utility is enhanced by the use of HIT and clinical decision support, both which drive improved adherence to evidence-based medicine. Strategies that have been promoted include direct payment for use of e-health technologies and payment for the process and outcome measures that leverage data sets generated by these technologies. Regardless of the strategy employed, a standard set of criteria and a publicly available certification process will be required.

Improving the Value Measurement of HIT

Health plans, clinical researchers, actuarial and other professions and industries interested in tracking healthcare expenditures need to understand the unique value that HIT provides. The measurement of this value in an incremental fashion will be critical in attracting ongoing investments to broaden system deployments, justifying system modifications to maximize ROI and supporting ongoing system improvements. Yet value measurement and quantification will be challenging. Among these challenges are risk adjustment, confounding variables such as benefit design changes, ongoing turnover at physician practices and a plethora of e-health record capabilities currently on the market. These challenges will require clinical trials similar to what a medical device might be put through in order to track efficacy and effectiveness. Standardizing a minimum functionality set reduces the variability of the effectiveness of the interventional group so that more compelling measures of value can be obtained. Without certification physicians who use glorified word processing tools or spreadsheets may be included in the analysis and reduce the refinement of the study.

Product certification of HIT products, including EHRs, is a needed and important requirement in the deployment of technology for use by physicians, patients and others in the healthcare industry. Organizations such as the Certifying Commission on Health Information Technology should be encouraged to rapidly deploy and make available a certification process for vendors seeking to deploy HIT solutions. The certification process is a central wheel in turning the industry toward greater use of technology. ■

weblink

Read about how combining financial processes with an EHR can significantly improve a hospital's economic performance in "Revenue Cycle Enhancement Associated with EHR Systems."

The Role of Centralization In Building the NHIN

Adopting a centralized approach to building their data infrastructure provides inherent benefits at each level of the NHIN.

[Matthew Quinn, Teradata, a division of NCR]

Centralizing data has been a key enabler for leading retailers, manufacturers and financial services companies to become "game changers" in their markets. Taking a centralized approach to their enterprise data supports the complex integration, data quality and decision-support needs of leading businesses like Bank of America, Kaiser Permanente, 3M, SBC, Wal-Mart and Harrah's Casino. With a centralized approach, it's all about getting the data right. From this foundation, thousands of users in their extended enterprise get their answers every day to questions on profitability, supply chain analytics and utilization.

The centralized approach has been implemented by many of the most admired organizations in and outside of healthcare because, in comparison to distributed approaches, it delivers the most business value, highest performance, most flexibility and lowest total cost of ownership (TOC) at the lowest risk. By building a flexible structure that contains all of the data at the detail-level from the beginning, the enterprise will be able to address new business needs as they are identified, without having to compromise or restructure the underlying data. As needs change and evolve, hierarchies can be easily changed without expensive rework of the foundation. Focusing on the data provides the starting point for a solution that is incremental, manageable and simplifies the enterprise rather than adding complexity to it.

Indeed, key benefits of employing a centralized approach include:

- Improved flexibility and lower TCO in integrating and maintaining disparate systems;
- Expanded analytical capabilities and data quality; and
- Improved security.

But the data for the entire National Health Information Network (NHIN) will most likely not be stored and accessed from a single, national, centralized data warehouse. While a centralized approach is technically and politically feasible for Fortune 100 corporations (and other nations' health information networks), it is technically but probably not politically feasible to have a single, centralized data warehouse for the United States.

Centralization, however, is both beneficial and – potentially – politically feasible at every level of the building blocks of the NHIN. Public, private and military health systems, regional health information organizations (RHIOs), public and private research and surveillance agencies, as well as federal- and state-level healthcare financing organizations would all benefit from taking a centralized approach with their data.

Organizations comprising the building blocks of the NHIN should seek to centralize to the highest level politically feasible. Because of the inherent benefits of taking a centralized approach (and the inherent limitations of taking a decentralized one), organizations at all levels of the NHIN should first seek to centralize data. In some instances, gaining acceptance of all involved stakeholders will not be possible. These organizations – by taking a decentralized approach – may choose to sacrifice capability, flexibility and cost of ownership for political expediency.

Defining the Centralized Approach

The centralized or enterprise data warehouse approach is characterized by a single, enterprise-level store of atomic-level detail data from all relevant source systems, using a normalized data model that allows for ad hoc discovery and drill-down analysis by multiple user groups.

The centralized approach can scale linearly to serve as the single, unified data infrastructure to support local, regional, organizational or even national interoperability and "single version of the enterprise" analysis.

Matthew Quinn is the healthcare program manager for Teradata, the data warehousing division of NCR. He is a graduate of the United States Military Academy at West Point and holds an M.B.A. from Colorado State University.

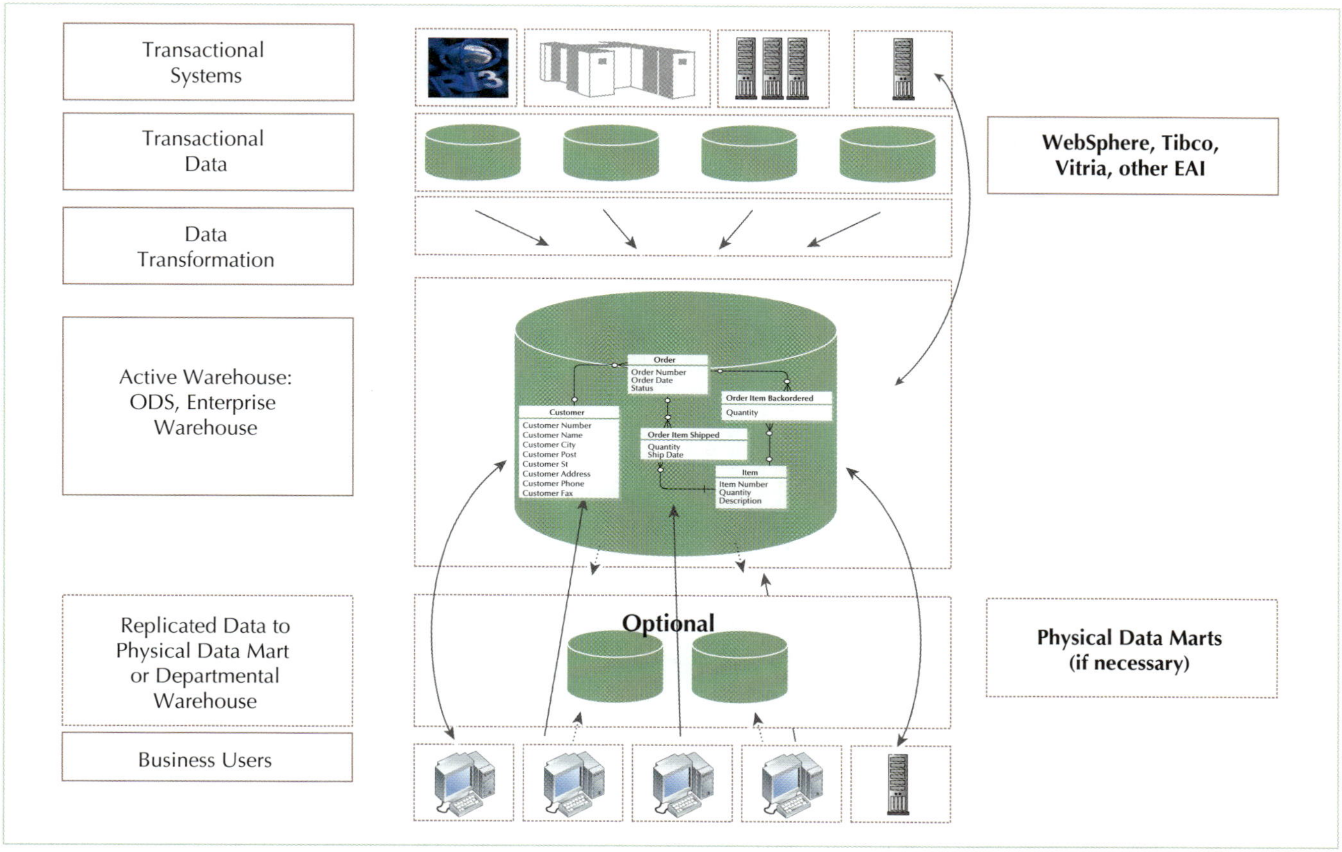

Figure 1 Centralized Topology

Components of the Centralized Topology

The components of this topology include (see Figure 1):

- **Transaction Systems and Data** are the "feeder" systems that provide data to the warehouse. In the context of the health system enterprise, these systems could include inpatient and outpatient EHR systems and the various enterprise and departmental clinical and administrative legacy "transaction" systems. In the context of a local or regional cooperative or RHIO, the feeder systems would be the participating organizations' EHR systems.
- **Data Transformation** consists of using industry-standard ETL (extract, transfer, load) tools to cleanse and move data from the transactional systems to the data warehouse. Common ETL tools include Informatica and Ascential.
- **Data Warehouse:** The heart of performance and scalability for the enterprise architecture is a massively parallel processing database engine. Better performance and linear scalability result from unconditional parallelism. The reason is the parallel database will split apart each SQL query spreading the workload across all of the units of parallelism available to it, thereby balancing the work of all the system resources. In order to offset these differences, conditional parallel databases will do a number of performance-enhancing tasks, including partitioning large tables, providing hints, reorganizing the data, de-normalizing the schema and distributing data across multiple database servers. A decentralized approach builds boundaries around the adaptability of the system, and causes the development and maintenance costs of the system to increase considerably.
- **Normalized Logical Data Model:** A normalized logical data model (LDM) is a blueprint that maps healthcare business processes and functions. Operational systems throughout the enterprise are mapped to the LDM and feed the data warehouse directly. Because a normalized model maps business processes and functions – and not legacy systems – it is application agnostic, able to work with any or all of an enterprise's applications.

Defining the Decentralized Approach

In contrast to the centralized approach, the decentralized approach maintains multiple, duplicate physical versions of the data in an enterprise. Typically decentralized architectures are built from the bottom up, bring together the physical data from the enterprise's source systems in a central hub and break the data into "marts" or subsets of the enterprise data to meet the analytic needs of various users.

Many legacy EHR systems employ a distributed or "hub and spoke" topology. This approach takes significant time and cost to implement and maintain, is inflexible in supporting system and user changes and – inherently – leads to limitations in analytical capabilities and complicates data quality issues. Figure 2 illustrates a typical distributed or hub-and-spoke topology.

Centralized Approach Benefits

Achieving the overarching goals of the Office of the Health Information Technology Coordinator – informing clinical practice, interconnecting physicians, personalizing care and improving population health – will require more than just being able to transact health information between and among healthcare stakeholders.

At all levels of the NHIN, achieving these goals will require the ability to flexibly, securely and cost-effectively bring together disparate systems, to gain insight from unconstrained analysis of massive amounts of atomic-level structured and unstructured information, and to activate this information in improving the safety, cost and efficiency of care.

The topology that an organization chooses will directly impact the cost, flexibility, analytic capabilities and even capacity to achieve these goals. Some of the benefits of choosing a centralized approach and some of the inherent limitations of choosing a decentralized one include:

Reduced Time, Effort and Cost in Integrating And Maintaining Disparate Systems

Unlike approaches that require building and maintaining interfaces between and among all of the applications in an enterprise,

What's wrong with this picture?

1. There are too many copies of the data. Will they all be the same?
2. There is too much latency – too long to get the data to the people who need it. Everyone sees different inconsistent points in time.
3. The solution is too complex. Every line on the chart represents an ETL process that requires life cycle maintenance.
4. The solution is too expensive. There are numerous components that lead to increased costs. Costs are often hidden in distributed organization.

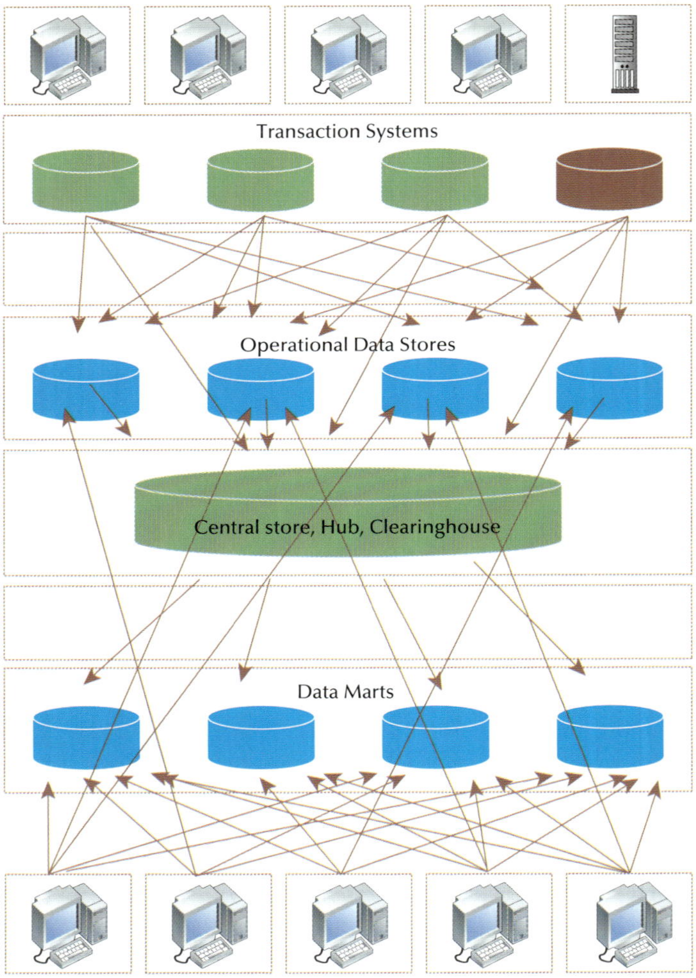

Figure 2 Hub-and-Spoke Topology and Issues

the centralized approach integrates disparate systems at the normalized logical data model level. This drastically simplifies the architecture, extends the life of legacy applications and supports the use of a variety of best-of-breed applications in the enterprise. Further, because integration takes place at the data model (versus between and among many applications), application changes do not typically require complex and expensive re-architecture of the system (and construction/changes to interfaces) to support them.

For a health system, this means that supporting (and making interoperable) the various enterprise and departmental systems (used by the various stakeholders in the system) that comprise the EHR is as easy as mapping each of these systems to the LDM. This is much quicker, simpler, less disruptive and less costly than mandating a single system/set of systems for enterprise use and/or establishing and maintaining/updating strict data standards among all stakeholders. Replacing legacy systems can occur at the pace of the organization's requirements and need not occur as part of a "big bang" up-front implementation.

Two key criteria for selecting a data warehousing approach at all levels in the NHIN will be the price performance, flexibility and TCO of that technology. The centralized approach has proven to be superior in both of these regards.

Each arrow on the topology diagrams in Figures 1 and 2 represent an IT process that must be implemented and maintained for the lifetime of the system. Each arrow represents dedicated staff, cost and risk. There are dramatically fewer arrows in the centralized topology than the distributed or hub-and-spoke one. Further, the centralized topology does not have arrows between and among the various feeder transaction systems. This means that, unlike in the hub-and-spoke model, replacing a legacy system or adding a new system does not impact each of the complex interconnection of interfaces in the hub and spoke.

In addition, the centralized topology eliminates all of the cost associated with the data marts and operational data stores in a hub-and-spoke topology – a huge component of ongoing IT costs.

Expanded Analytical Capabilities

Organizations collect and aggregate data to gain insight and achieve business value. The role of the enterprise intelligence designer is to minimize boundaries in achieving this goal. While the IT costs of choosing the wrong infrastructure can be great, the greatest cost of implementing the wrong architecture will be the opportunity costs that result from these boundaries. As much as 95 percent of future needs may be undefined

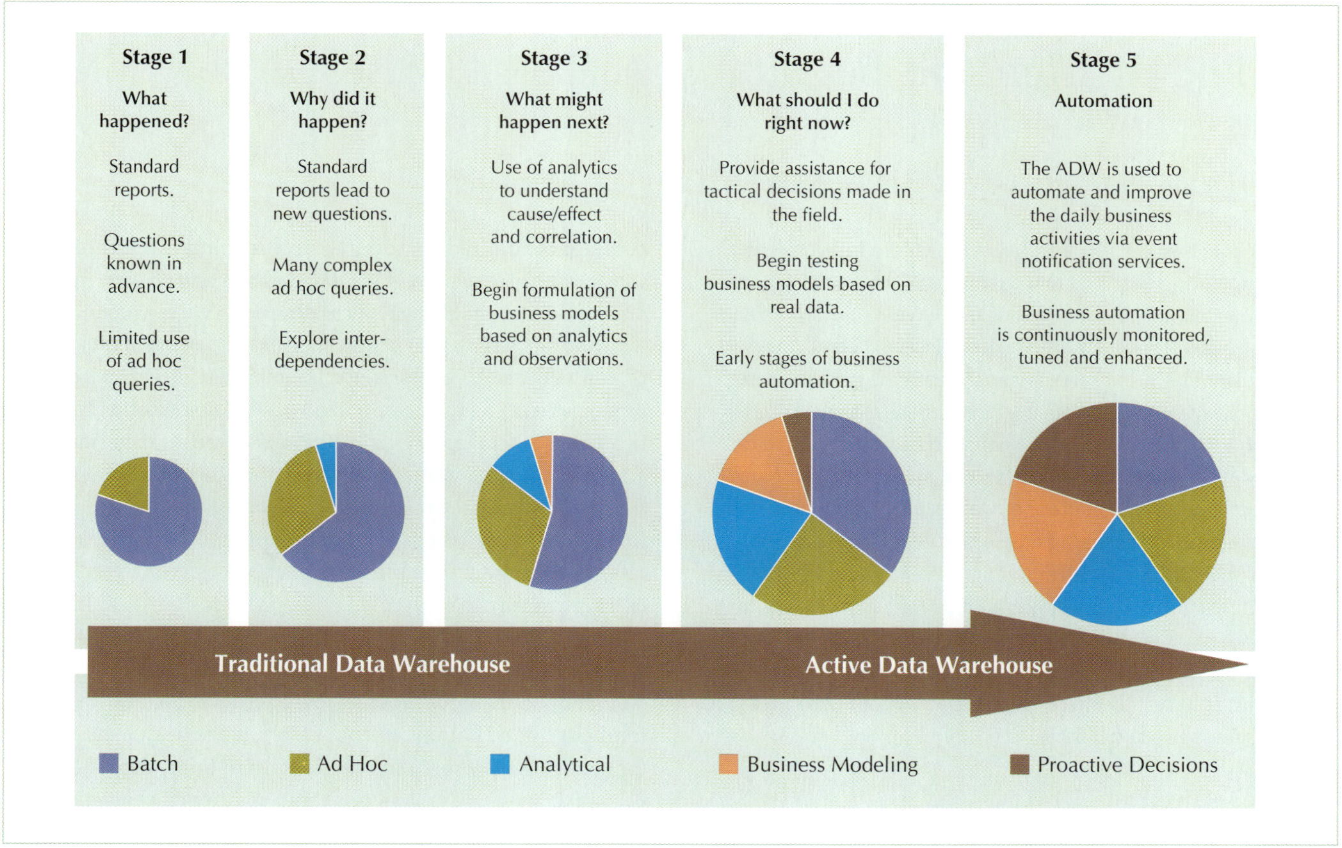

Figure 3 Evolving Toward Active Data Warehouse

early on. The key is continual expansion and flexibility. By building a flexible structure that contains all of the data at the detail-level from the beginning, the enterprise will be able to address new business needs as they are identified, without having to compromise or restructure the database. As needs change and evolve, hierarchies can be easily changed without expensive rework of the foundation.

The ultimate goal for informing clinical practice is to provide the full breadth and depth of insight of the medical community in a format that is useful at the point of care and for deeper clinical decision support. This requires a centralized topology and data warehouse technology that supports both horizontal and vertical views and the entire continuum (transactional, tactical and strategic DSS) of queries. OLTP or transaction-based systems (and associated distributed topologies) alone cannot support concurrent insight on these three types of queries.

Activating the Data

Figure 3 describes the evolution of data warehousing toward the goal of active data warehousing (ADW), where event-based triggering takes hold and the data warehouse takes on a mission-critical role in automating decisions and pushing insight to the frontlines of an organization. Two prerequisites for evolution toward ADW are having a central store of enterprise detail-level data and data warehousing technology that can support the extreme performance, scalability, availability and data freshness needs of this type of workload. Adopting a decentralized approach by extracting data from the central store limits this evolution and the ability of any database technology, no matter how robust, to evolve to this state.

Summarization, or making only a portion of enterprise data available at above the health system level, also limits the ability to accurately gain insight from data. Think of a bank producing a monthly bank statement that records checking account activity. If it summarizes the total amount of deposits and withdrawals, determining if a certain check had cleared would not be possible. That would require detail data.

Improved Security

A centralized data warehouse is much simpler to secure than dozens of heterogeneous data marts. Indeed many industry analysts and leading healthcare and financial services organizations agree that an enterprise data warehouse is the preferred implementation model, and among that model's many virtues is the fact that a centralized data warehouse's security is simpler and less expensive to manage, while providing higher levels of security.

Security and privacy are also major drivers of simplification. Imagine proving the implementation of a privacy policy to auditors when customer information is scattered among a dozen or more separate systems in a distributed topology. Data is dispersed, access control is difficult to prove and accuracy of privacy-related controls is difficult to ensure as the data is transported and transformed. Privacy and security policies are much easier to implement, manage, log and audit when there is only one copy of the data and one physical place it is accessed.

Where in the NHIN Does Centralization Make Sense?

As we have described, taking a centralized approach to building the data infrastructure provides cost and capability advantages over alternate approaches. Consequently organizations at all levels of the NHIN – from the health system on up should seek to take a centralized approach wherever politically feasible. Centralizing data requires a greater level of trust and cooperation among the stakeholders in an organization than a structure in which organizations only share an extracted portion of their data. Gaining this level of cooperation is simplest in centrally led organizations (in healthcare and otherwise) and most difficult in settings where intense competition or distrust exists among stakeholders. Organizations must weigh the benefits of taking a centralized approach against the ability of the stakeholders in the organization to cooperate and the cost and capability tradeoffs of a decentralized approach against the political expediency of not physically sharing data.

Commercial Health Systems and Networks

The centralized approach is both beneficial and politically feasible for the nation's for-profit and not-for-profit health systems. Even for national-scale organizations like Kaiser Permanente and HCA, despite the regional or local orientation of the stakeholders in these organizations, if the leadership of an organization seeks to gain both universal EHR adoption and a "single view of the enterprise" among the various institutions, clinics and individual physi-

By building a flexible structure that contains all of the data at the detail-level from the beginning, the enterprise will be able to address new business needs as they are identified, without having to compromise or restructure the database.

cian practices in the organization, then the centralized topology would be both politically and technically feasible.

ASP EHR Vendors

A growing trend among EHR vendors is to outsource hosting of EHRs for multiple providers to a single application service provider, or ASP. Centralizing the data for all clients that such a vendor serves simplifies system management and interoperability and provides the capacity for collaborative analytics not possible with physically separate data structures.

Federal Health and Military Health System Interoperability

The centralized approach would meet the goal of coordinating and making interoperable the various federal health information systems (e.g., VA, MHA, IHS). The hierarchical leadership structures of federal and military health systems are conducive to the cooperation required for physical data sharing. While EHR adoption among these organizations is far greater than among non-governmental institutions, the systems, standards, metadata and progress in implementing these systems varies greatly. The effort that would be required to link all of these systems using interfaces would truly be monumental (to mention nothing of the effort required to maintain this infrastructure). Centralizing the data for each of these systems would speed enterprise interoperability and greatly expand analytic capabilities.

Local, Regional and Rural Health Cooperatives and RHIOs

The building blocks of the NHIN will be local, regional and state level cooperatives and RHIOs. These organizations will be composed of the payers, providers, purchasers and others that share the goal of improving the quality, safety and efficiency of care delivered in a region. If a close enough level of collaboration and trust exists among the various stakeholders in a community or region such that they feel secure in physically storing their clinical data together (while, of course, providing organization and role-based access control measures to the data), they can concurrently achieve EHR adoption and interoperability. While several state RHIOs have announced that they will be pursuing a centralized approach in building their data infrastructures, this approach might be particularly attractive for a group of, for example, underserved or rural healthcare organizations that seek to gain the benefits of EHR adoption while sharing the cost of implementation, maintenance and interoperability with other organizations.

Research and Surveillance Agencies

Implementing a centralized approach would help achieve the goal of unifying public health, research and surveillance architectures. The centralized approach is unsurpassed in supporting integration of massive amounts of data from multiple systems into a "single version of the enterprise" and pushing analysis of that data out to the appropriate stakeholders in time to take action (activating the data.) Having detail-level data would allow the optimal use of neural network and other predictive modeling technology to improve the accuracy of analysis and reduce the occurrence of "false positives" inherent in summary data.

Moving away from a centralized model for unifying public health infrastructures introduces data timeliness and quality issues. As in business, this speed to insight is especially important in the context of public health, where hours can mean lives.

Studies by Rand and others have found the dissemination and practice of best-available evidence is woefully slow and inconsistent. A solution to the goal of accelerating research and dissemination of evidence should thus address the dual issues of gaining insight from data and integrating that insight into the workflows of clinicians in the field.

Centralized warehouses designed for answering any question at any time without the associated time, effort and cost of replicating and analyzing data outside of the warehouse (i.e., building a dedicated data mart), free clinical researchers from technological limitations in gaining insight from their data. And having detailed – atomic level – data available for analysis does not force researchers to limit the scope of their data and analysis before they begin (as is common in the decentralized approaches that advocate separate data subsets or "marts" for reporting and analysis).

Conclusion

While centralization of the entire nation's healthcare data is technically feasible, the political feasibility of such an architecture is probably unlikely. Instead the stakeholders that compose the "building blocks" of the NHIN – organizations at the health system; local, regional and state cooperative; RHIO; and research and surveillance agency levels – should consider and adopt a centralized approach except where this approach is not politically possible.

As many of the world's largest and most prestigious companies – inside and outside of healthcare – have proven, the benefits that they have realized by taking a centralized approach would not have been possible without having a single version of their enterprise data. ■

weblink

Read about the role of government in implementing EHRs in "Newt Gingrich Advocates the Creation of a 21st Century Intelligent Health System."

Collaboration: An Essential Element Of the Regional Exchange

Developing a functional EHR is not possible unless the constituents involved work together to determine its scope, how it operates, security measures, means of funding and governance.

[Mary E. Edwards, Accenture]

Collaboration is increasingly required to make the next set of fundamental shifts in the nation's healthcare system. For the last decade, significant progress has been made in improving the efficiency and effectiveness of the administrative aspects of care delivery and reimbursement within organizations. Payers have increased automation of claims and care management processes. The ability to exchange electronically the information necessary to conduct common transactions has been, in the main, achieved.

While the healthcare system continues to lag other industries, much progress has been made in digitizing key information within the provider domain as well. EHR systems are in the later stages of adoption in provider systems and there is a real trend toward EHR in the ambulatory setting. While it will take time for the healthcare industry to become as fully automated as, say, the financial services industry, the next "generation" of automation is already upon us.

Over the next decade, the focus will be to increase efficiency and effectiveness of care ***across*** organizations. In order to achieve a more integrated, better informed and, therefore, higher quality of patient care, the ability to readily exchange information about care itself needs to be achieved. Regional exchanges are emerging as the vehicle for this exchange.

A regional exchange, or regional health information organization, is a collective term for the system that enables certain information stored in medical records to be made available – in a bounded region or geography – for a predetermined set of constituents to share. These exchanges facilitate improved insight at the point of patient care by facilitating access to EHR data across the variety of care constituents that may be involved in patient care.

Such an exchange is not possible unless these constituents work together to determine its scope, how it operates, security measures, means of funding, governance, capacity for expansion and the process by which to educate and obtain feedback from the community using it. Success must be engineered through a cooperative effort that delivers value to each constituent.

Constituents of the Regional Exchange

The constituents of a regional exchange include all the players in the care management process: patients, physicians, hospitals, inpatient and outpatient services, independent labs and test centers, home health agencies, insurance agencies and others. All groups that would benefit from having insight into a patient's history – those who would modify or improve patient care based on having access to what happened to that patient yesterday or last week or last month – are constituents. Because of the fragmented nature of the healthcare system, constituents have a poor track record of self-organizing to forge change within the healthcare system (see Figure 1).

Payers are emerging as an organizing focal point – in some communities because they are seeing regional exchange as a way to dramatically improve the quality and reduce the cost of care and in others because they presume they will be "invited" to fund the lion's share of such efforts. Payers also have, by and large, a much more sophisticated understanding of the infrastructure required for such an exchange. Given that trust levels between payers and (all types of) providers have never been high, there are some challenges inherent in creating the collaboration needed to achieve a regional exchange.

Why Is Collaboration Required?

Collaboration is essential in the conceptualization, development, deployment and ongoing evolution of a regional exchange.

Mary E. Edwards, a partner in Accenture's Health & Life Sciences practice, has over 20 years of industry experience through various positions in the healthcare and life insurance sectors. Her work focuses on facilitating strategic market-based initiatives including payer-provider collaborations to improve administrative and clinical processes, and to promote and encourage EHR and eRx development and deployment.

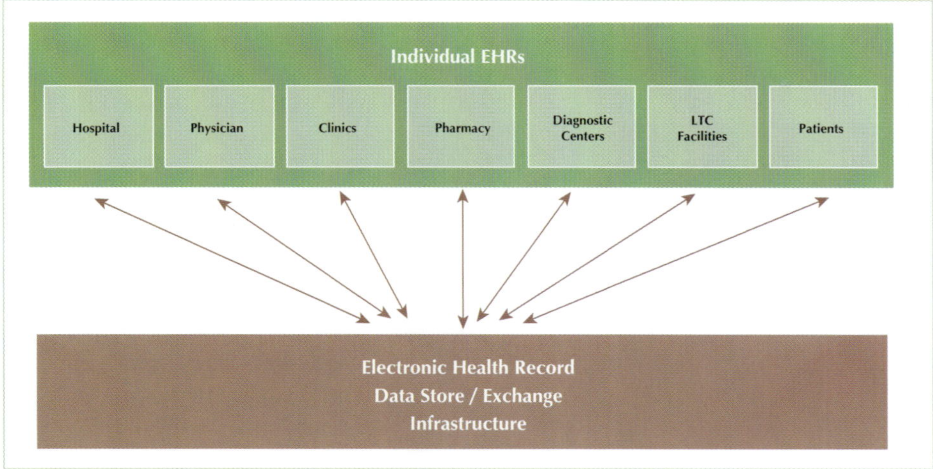

Figure 1 A Regional Exchange

Shared vision for how and what the exchange will facilitate is key to success. There is no single provider, payer, lab or patient, for that matter, who is the exchange. Even if an intermediary develops an exchange solution, t is likely that solution will also be the function of collaboration. Issues requiring collaboration include:

- **Governance** – How will the exchange be overseen? Who, or what body, will be responsible for setting the direction of the exchange?
- **Funding and Economic Model** – Who will fund the exchange initially and longer term? Will the exchange be self-funding? How will ongoing revenues be generated and managed?
- **Ownership** – Who owns the solution? It is possible, but unlikely, that a commercial entity will emerge with a solution. It is more likely that a collaboration will yield a solution that may be extended to (and therefore commercialized in) other communities. How each of the constituents "own" the intellectual and other more tangible capital and how they would "participate" in commercializing the solution needs to be addressed.
- **Operating Model** – Who will manage the exchange on a day-to-day basis including security and access management? How will business processes, policies and procedures be architected, implemented and monitored?
- **Deployment and Adoption** – How will the exchange be deployed? Who will be responsible for the activities that drive adoption? How will adoption be monitored? What feedback mechanisms will be used?
- **Practice Evolution** – How could care management processes change to take fullest advantage of the exchange? How will the exchange identify and/or enable providers to understand the impact on care management processes? How will ongoing improvement opportunities for the exchange itself, and corresponding improvements to care management processes, be identified and deployed?

How Can a Productive Collaboration Be Achieved?

While not an exhaustive list, the above highlights some of the more difficult areas to address. Collaboration projects of this complexity tend to require learning, discussion and iterative decision making over a period of time. In such efforts it becomes quite difficult to ensure that decisions build upon each other, rather than decisions continuously recycling. In order to be successful in this type of collaboration, consider these operating principles:

- **Make sure the right types of people are involved.** There will be technical, operating and business model considerations. Having the right skill sets focused in the right areas is paramount.
- **Make sure the people involved are decision makers – or are empowered to make decisions.** This will reduce frustration and ensure that momentum can build and be maintained throughout the collaboration process.
- **Create a work group mentality vs. a committee mentality.** Work groups need to produce deliverables. Groups with a committee mentality tend to have unlimited ability to keep things from happening and no apparent ability to get anything done.
- **Form work groups with well-defined scopes and completion criteria.** Just because the process is collaborative doesn't mean that every person has to be involved in every decision. Work groups should be formed to address specific scopes of work relative to the exchange. And as importantly, it should be clear what constitutes the work group being finished. Completion criteria will ensure the work group performs to the requirements and can be disengaged when the requirements are met.
- **Structure the collaboration in large blocks of time for specific work products.** Structuring eight-hour working sessions once every four weeks, for example, will yield much greater benefit than assembling the same group of constituents for

weblink

Learn how implementing a national EHR system will happen through a series of independent community-wide efforts in Clem McDonald's Q & A.

two-hour sessions once a week for four weeks. Ensure that the working sessions are well-designed to achieve needed outcomes.

- **Insist upon face-to-face participation.** Over time, virtual participation may be able to be accommodated; however, development of trust and group norms needed for success will be achieved more quickly and more firmly through in-person exchange.
- **Focus on gaining value as quickly as possible.** Start small and do something manageable with a limited scope and, therefore, a limited number of constituents. Beginning with a limited pilot or demonstration project can do a lot to prove out a concept while minimizing expenditures. It can provide the laboratory needed for the human dimensions of the exchange as well as the technical elements. Most importantly, it will likely lead to a larger implementation vision more quickly than those that aim to achieve the entire vision at once.

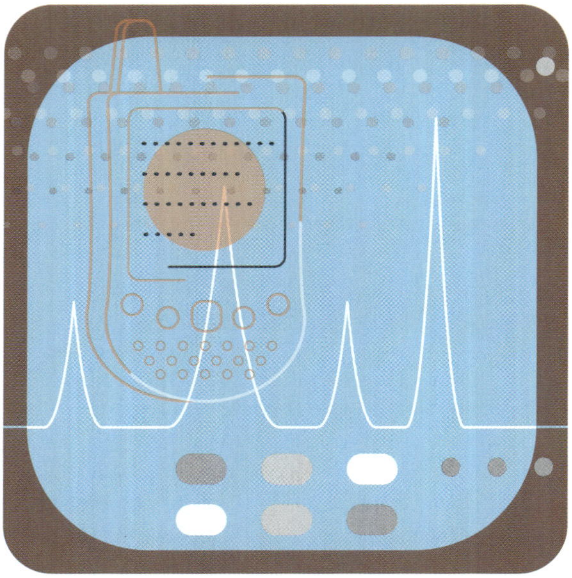

- **Consider third-party facilitation and support.** It will be difficult for any one organization not to be seen as "working an agenda" – even if they are not. This perception alone can cause significant fits and starts to the collaboration. An independent third party can ensure that this dynamic is not an issue for the collaboration. Most importantly, a third party can ensure that each interaction is structured for success, issues are raised and resolved in a timely manner, work groups are coordinated in the context of an overall workplan and timeline and progress is continuous.

Summary

The regional exchange can yield benefits to all constituents of the healthcare system, improving quality of care, increasing efficiency, eliminating duplicate testing and treatment and lowering costs. But in order to provide those benefits, the exchange must be properly designed and implemented, with suitable security measures, a system of governance, a means of funding and methods to encourage and monitor usage. Those design features can only be achieved through collaboration among the patient, provider and payer communities. Collaboration among these traditionally antagonistic groups requires outside facilitation in a setting that allows participants to get to know one another and build trust in each other's motives. Establishing such a collaborative approach between empowered decision makers who develop and stay true to a business case can deliver a win-win situation for all involved. ■

In order to provide those benefits, the exchange must be properly designed and implemented, with suitable security measures, a system of governance, a means of funding and methods to encourage and monitor usage.

- **Establish a business case and stay true to it during implementation and when measuring success.** Regional exchanges are intended to drive value to the healthcare system and, ultimately, to the patient. Defining that value at the outset is the most important step toward achieving it. There will be areas of the business case that are difficult to quantify; however, it will still be important to identify where value is expected and, often, proxy measures can be used as representative of a benefits stream.

The Healthcare IT Security Difference

Why are healthcare organizations interested in security issues?

Healthcare organizations are faced with ever-increasing volumes of communication via email and other electronic means. Physicians, pharmacies, laboratories, third-party administrators, care managers and others are all sending a variety of information to patient care organizations, and expecting communication in return. Imaging reports, X-ray images, lab results, scheduling confirmations and many other types of communications are now routinely disseminated to appropriate parties.

At the same time, HIPAA-based requirements for privacy and security of protected patient-specific health information (PHI) are backed by fines and prison terms for breaches. In practice, the threat of legal action by patients claiming harm from exposure of their data, as well as unfavorable publicity, could prove at least as injurious to patient care organizations.

What is needed is a simple, cost-effective, low-overhead and, most importantly, easy-to-use secure messaging solution that can ensure the privacy of PHI and enable healthcare organizations to return their focus to providing the very best healthcare services.

Voltage Security provides solutions that allow the healthcare industry to meet privacy concerns head on. Voltage's Identity-Based Encryption (IBE) secure messaging platform provides a way to encrypt and send secure electronic patient and physician information without certificates, passwords or the complexity of PKI.

As healthcare-covered entities implement HIPAA security requirements, Voltage solutions enable healthcare organizations to address all the technical safeguards of a HIPAA-compliant secure messaging system:

- **Access Control** – Confirms the person sending/receiving/accessing the data is who he says he is. In addition, the Voltage solution is centrally managed for emergency access procedures.
- **Audit Controls** – Logs all user activity so that organizations can prove the message was sent securely, identify suspect data access activities and respond to potential weaknesses.
- **Integrity** – Through digital signatures, verifies the message reached its recipient unaltered and unchanged.
- **Person and Entity Authentication** – Leverages users' identities (email address or network log-ins) to confirm the sender is who he says he is – the server will automatically stop issuing private keys if the identity is compromised.
- **Transmission Security** – Voltage's IBE enables data to be protected/encrypted without the need for certificates. All messages are guaranteed to be transmitted securely, and digital signatures are used to authenticate the origin, the content, and the integrity of an email message.

Voltage's secure messaging platform is easy for people to use, it's easy for IT shops to manage and it's easy to integrate into other systems and processes – ideal for the healthcare provider or payer interested in meeting government regulations or just safeguarding PHI. Fundamentally, ease of use is of preeminent importance to customer-focused organizations and will only become more important over time. This is particularly true in healthcare organizations, where IT staffing for network management and user support is a perpetual issue and where average users face busy workdays, relatively low levels of computer familiarity and multiple demands on their attention and awareness.

Voltage Security, a rapidly growing provider of messaging security solutions, remains fervently committed to the future of communications in healthcare. For more information, go online to www.voltage.com, or call 650.543.1280 today. ■

Voltage security

Voltage's secure messaging platform provides a way to encrypt and send secure electronic patient and physician information without certificates, passwords or the complexity of PKI.

Sathvik Krishnamurthy
President and CEO

Guido Appenzeller
Co-Founder and CTO

Terence Spies
Vice President, Engineering

Wasim Ahmad
Vice President, Products

Voltage Security, Inc.
1070 Arastradero Rd.
Palo Alto, CA 94304
Phone 650.543.1280
Fax 650.543.1279
info@voltage.com
www.voltage.com

Business Contact
Scott Edgington
Senior Vice President
WW Sales & Field Operations
Phone 650.543.1280
info@voltage.com

Federated and Centralized IT Architecture Models for Portable EHRs

Approaches to IT architecture to support the goals of portable EHRs have been discussed throughout the healthcare industry.

[John Quinn, Accenture]

The two main high-level architectural models – federated and centralized – are in development or already implemented in various configurations around the world. However, the U.S. healthcare industry faces unique constraints on how information can be organized and shared, which will shape the particular features of either model.

The desire to improve physician access to information and to increase patient safety, at the same time lowering costs, is driving a sharp rise in interest and activity among physicians and healthcare organizations in developing and creating health information networks. This growing and urgent need to access or transfer EHRs reliably and quickly requires first recognizing at a high level the range of intended uses for a portable EHR:

- Viewing summary demographic and clinical patient information;
- Viewing specific details behind the summary information; and
- Importing information ranging from a summary nature to all records available electronically from a number of different source computer systems.

Currently fewer than a dozen health information networks, or healthcare information exchanges (HIE), are operational, in development or even in an advanced planning stage. Serious planning of regional health information organizations (RHIOs) has only begun within the last two years, with national interest signaled by President Bush's 2004 State of the Union address. Previously, and to this day, the only working example of a RHIO and regional exchange is the Indiana Network for Public Care (INPC) in Indianapolis.

Two Models

The architecture of existing and proposed exchanges revolves around either a model where participants keep their own data but make them accessible within the network, or a centralized infrastructure that keeps a copy of the data.

These two different approaches are generally referred to as either a "federated" architecture (a highly distributed approach), or the more traditional "centralized" data services approach. Of course depending on the particular set of parameters a particular platform needs to meet, an almost infinite set of possible variations exists on what are really two general themes.

The Identity Issue

Regardless of the exchange architecture chosen, the U.S. faces a significant challenge in trying to correctly identify over 300 million individuals using mechanisms such as name, address and other demographic identifiers. At best, this is a difficult undertaking; at worst, any errors resulting from omission or misidentification can seriously endanger a patient's safety. Clearly correct patient identification needs to be assured at all levels.

However, this is not as simple as it sounds. While patients must be identified, it is not politically possible to implement a simple approach such as a new, nationwide patient identifier or patient identity card. In the U.K., with England having over 60 million participants in the National Health Service (NHS), an NHS identifier for each patient has been a reality for almost 60 years. In the U.S., even a proposal for a national identifier has brought swift legislative action to prevent it. Contrary to what many believe, the Social Security number (SSN) is not a national identifier; nor can it become one under existing law. Even using the SSN as a local identifier has been seriously discouraged over the past few years. For example, California's CA SB 168 mandate dictates that a SSN cannot be sent on any document through the mail (including email) to members.

John Quinn is chief technology officer in Accenture's Provider, Health & Life Sciences practice focusing on emerging health care information systems technologies. He has over 29 and 32 years' experience in the healthcare and computer industries respectively. He has participated on the HL7 board of directors since its inception 18 years ago and has served as the chair of its technical steering committee for the last 14 years.

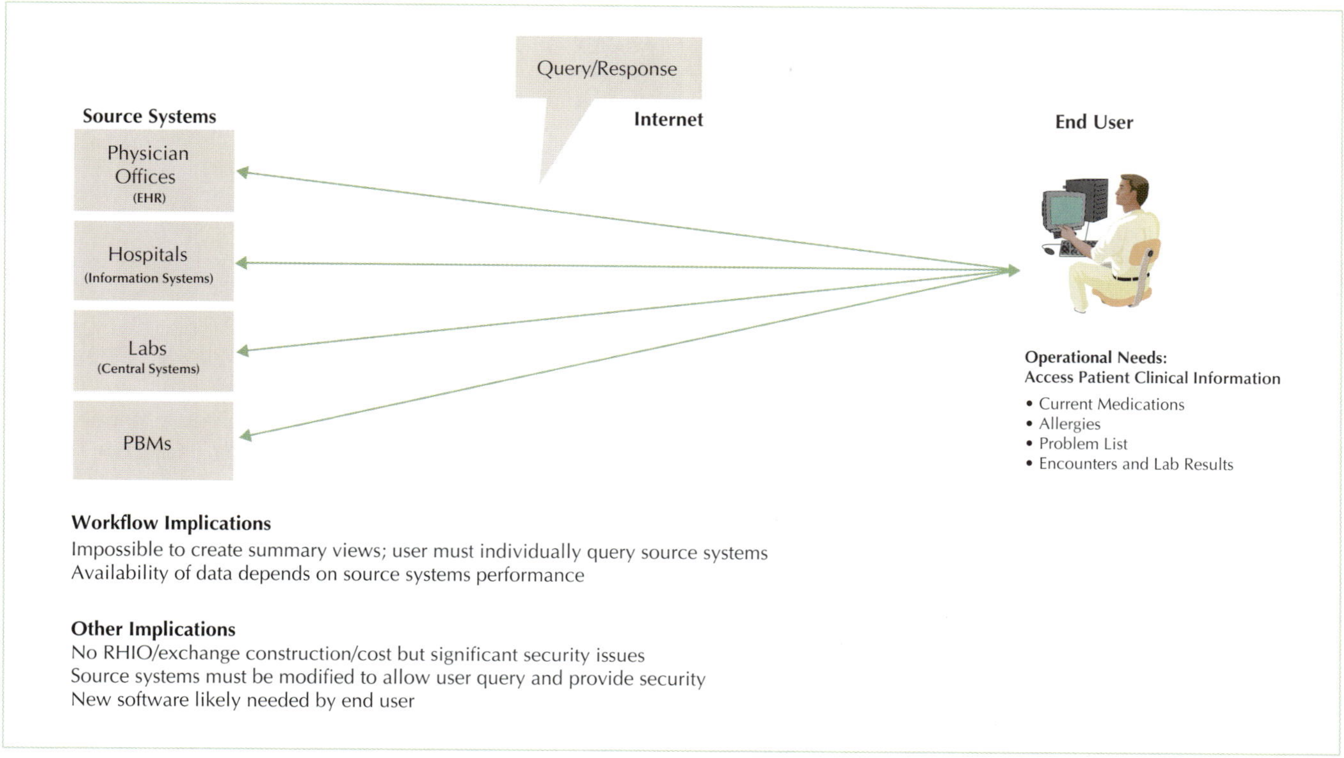

Figure 1 Disconnected Exchange Model

Assuring the positive identification of a patient – anywhere in the U.S. or around the world – without the use of a "health identifier" is an additional technical hurdle for an acceptable electronic health record system (EHRS) architecture.

The efforts to define, develop and implement an efficient and reliable HIE model must support industry recommendations/guidelines while also addressing patient identity questions – and the ensuing privacy and security issues.

Federated Models

Because of its straightforward architectural layout, the federated model found initial favor within the U.S. Department of Health and Human Services and with many who embarked on regional exchange planning in 2004, and is actually being planned as the model for a national infrastructure in the Netherlands. However, recent consideration and experience with other models has caused industry interest in the U.S. to shift.

Disconnected Exchange Model

The first example is a pure federated architectural approach – the disconnected exchange model – based on an attractively simple concept: "me," and the rest of the world. There is no need with this model for a health information organization and it does not require the implementation or maintenance of an information exchange system. The end users control their own data at all times and electronically query other source systems on the network individually for further patient information.

This approach is directly analogous to the way most of us use a browser to query the Internet for information. Figure 1 illustrates the "extreme" model. It is not at all clear how patient identity, privacy or directory services are managed in this approach.

The disconnected exchange model is a federated architecture where source systems are accessible to the end user individually through log-in screens or direct queries. Each source system within the network must be modified to source system queries and provide their own log-on services, privacy and security.

However elegantly simple the diagram of a disconnected exchange may appear, fundamental data security issues are unresolved, and further disadvantages remain. From a work-

weblink

Read how Intermountain Health Care is fulfilling its objective of a unified longitudinal medical record in the Q & A with Mark Probst.

flow perspective, it is not at all obvious how to create a summary view of a patient's medical history and – more importantly – it assumes that the user knows where to log in to find the corresponding patient information. This means the user, or a proxy (such as an application on the user's local computer system) must query each of the source systems individually. The only possible connection to a national health information network (NHIN) is from each source system that is tied to the NHIN. And finally, for the user, it would be difficult to import the patient data located at a source system to the user's local system.

For the end user, the availability of patient data also depends on source system performance and availability requiring a remote log-in (over the Web) capability and a functional security procedure for all potential users. Extending the privacy requirements to all possible users is a prodigious, if not also an obvious, programming challenge in itself. Today most IT systems experts consider the disconnected exchange model a "technology baseline" rather than a practical approach.

As the name implies, the practical and regional federated exchange model makes the federated architecture more practical by integrating an information exchange platform.

Practical and Regional Federated Exchange Model

As the name implies, the practical and regional federated exchange model makes the federated architecture more practical by integrating an information exchange platform (see Figure 2). For example, the new cross-document sharing (XDS) profile developed by Integrating the Healthcare Enterprise provides a conceptual base on top of which an exchange might be built. (IHE is an initiative of RSNA and HIMSS that promotes the coordinated use of established standards such as DICOM and HL7 to address specific clinical needs.) Systems developed in accordance with IHE communicate with one another better,

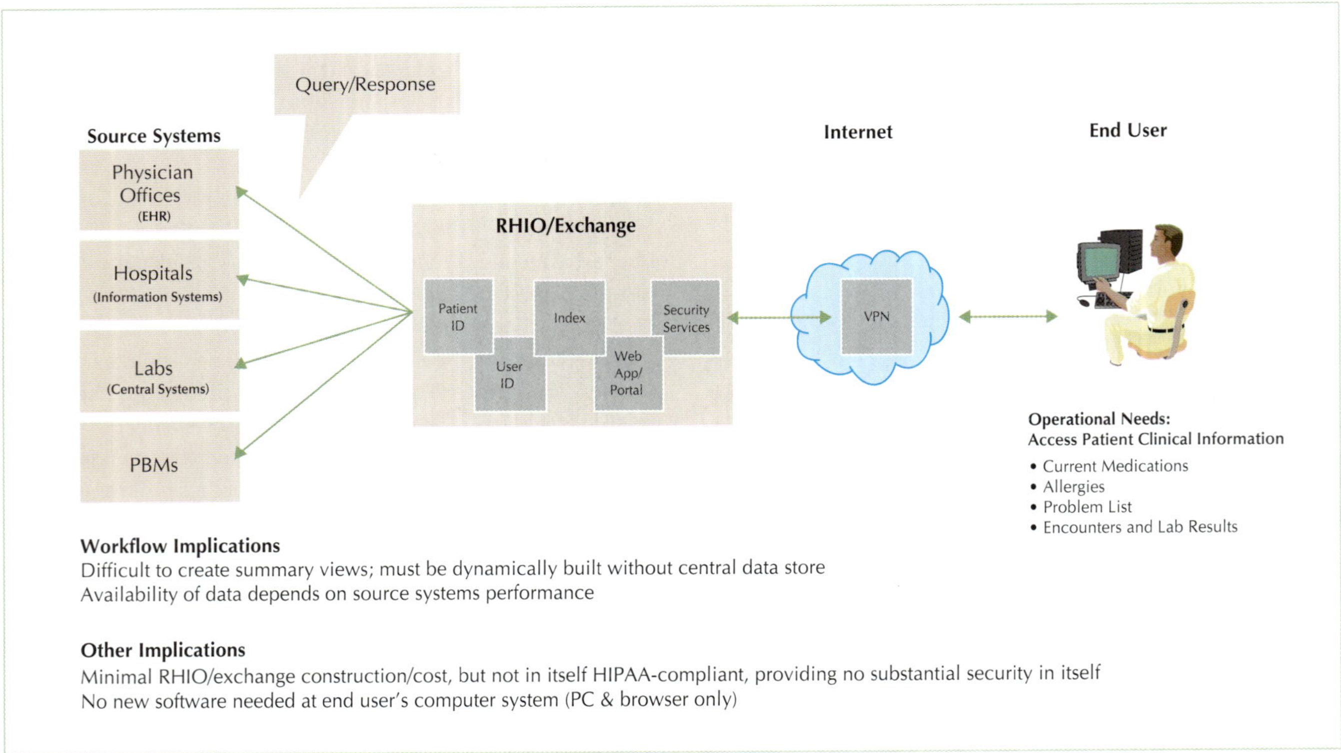

Figure 2 Practical Federated Exchange Model

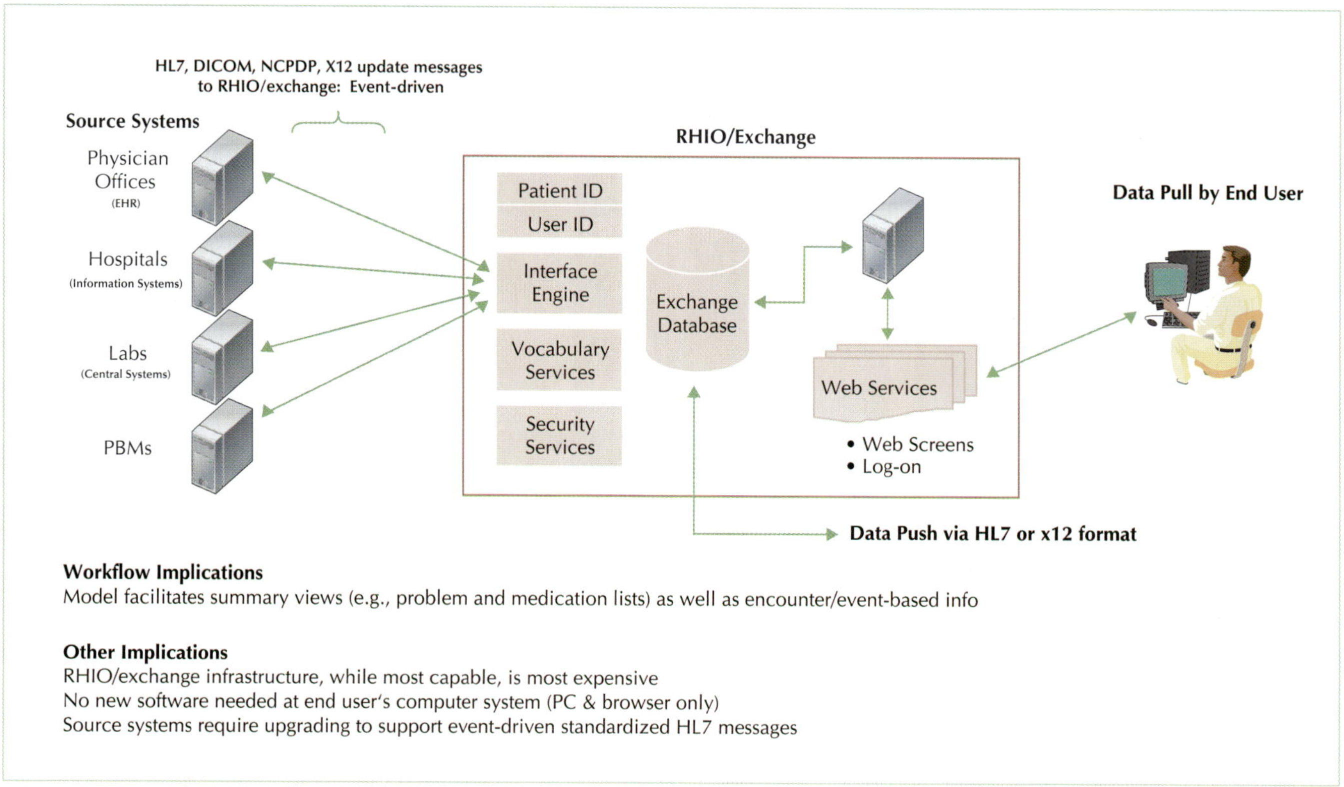

Figure 3 Pure Centralized Regional Exchange

are easier to implement and enable healthcare providers to use information more effectively. The XDS profile grew out of the DICOM standard and evolved at the RSNA. It is funded and managed by ACR/NEMA, RSNA and HIMSS.

In the practical and regional federated exchange similar to the disconnected exchange model, direct access to patient information can be created, using technologies and implementation guides such as the relatively new HIMSS IHE Integration Profile for cross-document sharing (XDS). The XDS implementation profile from IHE is an attempt to bring Napster-like capabilities to an EHRS infrastructure (i.e., quick exchange of relevant information collected from a broad network). Relying on underlying standards, XDS is an implementation approach that describes how HL7, DICOM, NCPDP and Web syntax standards such as XML can be used. It's important to remember that XDS is not a data, messaging or vocabulary standard, nor does it have a consensus-driven balloting process required by the American National Standards Institute (ANSI). Nevertheless it is an important first step that can be further developed to give us the means of connecting and cataloging the diverse information available into a regional exchange.

From a workflow perspective, it is still difficult (or potentially impossible) for the user to create summary views of patient information. Because there is no centralized data storage, this view must be built dynamically through a query of each source system. This assumes performance and functional capabilities of the targeted source systems such as:

- Domain Index registration of available documents for viewing;
- Queries indexed by the domain index server;
- Queries to retrieve documents from original source systems; and
- Availability of HL7 CDA queries on the source system to support electronic documents of structured clinical information.

The construction (and associated costs) of a regional exchange platform is less expensive than the following centralized approaches. But the practical federated model will have difficulty meeting HIPAA compliancy regulations.

Within the federated models, the practical regional federated is considered a more realistic – and "doable" – architectural approach when compared to the disconnected exchange model.

Centralized Models

The heart of the centralized model is a central database. In technical terms, this architecture is the easiest to understand; the user simply accesses the local central database, "checks out" the corresponding patient's information and then potentially returns that information to the database (information can be amended, but not changed or deleted). However, assimilating records for over 300 million patients (in the U.S.) into a single, structured database, ensuring correct patient and user identity and ensuring privacy – all with acceptable performance – seems an insurmountable challenge. On a slightly smaller scale (1/5 as large), the NHS in the U.K. is working on just such a centralized architecture for all of its 60 million citizens in England.

A single central database for the entire country is not under consideration in the U.S. Rather, a more likely approach foresees interconnecting all regional exchanges through some form of intelligent digital network.

Pure Centralized Regional Model

The pure centralized regional approach uses a central exchange database to store and provide patient information in a regional exchange. This information is obtained from the source systems and enables user queries – thanks to added functionalities in the exchange that can support key procedures such as patient and user identification, security and patient identity services.

Patient information is transferred from the source systems to a central exchange database. All key functionalities are provided centrally (such as patient ID, user ID, interface engine, vocabulary services, security services, Web services, etc.), enabling patient chart summaries (see Figure 3).

From a workflow perspective, this is a robust model that can facilitate summary views such as problem and medication lists, as well as encounter and event-based information. Data can be moved into the user's system as well as simply viewed (both push and pull of data).

However, this more efficient RHIO/exchange infrastructure is more costly than previous models. The centralized regional architecture model needs no software applications added on the user's system to simply view data (PC and browser only). However, application software will be required to support event-driven messages and queries that can populate exchange and the user's local EHR.

A single national central data repository would add unnecessary expense and risk to the NHIN and is probably beyond current information and database technology anyway. Putting all patient information into one database also heightens fears about privacy, security and the likelihood of illicit access. These political implications make this model of a national central exchange likely unfeasible for the U.S.

Distributed Central Exchange Hybrid

With technical benefits similar to the pure centralized regional approach, the distributed central hybrid model is able to manage the various security and privacy issues while providing a reliable source of patient information. A short description of the

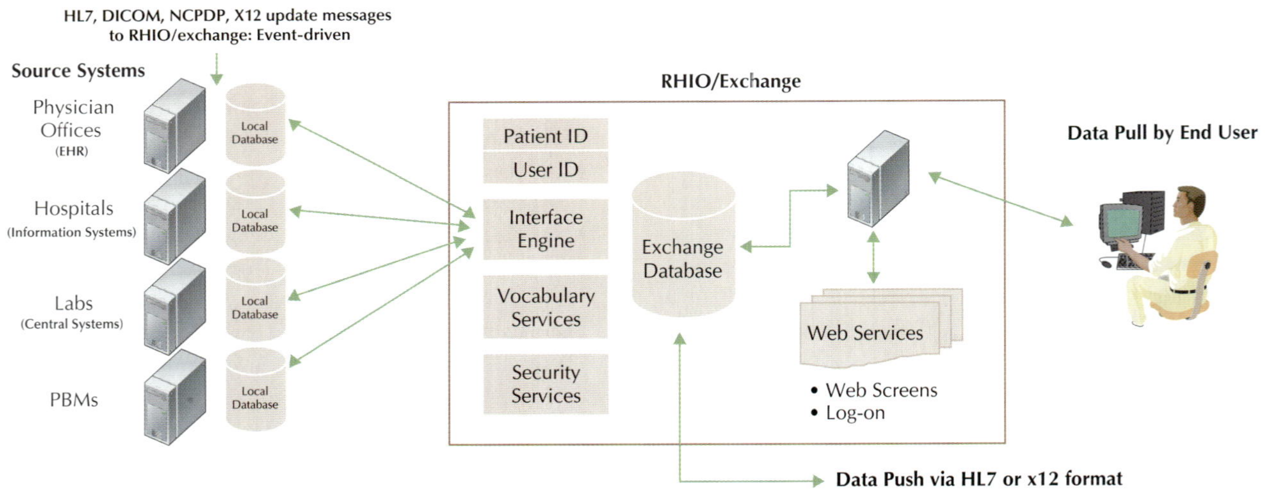

Workflow Implications
Data less available to end user as control is lost over distributed databases/servers

Other Implications
RHIO/Exchange infrastructure comparable to central model in terms of expense
No new software needed at end user's computer system (PC & browser only)

Figure 4 Distributed Central Exchange Hybrid Model

INPC – Contents	INPC – Participants
In the system: ▪ 1.3 million patients, 5 million registration "events" ▪ 24 million orders ▪ 489 million coded results ▪ 12 million dictated reports ▪ 8.8 million radiology reports ▪ 25 million prescriptions ▪ 480,000 EKG tracings ▪ 45 million radiology images Added per year: ▪ 600,000 ambulatory encounters ▪ 50,000 inpatient encounters ▪ 45 million radiology images	In the system: ▪ 22 hospitals from the 5 major hospital systems (99% of non-office care) ▪ National and regional laboratories ▪ All four homeless care systems ▪ Public health departments (county and state) ▪ Approximately 50% of ambulatory practices

Figure 5 Characteristics of INPC (Source: INPC March, 2005)

INPC at the Regenstrief Institute (see Figure 4) takes a look at a current operational network based on this model.

The distributed central exchange hybrid is very similar to the centralized regional approach. This hybrid architecture features additional shadow servers associated with each source system. It provides some advantages of data ownership, but with reduced data availability, because the control of the shadow servers may remain with the source system organization.

The hybrid model gives each organization some level of control over their clinical data, while providing access to the regional exchange. End users, in turn, can view and (optionally) import copies of the patient information into their local EHR.

The Regenstrief Model (INPC)

One of the best examples of an operational network based on a centralized architecture model is found at the Regenstrief Institute in Indianapolis.

Closely affiliated with the Indiana University School of Medicine, the Wishard Memorial Hospital and Clarian Health, researchers at the Regenstrief Institute have developed a healthcare network for the capture, analysis, content and delivery of medical information needed by patients, their healthcare providers and policy makers.

The INPC links a large community medical record system to three hospital emergency departments, 50 community pharmacies, 10 clinics, four health maintenance organization offices and 12 homeless care sites in Indianapolis. The INPC relies on the Regenstrief Medical Record System (RMRS) as its centralized clinical data repository.

One of the largest medical record systems in the U.S., with 3 million patient records, RMRS is a clinical database (including laboratory results, radiology reports and images, pathology reports, dictated reports, ADT data, electrocardiograms, vital signs, etc.) that receives inputs from a wide variety of sources and converts them to data standards such as HL7, LOINC and other standard codes. These data are used to deliver a variety of services, such as electronic laboratory reporting for public health, creating a clinical data repository and clinical messaging for the hospitals and other providers. Figure 5 summarizes some of the characteristics of INPC.

Summary

Growing national interest has increased healthcare industry focus on two different general approaches to IT architecture for regional exchanges – federated and centralized. The federated model is a highly distributed approach that avoids the extra cost of a regional exchange platform, but without a patient information summary, fundamental data security and patient privacy issues being unresolved. The centralized model uses a central database (regional with optional local copies) and manages the various security and privacy issues, albeit at a higher cost. The Regenstrief Institute is an excellent operational example of a central exchange hybrid model regional architecture.

While much work still needs to be done to educate the public about the benefits and necessity of an efficient health information exchange, our experience and evaluation of numerous projects points to a hybrid version of a centralized regional model as the most promising for the U.S. Regardless of the architecture model chosen, there is a need for ongoing intervention studies to measure the efficiency of the network, to resolve the related safety and privacy issues and to deliver a consistent and reliable improvement in healthcare quality. ■

EHRs in Spain: An Assessment

Confronted with a heterogeneous political and technological landscape, Spain is now taking steps to establish the parameters for EHR implementation.

[Baltasar Lobato, Accenture]

The Spanish healthcare system is based on the principles of "universalidad": global coverage, equality and a decentralized structure. The Spanish healthcare scenario is highly fragmented, organized by each of the 17 "autonomous communities" (roughly equivalent to states in the United States, with wide legislative and executive autonomy and their own parliaments and regional governments) across Spain, each with full healthcare services management and decision-making capabilities. The central government's Ministry of Health and Consumption plays a leading role in coordination and inter-territorial compensation, defining the healthcare policies applicable to the 17 autonomous communities.

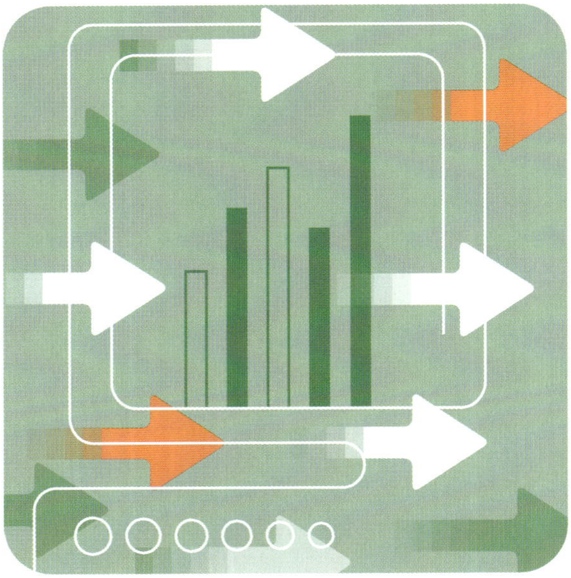

Similar to the National Health Service (NHS) in the United Kingdom, the Spanish system is based on a national health service model, mostly financed with public funds (accounting for nearly 90 percent of national spending in health-related services), and complemented by working agreements with private healthcare services.

There is also a growing private healthcare market, accounting for the remaining 20 percent of national spending. Three private health insurance companies, sharing nearly 80 percent of the private market, dominate the private healthcare area. These "big three" maintain their own small- and medium-sized healthcare center networks and medical benefit companies that reimburse medical expenses. They support the emerging hospitals networks – private healthcare organizations (such as hospitals and clinics) that contract surplus capacity to the public healthcare sector.

As with the healthcare industry, the IT systems in the healthcare organizations are characterized by heterogeneous, immature technological environments with investment rates of less than 1 percent. This situation has strong growth potential, with several upgrade initiatives focused on information consolidation/centralization, increased access for the patient, expanding computerization to clinical practices and implementing an EHR standard.

With respect to health information systems and EHR on a national level, the Ministry of Health and Consumption maintains a centralized database of citizens' information, including a national repository of basic data on hospital admissions and discharges (CMBD). The CMBD is fed with information from all 17 autonomous communities, as well as from the private healthcare sector. Based on the number of patient names and contacts with healthcare providers (not yet, however, on the type and quality of the contact), the CMBD determines the amount of the subsidy paid out to each autonomous community by the Ministry.

Baltasar Lobato is a senior manager with Accenture. He is a general practice physician with experience in hospitals and primary care centers. His consulting background includes work with public and private health services, insurance companies and health providers.

EHR Approach and Objectives

The basic concept behind the coming EHR implementation in Spain is a template that contains a patient's complete health history, with all information generated by healthcare professionals providing any level of healthcare.

The increasing mobility of people and the "local" generation of records throughout an individual's life affect not just the health centers, but also national and European policies. This is why the Spanish healthcare system considers EHR as a group of reports scattered in different locations, virtually associated by sequence links coordinated through a single patient identification code. The database systems storing this information should be "open" and interconnected through large capacity communication networks to enable EHR access both by patients and physicians over the Internet (and incorporating security and privacy functionalities).

... it is necessary to define and reach a consensus on the necessary standards that make a modern EHR system possible, and make it accessible from any location – fulfilling the needs both of patients and physicians.

Given the fragmented healthcare structure and the need to link clinical information from all autonomous communities, the Spanish Healthcare Information Society (Sociedad Española de Informática Sanitaria, or SEIS) has set three EHR functions:

- Help promote and maintain patient health and safety;
- Function as a legal document; and
- Provide a source of knowledge for research and education.

Current Situation for EHR

Bearing in mind the healthcare industry's technical heterogeneity, the baseline situation for EHR implementation in most of the 17 autonomous communities can be generally characterized by:

1. The consolidation of a healthcare card system (mostly based on a magnetic band without clinical data) and a patient ID card. These systems are complex and complete (covering 98 percent of the population) and include a patient's administration information as a prerequisite to EHR implementation.
2. Hospital environments with ERP systems (human resources, financial, logistics and maintenance) and patient management (HIS-ADT, mostly standard packaged solutions provided by vendors such as HP, Siemens, Novasoft or SAP), consolidated with approximately 100 percent coverage. Specialized outpatient care relies on the hospitals and shares the same information systems. Computerization in departmental areas is achieved with HIS-integrated systems at the local level (RIS, PACS, laboratories, pathological anatomy, etc.). The technological environment is decentralized and client-server based, making information sharing and remote access difficult. Autonomous communities generally maintain showcase "excellence hospitals" where new management models are developed and latest-generation technology EHR systems (intra-hospital) have already been implemented.
3. The *Centros de Salud* (primary healthcare centers) are nearly 100 percent computerized, with patient information, clinical management and EHR (standard packaged solutions, developed at the national level by vendors such as Stacks and Novasoft) capabilities. The IT architecture is characterized by distributed client server environments that hamper the transfer of patient clinical information to other primary healthcare centers or hospitals.
4. Initiatives to integrate primary and specialized healthcare systems, primarily for patient appointments and the request and receipt of diagnostic tests. In certain autonomous communities, patients are given access to appointment systems to make it easier for them to manage their queries. These initiatives represent the first step in the consolidation of relevant clinical information and EHR implementation. Given the heterogeneous nature of the IT environments, enterprise application integration-based solutions were selected (such as Biztalk, Tipco or Rhapsody).
5. To enable EHR implementation, large functional and technological transformation projects are under way. These involve system centralization/consolidation, with Internet technology

weblink

Read why physicians will adopt a change in clinical processes in "Securing Physician Adaptation and Adoption of EHR" in this book and at www.hctproject.com

at the primary and specialized healthcare levels, the definition and convergence of HL7 and IHE-based integration standards, XML messaging and Web services.

6. Similarly fragmented development and progress in the private healthcare sector, although EHR implementation initiatives focused on providing citizens with access to their clinical data (appointments, discharge reports and test results) exist.

Funding of both public and private projects is generally undertaken by the corresponding organizations launching these projects.

Remaining Challenges

The technology for EHR implementation has been available in the autonomous communities for some time. Nevertheless, it is necessary to define and reach a consensus on the necessary standards that make a modern EHR system possible, and make it accessible from any location – fulfilling the needs both of patients and physicians.

In Spain, EHR implementation is a government mandate and is regulated by the Health Care Law and Law on Protection of Personal Data (LOPD). But in contrast to conventional paper medical records, an EHR is more demanding and requires greater legal and technical guarantees with respect to physical and logical security.

Factors for Success

The creation of a patient master file should be considered first. This file should be unique and common for the entire organization, containing basic patient data and ensuring secure patient identification throughout the entire healthcare network. Automated update and replication mechanisms are needed to maintain current records on all relevant systems.

It is also advisable to consider global standard clinical encoding solutions that cover the patient's entire clinical history and enable system interoperability – to eliminate the existing barriers for information transfer between heterogeneous systems.

Finally, by guaranteeing information security from the solution design origin, ensuring data integrity, confidentiality and availability from the patient and physician perspectives:

- The healthcare professional has the right to access the patient EHR by creating the corresponding access profiles;
- The patient's express consent is needed to share information with healthcare professionals; and
- The patient has access to check his/her clinical records.

Moving Forward

Achieving EHR implementation in each of the autonomous communities can be enhanced by significant corporate projects, where change management is a key element and more relevant than technology. Change management will establish mechanisms to guarantee the quality of deliverables, ensuring that these meet requirements and are aligned with the overall corporate strategy.

Achieving EHR implementation in each of the autonomous communities can be enhanced by significant corporate projects, where change management is a key element and more relevant than technology.

EHR implementation is directly related to the level of technological development. This means all involved agents should meet and exceed a "technology threshold" to ensure success, and avoid a situation where one agent is technologically advanced (such as primary healthcare) and another does not meet the minimum requirements (such as specialized healthcare). Therefore, EHR implementation must be approached globally, and not begun through a single agent.

Summary

Heterogeneity and the standardization difficulties are key characteristics of the Spanish healthcare environment. Generally functionality and service suffer when systems are standardized at any price. Consequently, these heterogeneous systems should be integrated through service-focused architectures, integration platforms and integration standards. Using standard solutions with open systems will make it possible to benefit from the knowledge and experience of others.

EHR implementation in Spain will require a high level of technology and human commitment. This implies managing the resources needed to achieve a functional and reliable EHR system. The autonomous communities will take the initial steps toward this ultimate goal during the next two to three years. ■

3

Improving Clinical Outcomes

Implementing EHRs allows healthcare providers to offer safer and more consistent care to patients. They play an important role in improving the ability of the U.S. health system to better advance national best practices that are shown to enhance outcomes. Building upon the knowledge gained from clinical data, organizations can adopt process, workflow and culture changes that make performance improvement an automatic result of daily operations.

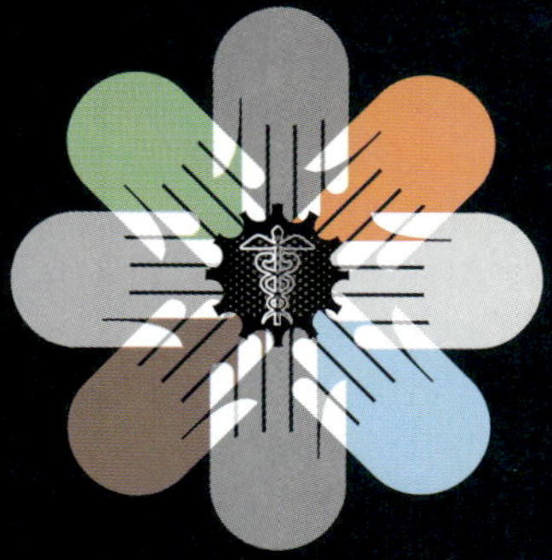

3

EHRs Drive Dramatic Change in Clinical Practice

Embracing all levels and types of clinical practice, EHRs provide real-time access to key patient data, optimize scarce resources and enhance collaboration along the entire care continuum.

[Manuel Lowenhaupt, M.D., Accenture] [Lawrence M. Hanrahan, M.D., Accenture] [Scott J. Cullen, M.D., Accenture]

EHRs (electronic health records) drive dramatic, positive change within clinical practice. By improving information and knowledge exchange, they make it possible for clinicians to act more proactively and collaboratively.

A multitude of legacy systems hold a wealth of information about patients and their care. Payers, providers, patients and supporting vendors all "own" a piece of the puzzle. Integrating their systems for bidirectional connectivity creates an interactive umbrella covering vast amounts of information and data.

With bidirectional access, everyone involved in patient care benefits from current and retrospective data. The emergency room physician, for example, can review information already collected by the primary care physician and specialists, and the primary care physician can maintain up-to-date information about the patient's status in acute, post-acute and home-care venues. Great potential exists for enhancing all levels and types of clinical practice but, in practical terms, what are the obstacles to EHR implementation and meaningful interoperability?

What Are the Roadblocks?

To make EHR work in a highly fragmented market, the various venues must come together at the information and data level, because the patient can be anywhere along the care continuum at any given moment. Aligning data access, input and retrieval creates a seamless virtual system that leads to a consistent standard of care and the best outcomes.

Diverse systems and a lack of standardization challenge implementation of EHRs. Literally hundreds of vendors populate the market. Many focus solely on segments. Most offer desktop, remote and wireless integration, but not all offer a portable device or one with full functionality. Although the marketplace for EHR applications and products has consolidated, only a fraction of the hundreds of vendors offer meaningful solutions and even fewer may address specific clinical needs. In addition, physicians, acute-care facilities, post-acute care venues and home-care providers - as well as their suppliers - remain invested in their legacy approaches and systems, which may or may not accommodate interconnectivity.

Other roadblocks to implementation include the cost and technical challenges related to modifying or creating new systems, complying with evolving standards, navigating antitrust and other legal issues and the generally arduous processes of systems selection and decision making.

In addition, as clinical information systems improve, expectations for those systems increase exponentially. Physicians, in particular, tend to seek out "the next best thing," looking for ways to improve workflows. Remote information retrieval, for example, makes it possible to access X-rays from home, so why not retrospective data from specialist visits, too? In essence, the expectation and satisfaction cycle shrinks every day as more clinicians adopt - and want more from - new processes. That makes it more and more difficult for any system to satisfy its users.

What's on the Market?

The hundreds of vendors who offer EHR products include small companies with specific capabilities and large medical information systems providers. Each offers different capabilities for handling key requirements, depending on the size(s) of the businesses

Manuel Lowenhaupt, M.D., is a partner with Accenture and the national practice leader for clinical transformation. He is internationally noted for his work in clinical effectiveness, care management and clinical informatics, with experience in organizations in the United States, Canada, Europe and the Far East. **Lawrence M. Hanrahan, M.D.,** is a senior manager with Accenture and a national resource for physician adoption strategies and clinical transformation. Dr. Hanrahan is internationally noted for his strategic and operational work with academic medical centers, hospital systems and post-acute care venues. **Scott J. Cullen, M.D.,** is a manager in Accenture's Provider, Health & Life Sciences practice and has more than 15 years' experience in the healthcare industry, both as a practicing clinician and software developer.

it targets. For example, some vendors offer implementation assistance while others do not.

In general, physicians want EHR tools that provide clinical value, are easy to access and do not slow them down. From their perspective, a desirable system:

- Uses the same or less time in clinical care per patient;
- Does not encroach on nonwork time;
- Allows easy entry of orders with little training;
- Provides useful access to current clinical information, such as lab and pathology results, diagnostic studies, vital signs, current orders and history;
- Can be accessed from home, hospital, office or elsewhere;
- Provides one-stop shopping with a single sign-on for all tools;
- Allows access to useful reference information;
- Enhances Part B documentation and coding; and
- Improves patient safety.

At the most basic level, some products offer limited clinical note-taking capability, together with e-prescribing, some document image management, clinical results tracking and messaging, and the ability to view lab results and dictated reports. Further up the scale, other products offer "charting systems" with complete clinical notes and some alerts and decision support. This level of functionality usually incorporates limited coding methodology and a limited summary of clinical results.

Some products provide more complete electronic medical record (EMR) functionality, with a full charting system, including automated coding and drug alerts, as well as access to a limited national knowledge base and clinical decision support. This level includes limited formulary compliance and a summary of clinical results. At about 40 percent of the cost of full EHR capability, this approach tends to be the most popular.

At the full EHR level, in addition to meeting charting system and EMR requirements, the product provides national drug and clinical alerts, access to national clinical protocols and guidelines, a third-party clinical knowledge base, clinical decision support, information about clinical standards and a physician-specific summary page with workflow. This highest level of functionality also includes multi-health plan health-maintenance rules, direct patient interaction and other capabilities.

The costs of various products vary, depending on their ability to meet these requirements, including one-time capital and operating investments and ongoing operating costs. Financing options range from governmental programs and payer subsidies to employer/business coalitions and fee-for-service approaches. Implementation time frames depend on the level of service needed and prioritization of modules.

What Does It Mean?

EHR implementation offers great promise for clinical practice and care management. Fortuitously, as order entry drives direct use of electronic interfaces, more and more physicians engage in such processes and see the benefits. (Most studies indicate that being able to view results and other patient information strongly influences adoption, as does the ability to involve patients in their own care management.) Participation by more physicians – and the accompanying benefits of expanding adoption – will drive EHR implementation exponentially.

EHR breaks down the arbitrary silos between care venues, all operating independently and not fully communicating. By eliminating such barriers, clinicians can collaborate across the entire care continuum. In addition, such care takes place in an environment of automated checks and alerts built on evidence-based algorithms. Outcomes improve dramatically when clinicians, caregivers and patients interact based on objective information.

This highest level of functionality also includes multi-health plan health-maintenance rules, direct patient interaction and other capabilities.

Other factors further enhance patient safety and outcomes. Critical information handovers are better managed, such as those involving admissions, discharges and transfers from one hospital, physician or caregiver to another. Key data doesn't get lost in the shuffle and can be accessed by everyone. Typical failure points are minimized, such as information loss between shifts, units, venues and clinicians.

In addition, e-prescribing made possible by EHR reduces error rates in the ordering process and the reading of orders by physicians, pharmacists and nurses. Dosage verification ties objective algorithms to current medications, disease states and laboratory values, and flags abnormalities or contraindications.

EHR also integrates tracking of patient compliance with directives. This drives optimal use of (and reduces physician liability for) medications, interval lab testing and discharge instructions for follow-up visits.

EHR augments workforce planning by reducing redundancies and optimizing the performance of physicians, physician extenders, nurses, technologists and administrative personnel. Access to diagnostic and therapeutic information, as well as a central repository for patient and care information, dramatically enhances productivity across the spectrum. Typical business processes become more standardized for greater efficiency. Key improvements can be realized in scheduling, for example, by allowing up-to-the-minute access to patient information and enabling immediate documentation, prescribing and billing.

With peer-reviewed online decision support, and disease-appropriate prompting for medications and testing, EHR can integrate formerly fragmented disease management models. This results in improved coordination of services, without an added burden to the primary care physician, and enhances patient understanding of the long-term benefits of disease management. With better documentation and decision support at the time of service, physicians and other providers see dramatic improvements in risk management, particularly in rapidly growing "failure-to-diagnose" malpractice claims.

EHR implementation, with its inherent capabilities for enhanced communication and access to information, will surely lead to even greater increases in patient satisfaction.

Finally, many studies have shown that email communication between patient and physician and improved patient access to information via the Web increase satisfaction both for patients and providers. EHR implementation, with its inherent capabilities for enhanced communication and access to information, will surely lead to even greater increases in patient satisfaction.

What's Next?

Prioritizing needs, starting small and achieving early and continuous success help realize the potential clinical benefits of EHR implementation, but true success depends on physician adoption. Engaging physicians early in design and implementation phases, focusing on practical workflow and operational needs, and using physician champions as leaders and communicators will ensure that the result centers on real patient care.

A Case Study
Mr. Davis and His Diabetes

With EHR-Optimized Care

Mr. Davis visited his primary care physician for a routine yearly physical, *prompted by a letter from Dr. Jones' office's EMR system,* which tracked health maintenance intervals based on the fact that Mr. Davis is diabetic.

Prior to his visit, *labs were ordered through the integrated ordering system,* prompting HgbA1c, LDL orders by Dr. Jones. The system also *reminded him that Mr. Davis had not had an eye exam* in the past year. Mr. Davis went to the lab a week ahead of his appointment and had his blood drawn, based on a telephone reminder from Dr. Jones' office on the previous day.

On the day of his appointment, *the EMR system prompted the medical assistant at the office to collect a urine sample* for microalbumin. The screening showed a significant positive result, which was *entered into the system by the testing device* prior to Dr. Jones entering the exam room.

Dr. Jones explained some of the findings of his lab tests to Mr. Davis. "Tom, I'm seeing some warning signs of early kidney problems, and your cholesterol could be better," he said. "Your blood pressure was also a little above normal, and for a diabetic, that's a real problem. I'm going to put you on something called an ACE inhibitor, which will help protect your kidneys as it lowers your pressure. In addition, we'll need to get on top of that cholesterol with some Zocor. Both medicines are once a day, so you shouldn't have any problem taking them. We'll follow up in a month or so and make sure that you're not having any problems."

Dr. Jones *handed Mr. Davis several brief educational printouts from the EMR* that described diabetic complications and potential side effects of the meds he had *prescribed electronically*. Mr. Davis also received a lab slip for blood work to be done the following week for serum potassium and LFTs, as *prompted by the EMR when Dr. Jones prescribed Zocor and Zestril.*

One week later, Dr. Jones *received notification from the EMR of a high potassium level from Mr. Davis' follow-up lab draw.* He called his patient and discussed Mr. Davis' diet, discovering that he had been eating three bananas daily on the advice of his neighbor. Dr. Jones told him to cease the Zestril and bananas for three days and have another blood test, *ordered directly through the EMR*. Follow-up testing showed a normal potassium level, and Mr. Davis resumed his Zestril (though not his bananas) without incident.

Six months later, *Mr. Davis emailed Dr. Jones* to report that his first toe was becoming mottled and the nail bed reddened at the corner. *Dr. Jones immediately called him, making an appointment for him that day through the office EMR scheduling model.* Mr. Davis arrived that day and was admitted to the hospital for IV antibiotics for 24 hours, and then set up for home IV therapy for the next 10 days through VNA, *all ordered online through the EMR.* As Mr. Davis had an allergy to penicillin, *the EMR warned Dr. Jones that Mr. Davis' original Unasyn prescription needed to be changed, and offered Clindamycin and Ciprofloxin as alternatives.* Mr. Davis went home the following day and visited the office twice during the course of treatment. He did well and was back to playing golf in three weeks.

Six-monthly visit reminders were sent to Mr. Davis by the office EMR system via email and he was generally compliant with visits, having periodic HgbA1c, LDL, microalbumin and retinal exams. With aggressive weight and nutritional counseling, as well as the addition of Glucophage to his medication regimen, he reduced his BMI (body mass index) from 31 to 25 over a two-year period, and was able to increase his physical activity appreciably.

Four years later, interval retinal exams showed some small hemorrhages, which were treated with YAG laser. Mr. Davis continued to have more frequent ophthalmic visits but experienced no significant loss of visual acuity over the subsequent decade.

Without EHR-Optimized Care

Mr. Davis has been taking Glipizide for the past six years and has seen his primary care physician Dr. Jones only twice in that time, even though he has been reminded at each visit to come in every six months. Because of its paper-ledger system, however, Dr. Jones' office can only schedule three months in advance and Mr. Davis forgets to set up his appointments. Mr. Davis' medications have been refilled as a matter of course because Dr. Jones would rather he be taking them than refuse to fill them because he hadn't been seen in the office.

It has been two-and-a-half years since Mr. Davis had an HgbA1c test and at that time, the result was high. Dr. Jones advised him to increase his medication to the maximum 20 mg daily and exercise more, since he was gaining weight. He received a lab slip for follow-up in three months and was told to call the lab for an appointment, but was too busy to call and forgot after one week.

A year later he noticed that his big toe was becoming darker and showing some discharge on the sock. After a week, when it began to smell foul, he became alarmed and called Dr. Jones. Since the schedule was full, he could not be seen that day and was told to go to the emergency room. There he neglected to mention his diabetic status to the ER physician, who debrided the nail bed and started him on oral Keflex.

Two days later, his toe had turned black and his entire foot was red and swollen. He returned to the emergency room and was admitted, after calling Dr. Jones again. A surgeon saw him and started him on Unasyn, obtained an X-ray which showed bone involvement and scheduled him for surgery. He had not been admitted before and had no allergies on file in the hospital since the surgeon was unfamiliar with him. Within two hours, Mr. Davis was short of breath and flushed. The surgeon diagnosed an allergic reaction and administered treatment, changed the antibiotic and transferred Mr. Davis to the ICU for stabilization.

Surgery was delayed for three more days while Mr. Davis recovered, but finally resulted in a fore-foot amputation, due to metatarsal osteomyelitis. Mr. Davis was transferred to SNF for a week of wound care, and then home. He had a special orthotic fitting and was mobile with crutches after one week.

While he had been hospitalized, his labs showed decreased creatinine clearance and increased cholesterol levels. He was started on Zestril and Zocor in the hospital before discharge. Due to his new mobility issues, however, he was unable to get to the lab for follow-up blood testing.

At two weeks following his operation, he complained to his wife of palpitations, and she called Dr. Jones. Dr. Jones suggested ambulance transport to the emergency room. On arrival, Mr. Davis discovered he had forgotten to bring his medications and could not recall the names, telling the staff, "One is for my heart, and I don't know what the other one is for." His EKG immediately demonstrated sharp T-waves suggestive of hyperkalemia. His serum potassium was 6.2.

Mr. Davis was admitted to the ICU again and started on Kayexalate, but had an episode of chest discomfort within two hours. His treating physician decided on emergency hemodialysis. A Tenkoff cath was started and dialysis successfully lowered his potassium level to 3.4. He had a complete cardiac workup, including stress testing, which was equivocal, and was sent for catheterization due to his multiple risk factors and diabetic status. This showed one area of 50 percent stenosis of the LDA (left anterior descending) coronary artery of his heart and 75 percent ratty stenosis of the circumflex artery of his heart, neither lesion amenable to PCTA (percutaneous coronary transluminal angioplasty). He had no enzyme elevations, however, so it was decided that he would be managed medically and closely followed.

After three days, Mr. Davis returned home on daily aspirin, Zocor, Zestril and Glucophage, and was instructed to follow up with his primary care physician. He became dramatically less active at home, due to anxiety over his "heart trouble," and continued to gain weight. He had one post-discharge visit with Dr. Jones, who explained that he needed to return every three months to have his blood tested. Dr. Jones further instructed him to schedule a visit with an ophthalmologist, which he did for two years. He only saw Dr. Jones twice in that time, and often did not get his lab results after testing because he was given orders at each visit, rather than beforehand, and did not receive reminders for visits and regular testing.

Four years later, Mr. Davis' BMI had reached 33, and he was less active due to his weight and diminishing eyesight. When he was unable to read the newspaper clearly, even with his glasses, he again saw the ophthalmologist, who noted severe retinopathy, functionally unimproved by laser treatment. He was certified legally blind and lost his driver's license, much to his wife's initial relief, but with less opportunity to attend follow-up appointments, visit with friends and build on his already diminished activities, Mr. Davis became depressed. At 67, he became essentially home-bound, and even less compliant with treatment and follow-up visits than before. ■

Clinical Intelligence

Enabled by EHRs, clinical intelligence holds the key to bringing large-scale data into the process of continuous quality improvement.

[Scott J. Cullen, M.D., Accenture] [Wendy L. Wilson, M.D., Accenture]

Access to information is at the very core of medical practice in the modern age. Ironically, medicine has lagged significantly behind most other fields in the type of data awareness and evidence-based feedback by which other industries live and die. And patient-specific information that individual providers need in order to provide quality care is only a part of what is needed.

Pressure from quality-oriented groups such as Leapfrog and IHI, as well as impending payer initiatives on pay-for-performance, have begun to highlight the serious drawbacks in most provider organizations' ability to access, analyze and implement change driven by clinical information. Many studies of outcomes have used billing data, always a crude tool at best and rarely an accurate reflection of what care has been provided. Adhoc studies of limited duration and scope in real clinical data are either prohibitively expensive, or so narrow as to be difficult to generalize.

Gaps in Information and Knowledge

Even in organizations that have robust clinical information systems in place, extracting meaningful data from them for examining the quality of care is extremely difficult; these systems are designed to be patient- and provider-centric – the architecture of a true reporting tool that gets at process information and aggregate data was never part of their initial design. One can easily ask the question, "What was Mrs. Jones' potassium over the past month?" but getting to, "How many patients with a potassium of 6.0 received a repeat lab and/or timely treatment in the past six months?" is another type of question entirely - one that few clinical systems are designed to answer without an extensive adhoc query which, if even technically possible, would have a significant impact on the system's real-time transactional performance.

It has become clear that there are not only a great many unanswered questions to address, but an even greater number of unasked questions. One of the hallmarks of clinical intelligence (essentially what other industries call business intelligence, as applied to clinical data and processes), is that there is often the unanticipated result of finding answers to questions that we didn't even know enough to ask, sometimes referred to as knowledge discovery.

Foundations of Clinical Intelligence

Continuous quality improvement through clinical intelligence is not merely about finding answers, however. The amount of effort and expense required to implement such a system is only rewarded when the information gathered will have an impact on the processes that drive the organization. Using clinical intelligence to drive quality improvement is a circular process which rests on three critical elements:

- Identification of the proper measures to apply
  - Using real data on outcomes, rather than surrogate process measures, where possible;
  - Center for Medicare and Medicaid Services and private pay-for-performance indicators provide a starting point; and
  - Reiteration: As answers come back, using this information to ask questions with more precision and power.
- Data
  - The quality of data collection, its reliability and granularity, will be the cornerstone of any clinical intelligence initiative;

Scott Cullen, M.D., is a manager in Accenture's Provider, Health & Life Sciences practice and has more than 15 years' experience in the healthcare industry, both as a practicing clinician and software developer. His areas of focus at Accenture include health package implementation, clinical transformation, business intelligence and health exchange development. **Wendy L. Wilson, M.D.,** is a senior manager with Accenture. She has over 20 years' experience in healthcare. Her work as a consultant has been diverse and has extended both across payers and providers, most recently including clinical intelligence, outcomes, care management and payer-provider collaboration.

  - As compliance with standards such as Health Level 7 (HL7) and LOINC increase, the interoperability and quality of data will improve as well; and
  - The breadth and depth of the data gathered will have an exponential effect on the quality of information generated.
- Action
  - Implementing clinical intelligence will be an initially expensive effort, both in financial and political resources. Organizational leadership must see the clear benefits and make a commitment to an evidence-based approach to patient care at the management level; and
  - Technology is merely an enabler of the processes in any healthcare organization. Information generated by data warehousing will have no effect unless the organization is willing and able to align its behavior with the evidence, once presented.

Leading Practices

Several leading practices come to the surface in the course of examining organizations that practice clinical intelligence:

- **Information Leads to Action:** Data gathering must be clinically relevant and lead to changes in practice within the organization. Changes in practice which result from identifying areas of improvement in clinical processes should result in measurably positive outcomes.
- **Ongoing Measurement:** The process of measurement should be circular, closing the loop and driving further improvement.
- **Enterprise-wide Data:** The collection of data should encompass the widest possible scope within the organization if it is to be most useful. Oftentimes seemingly unrelated systems, when data is combined and analyzed, will reveal relationships key to the understanding of process gaps and inefficiencies. In addition, as our ability to draw from a wider pool of data increases, the closer we get to being able to measure real outcomes, rather than surrogates.
- **Clinician Governance:** The process owners must decide how data is collected and interpreted. No effort at standardization or reporting can be successful unless the data means something to those who will use it. IT professionals must yield their traditional ownership of "all things data" to an unprecedented level of clinical oversight to ensure that the data becomes actionable information.
- **Self-Service:** Ideally users should be able to access current information on their own performance and on those who report to them through standard views, such as "dashboards," but also through adhoc or custom views of the data, where appropriate. Physicians have long recognized and valued the evidence-based approach to providing care, but have had limited access to specific feedback about their own performance.

Where It Works

One example of an institution which demonstrates many of these key practices is Intermountain Health Care (IHC).[1] IHC has an extremely robust quality infrastructure, with areas of focus across

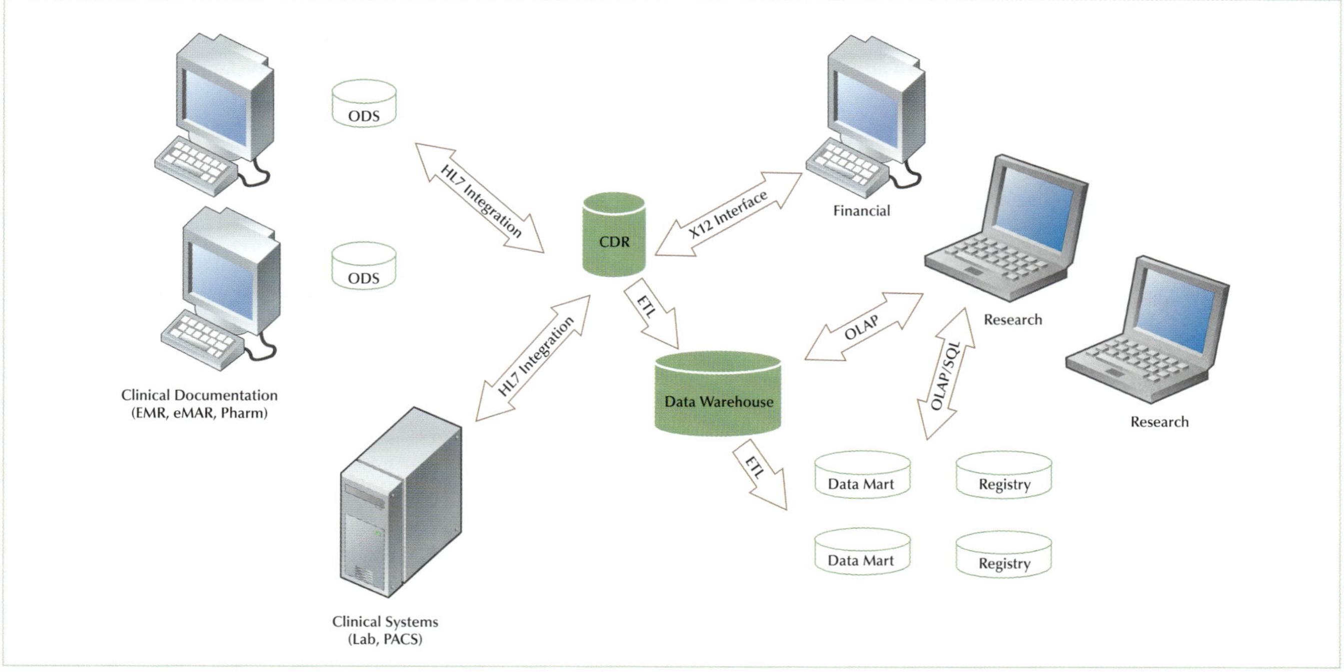

Figure 1 An organization's data infrastructure includes a CDR that allows for access to clinical data transactions.

the entire 19-facility system, examining processes both in inpatient and outpatient realms. Their data infrastructure includes a clinical data repository that connects their facilities and allows for access to clinical data transactions (patient visit documentation, medications, problems lists, etc.), across the enterprise (See Figure 1). In addition, this repository feeds a data warehouse, designed for reporting capability, research and knowledge discovery.

Among their primary care initiatives are measures programs in diabetes, asthma, depression, pneumonia and congestive heart failure. Within the Diabetes Care Management System, they extract a registry of more than 25,000 diabetes patients from the data warehouse and follow diabetes longitudinal care measures including cholesterol, hemoglobin A1c (HgbA1c) and urine microalbumin screening. Every primary care provider in the organization gets a quarterly report on how well their specific patients are doing in these measures over time, as well as a comparison to their colleagues' performance. This has been powerful medicine. In the four years between 1998 and 2002, they saw improvements of 25 percent in some of these measures, with plans to expand the program yearly and increase clinician's access to real-time, clinically focused data.

Another excellent example of the use of clinical intelligence at IHC involved the study of induced labor.[2] IHC extracted data on 85,000 live births from its data warehouse and looked at the timing of induced labor for women from 37 to 39 weeks of gestation and later, comparing Bishop scores (a measure of cervical readiness for labor), and outcomes for neonates and the likelihood of emergency cesarean section. Conventional wisdom among physicians practicing obstetrics was that there was no negative impact from pharmacological induction after 37 weeks, provided the cervix appeared to be receptive. Their ability to extract data on neonatal admissions to the intensive care unit and rates of C-section demonstrated otherwise, however. They found a 4.1 percent increase in NICU admissions among children delivered by induction at 37 weeks, as well as a higher rate of these inductions going to C-section for failure to progress and other complications. They have since instituted tighter controls on labor inductions across the system, raising the threshold and asking for clinical indications to early induction.

Challenges in Implementing Clinical Intelligence

As illustrated in the IHC example, physicians' behavior has been shown in multiple studies to be highly responsive to data, both generalizable from clinical studies as well as specific feedback on their own performance. The caveat, however, is that there needs to be trust in the quality of the information. Access to data is essential, but not sufficient. There must be a perception that the right elements are being measured in the right ways, and that apples and oranges are not being confused with each other. This also relates to issues of standardization and data integrity which invariably come into question when clinicians are not principally involved in managing the process of data collection.

In order to build the infrastructure for clinical intelligence, disparate systems across the provider enterprise need to move toward a standardized set of vocabularies, data elements, policies and procedures so that integration of information can be achieved in a meaningful way. This is often a daunting task, and is a process of evolution, rather than revolution. Some information is easier to move to a structured data warehouse environment than other types, and will be warehoused first, but may represent too limited a set of data to be clinically useful until a critical mass of different systems are tapped. Among the barriers to this are cost, poor knowledge management and documentation in IT departments, inflexible legacy systems, and the failure to adopt standard terms and data elements so that the data is internally consistent.

Perhaps most critical to the success of any effort to implement clinical intelligence is a strong governance structure, from the executive suite down to the provider level. Without clear enterprise-level guidance on how to facilitate the process of moving clinicians and IT professionals toward agreement on standards and procedures across the institution, very little will be accomplished, at very great expense. In addition, an ongoing joint working group of IT and clinician leaders is necessary for the maintenance and integration of constantly evolving dictionaries, processes and standards. A centralized knowledge management system for use by this group in designing modifications, tracking history and avoiding redundancy is indispensable. And finally there needs to be a group of clinicians and administrators with the power and will to redesign workflow in response to their examination of the resulting data. Often this will involve changes to existing clinical information systems, such as alerts and design changes, as well as work process revisions, such as timing the administration of antibiotics or moving patients through the facility.

Conclusion

Though the challenges are significant, the pressures on healthcare organizations of all kinds to measure their own quality of care are only accelerating. In the competitive environment, key differentiators will be based on publicly available data. Some private payers have already begun to demand proof of quality in what they are paying for, and Medicare will soon be doing so. As large institutions move away from paper as an information vehicle, they are confronted with the opportunity to leverage the new electronic medium to meet these demands. There is just no other way to do so in many cases. But clinical systems designed for real-time care provision will not be able to fill this need. A robust clinical intelligence architecture that is designed to extract aggregate data and use it effectively will be essential, as medical care emerges from the dark ages of information management. ■

Endnotes

1. Journal of Managed Care Pharmacy, *Vol. 9, No. 6, 553-8.*
2. Desert Morning News *(Salt Lake City), Oct. 20, 2003.*

Integrated Information Solutions for the Healthcare Industry

THOMSON™

Today's healthcare executives face an increasingly difficult operating environment - cost pressures, regulatory scrutiny, expensive technologies, labor shortages and competition all threaten economic viability. At the same time, healthcare customers - health plans, employers, government and the patient - are demanding higher standards of clinical care through approaches such as "pay-for-performance" and quality reporting. Healthcare providers must carefully balance between these complex forces - challenges to financial stability and demands for demonstrably high-quality care - to be successful.

Information and knowledge management tools are essential keys to improving clinical and financial performance. Health system executives require information solutions to optimize resource utilization, drive revenue growth, control costs and improve clinical decisions. To fully leverage human, technological and clinical resources, health system executives must have proven clinical knowledge and analytical tools that translate information into action and results. Integrated clinical knowledge and performance management offerings from Thomson Healthcare provide a single-source solution that empowers healthcare executives and clinicians with powerful tools to manage cost and quality.

Better Information. Better Decisions. Better Outcomes.

Thomson Healthcare solutions optimize clinical outcomes by identifying and minimizing errors, decreasing waste such as unnecessary tests and procedures and increasing appropriate care while reducing treatment costs. A comprehensive suite of alerts, answers, protocols and interventions - covering drugs, disease, patient education, toxicology and laboratory information - provide robust clinical decision support for caregivers and patients.

Thomson's unique integrated clinical content features the broadest and deepest evidence-based knowledge available in the industry. Thomson is the only company to offer a unified information repository underlying this knowledge base to ensure consistent and standardized knowledge delivery across the enterprise and at every point of care - during diagnosis, dosing, ordering and treatment. Consistent clinical information that is integrated into staff workflows - instead of being derived from multiple, independent sources - is a key driver for enabling informed, uniform decisions and driving best practices. Information can be accessed in a variety of formats to meet the needs of clinicians: Internet, intranet, integration via clinical information systems and mobile devices provide point-of-need access throughout the care continuum. All stakeholders benefit from standardized, enterprisewide knowledge, including patients, doctors, nurses, pharmacists, students and other healthcare professionals.

Hospitals Can't Improve What They Don't Measure

Measuring, improving and reporting on clinical and business performance is critical for health systems today as revenue is increasingly tied to targeted measures. Thomson's performance management expertise, business management applications and data meet health systems' critical information needs at every stage of the business planning cycle. Thomson works with hospitals and health systems to identify the clinical outcomes, financial risk points and market conditions that impact the revenue cycle.

Comprehensive resources and tools support vital strategic and tactical business decisions related to growth planning, marketing, reimbursement, cost, return on investment and other financial performance metrics. As a result, providers are able to manage high-cost patients, renegotiate unprofitable contracts and uncover the workflow processes compromising revenue collection. Clinical analyses reveal the physician practice patterns fueling excess cost and contributing to suboptimal care. Market intelligence tools integrate diverse data to produce consumer profiles of utilization, lifestyle and buying habits to help planners understand service demand and target growth.

Measure. Empower. Improve.

Collectively, Thomson's integrated knowledge resources and performance measurement and improvement tools provide a powerful enterprise engine to deliver on demand, "actionable" decision support coupled with the ability to measure results and implement improvements. Below is a sampling of these solutions.

Decision Support for Medication Safety

- Avoid inappropriate drug selection (contraindication, interaction, costly, better option).
- Ensure appropriate medication administration (avoid wrong route, dose) and monitoring, and minimize adverse events.
- Facilitate compliance with Joint Commission on Accreditation of Healthcare Organizations (JCAHO) and Institute for Safe Medication Practices (ISMP) guidelines.

Expert Knowledge for Disease and Condition Management

- Deliver comprehensive, current, evidence-based, best-practice patient management protocols.
- Establish quality guardrails and safety net for care planning.
- Support interpretation & management of results for unfamiliar laboratory tests.
- Facilitate compliance with JCAHO and Centers for Medicare and Medicaid Services (CMS) care guidelines.

Educational Material for Patient Empowerment and Engagement

- Empower patients with understanding about their conditions, evaluation, treatment and self-management.
- Improve patient comprehension and identification of their medications and how to take them appropriately and monitor their effects.

Integrated Information Solutions for the Healthcare Industry

- Engage consumer and patient community with healthcare organization as a trusted source of information.
- Facilitate compliance with JCAHO patient education requirements.

Improved Strategic Decision Making

- Identify profitable service growth opportunities ahead of the competition.
- Assess competitive position by service line and market to identify opportunities and threats.
- Evaluate major investment decisions such as service location, facility expansion and technology purchase.

Enhanced Care Quality And Effectiveness

- Strengthen risk-adjusted clinical performance by highlighting specific areas for improvement.
- Enhance financial performance by addressing costly complications and practice variances.
- Improve patient safety through adverse event tracking and powerful root-cause analysis tools.
- Ensure timely, efficient and cost-effective reporting to JCAHO, CMS, The Leapfrog Group and other data aggregators.
- Understand the strategic implications of pay-for-performance initiatives.

Maximized Reimbursements

- Ensure accurate payment of claims.
- Identify revenue cycle risk points and processes that prevent denied claims.
- Facilitate the management and recovery of denied claims.

Building Partnerships For Global Success

Integration of Thomson Healthcare knowledge solutions into enterprise systems and applications is supported by partnerships with the top Healthcare Information System vendors. Thomson

Creating World-Class Evidence-Based Clinical Knowledge

Thomson Healthcare has been employing insights gleaned from guiding industry-leading clinical decision support initiatives to evolve into a premier provider of clinical knowledge solutions for healthcare organizations. Supporting this evolution are major enhancements in how Thomson Micromedex creates and delivers clinical content and supports its deployment. These include:

- Refined and thoroughly documented editorial practices, leveraging clinical writers, editors, medical librarians and advisory boards.
- Continuous review, analysis and synthesis of medical literature, evidence and peer-reviewed research literature is supplemented with authoritative clinical practice guidelines, expert opinion and the perspective of clinical practitioners to provide evidence-based, practical and authoritative answers and recommendations.
- Grading of both the quality of evidence and the strength of major clinical recommendations adds additional support for implementing evidence-based medical practices.
- Rapid, accurate turnaround from publication of new, practice-changing studies and events (e.g., drug withdrawals) to incorporation in Micromedex content; process is evolving toward real-time updating and dissemination.
- A leading-edge, enterprise-class technology infrastructure facilitates development of standards-based, patient-oriented content that is clinically consistent, internally integrated and highly granular.

The Development Process

More than 100 full-time clinical staff members, including physicians, pharmacists, nurses and medical librarians, are involved in the multi-step process to create and review the content in Micromedex's clinical knowledge products. Our clinicians are trained and experienced in a wide range of specialties including, but not limited to:

- Internal medicine;
- Oncology;
- Geriatrics;
- Pediatrics;
- Emergency medicine;
- Toxicology;
- Clinical pharmacokinetics; and
- Alternative medicine.

Our editorial staff is also trained in the identification of relevant literature and accepted literature evaluation techniques that assess methodological rigor and appropriateness of statistical analyses, as well as clinical relevance. These literature evaluation skills, in conjunction with clinical judgment, are employed throughout the content creation and review process.

Our content facilitates the practice of evidence-based medicine whereby the clinician can identify best practices and choose the most appropriate treatment plan for a specific patient.

Step 1: Identification of Literature and Topics for Inclusion

Senior Micromedex editorial staff consider many factors when selecting subjects for our clinical databases. Topics chosen for further research are based on ongoing review of the world's medical journals, customer requests, clinical judgment and recommendations, regulatory standards and compliance, national healthcare trends, FDA approvals, editorial board suggestions and policy changes in health and disease management from professional health organizations.

The foundation of our ongoing literature surveillance is an automated literature query designed and monitored by an internal medical library staff and senior editorial staff. Our literature evaluation process comprises three levels: surveillance, title and abstract analysis and deeply engages with vendors to seamlessly integrate its clinical knowledge solutions within each enterprise's key applications. These integrated solutions provide clinicians with point-of-care alerts and interventions that are both context- and patient specific.

Thomson also collaborates with customers to simplify and streamline the implementation experience - from concept to realizing benefits. Every Thomson customer has access to full integration, implementation, deployment and training services, streamlining the path to return on investment.

More than 3,600 hospitals in the U.S. and Canada, in addition to major health plans, employers, pharmaceutical companies and state and federal governments, use Thomson Healthcare's knowledge solutions daily. And over 93 percent of customers trust their decisions to Thomson by renewing the relationship annually. Thomson Healthcare draws on the substantial resources of the Thomson Corporation, an $8 billion global leader that has been providing integrated information solutions across healthcare, scientific, legal, regulatory, business and financial markets for more than 150 years. ■

full-text analysis. This three-step approach supports objective and systematic selection of the most important evidence-based research. Selected literature is prioritized and launched into our editorial workflow for content creation.

Step 2: Creation of Content

Primary literature identified in Step 1 is forwarded to a clinical writer to further assess the appropriateness of inclusion in our databases. This additional assessment is again based on accepted literature evaluation techniques and includes an analysis of methodological rigor, application of statistics and clinical relevance. If deemed appropriate for inclusion, the information is summarized in our proprietary, state-of-the-art content management system. Clinical writers adhere to internal style guides, policies and procedures to create accurate, consistent content.

Step 3: Internal Review of Content

An internal senior clinical staff member reviews new content. The review assesses clinical accuracy and relevance as well as adherence to internal style guides, policies and procedures.

Content creation and review is an iterative process by which the reviewer provides feedback to the writer. Content may cycle through the creation and review process several times before moving to the next step. This promotes continuous learning and serves to ensure our content is of the highest quality. The chief medical officer is ultimately responsible for the content output by the editorial team. Our senior clinical staff and internal experts regularly meet with the chief medical officer to validate content decisions and to ensure inter-rater reliability within the group.

Step 4: Advisory Board and Expert Review of Content

Certain off-label indications for drug therapy as well as topics in specialized disease and toxicology subject areas undergo additional review by a Thomson advisory board or an expert reviewer.

Step 5: Final Clinical Review and Promotion to Production

An internal senior clinical staff member performs a final review of the content, taking into account feedback received from the advisory board or expert review. Content is promoted to production and is available for release in Thomson clinical knowledge products.

Our editorial staff is dedicated to the integrity of our information. By verifying every detail, they ensure the content is accurate, up to date and clinically relevant. This scrutiny instills confidence in clinicians who know they can put their highest trust in Micromedex clinical knowledge resources.

THOMSON™

Thomson Healthcare provides health systems access to decision support solutions that help build and monitor performance and improve quality of care. The Thomson companies' Micromedex and Medstat brands marry market intelligence and clinical knowledge with actionable alerts, guidelines, reporting tools and detailed analysis to ensure efficient and effective practices facilitywide.

Kevin King
President and Chief Executive Officer, Thomson Healthcare

Jeffrey R. Reihl
Executive Vice President
Thomson Micromedex

Carol Diephuis
Executive Vice President
Thomson Medstat

Clinical Decision Support Solutions
Thomson Micromedex
6200 S. Syracuse Way, Ste. 300
Greenwood Village, CO 80111
Phone 303.486.6400
Toll-Free 800.525.9083
Fax 303.486.6464
www.micromedex.com
mdx.info@thomson.com

Business Decision Support Solutions
Thomson Medstat
777 E. Eisenhower Pkwy.
Ann Arbor, MI 48108
Phone 734.913.3000
www.medstat.com

An Approach for Improving Business And Clinical Performance

To thrive and deliver optimal value, healthcare enterprises must address both the quality and business dimensions of performance.

[Jerome A. Osheroff, M.D., Thomson Micromedex]

Rising consumerism coupled with falling profit margins has produced a challenging dilemma for healthcare organizations: providing the highest quality care for the lowest possible cost. Today care is a product, payers and patients are customers, healthcare is a business and quality care is more than an ethical concern - it is an economic imperative.

And while hospitals, clinicians, health plans and purchasers have struggled to improve the quality of care and reduce medical errors following alarming reports from the Institute of Medicine and others, their "customers" don't see adequate change for the better. Indeed, roughly 78 percent of people say the quality of healthcare has stayed the same or gotten worse[1] - for good reason according to recent studies:

- In a study of 700 medical groups, only 75 (- 11 percent) scored in the top quartile on at least four out of six overall performance dimensions (e.g., care management, health promotion, disease prevention, physician turnover, use of electronic health records and financial viability).[2]
- More than 20 percent of patients admitted to intensive care units at Boston's Brigham and Women's Hospital experienced an adverse event, such as receiving the wrong dose of a medication. Twenty-four percent of these events were fatal, life threatening or potentially life threatening. About 45 percent of these errors were preventable.[3]

In addition, poor quality care also has a significant economic cost:

- A Food and Drug Administration study of hospital adverse drug events (ADEs) found medication error rates ranging from 2.4 percent to 6.5 percent per facility, resulting in an average cost of $2,257 per event.[4]
- Hospitals spend an average of $9,705 per 100 admissions in treating the effects of ADEs. A facility averaging 20 daily admissions could incur $708,100 in annual expenses.[5]
- The Managed Care Institute estimated as many as 28 percent of all hospitalizations, at a cost of $50 billion per year, are attributed to drug-related morbidity.[6]
- An Agency for Healthcare Research and Quality (AHRQ) study concluded that length of stay, charges and mortality resulting from adverse events (based on sampling 20 percent of U.S. hospitals) has significant financial impact.[7] Extrapolating the data to all U.S. hospitals suggests that 18 different types of medical injuries may add 2.4 million days of hospitalization and $9.3 billion in excess charges to the industry.

Clearly medical errors and poor quality care are expensive both in terms of human life and healthcare costs. As a result, organizations ranging from the federal government to the Institute for Healthcare Improvement, AHRQ, the Joint Commission for Accreditation of Hospital Organizations and the Leapfrog Group have made improving care safety and quality an imperative.

In response, many healthcare organizations are working hard to improve clinical performance by aggressively investing in such tools and practices as evidence-based protocols and guidelines, clinical decision support (CDS), quality assurance programs, patient safety initiatives, compliance measures and business decision support.

Increasingly healthcare organizations are making substantial investments in clinical information systems, in part to support these performance improvement efforts. Is this an effective strategy? The answer depends on how systems are selected and implemented.

Jerome A. Osheroff, M.D., chief clinical informatics officer for Thomson Micromedex, helps ensure that Micromedex decision support offerings are optimally responsive to clinicians' and patients' information needs. He is a fellow of the American College of Physicians and the American College of Medical Informatics and chairs the HIMSS CDS task force.

The (Potential) Value of Clinical Information Systems

Clinical information systems, particularly when enriched with decision support functionality, play a decisive role in improving business and clinical performance, the obvious benefits of which are better patient outcomes and decreased costs. Mounting evidence confirms this:

- Computerized medication administration decreases medication errors by 81 percent, and integrated pharmacy and clinical information systems decrease preventable drug reactions by 78 percent.[8]
- BlueCross BlueShield of Tennessee reported a $2.3 million average annual savings from health informatics programs in the three-year ROI study period. The number of its catastrophic cases decreased from 17,000 to 10,000. The number of cases per case manager per month dropped from 103 to 76. The average monthly savings per case manager increased from $116,000 to $291,000.[9]
- At CareGroup Health System, which operates several Boston-area hospitals, a computerized physician order entry (CPOE) system deployed in its Beth Israel Deaconess Medical Center has reduced drug errors by more than 50 percent.[10]
- Boston Medical Center's CPOE system reduced prescribing errors by 37 percent.[11]

Less obvious, but equally important, are other business benefits of clinical performance improvement enabled through information technology:

- Productivity: Reduced resource consumption (staff efficiencies, equipment, supplies) and streamlined daily workflows.
- Risk management: Targeted quality improvement initiatives ease exposure to legal liability and regulatory scrutiny.
- Patients' perspectives: Higher quality care translates into brand preference, which boosts a hospital's patient volume.
- Industry image: Demonstrable clinical excellence produces competitive advantage in terms of marketing, partnerships, staff recruitment and retention.

The sidebar summarizes the business benefits associated with the clinical decision support components of performance improvement efforts.

Value Not Fully Realized

Many organizations don't optimally address the symbiotic nature of business and clinical performance, or the enabling role that information systems can play in improving both these dimensions. For example, despite demonstrated successes, nearly 30 percent of electronic medical record/CPOE technology implementations fail, according to the Office of the National Coordinator for Health Information Technology.[12]

Many other organizations don't achieve anticipated benefits from information systems because of problems in the strategic, cultural, management or technical dimensions of their performance improvement efforts. For example, information for clinicians or patients that is intended to support clinical decision making may be unhelpful, inconsistent, delivered at inappropriate times or through a sub-optimal channel. Besides missing opportunities to help, financial consequences of poor decision support can include wasted time, money and staff or patient good will.

A Model for Effective Performance Improvement

A systematic approach to defining and achieving performance targets is essential.[13] A four-step process that utilizes sophisticated measurement and decision support tools in a continuous improvement loop can help ensure that organizations achieve their priority clinical and business goals.

Step 1: Identify

You cannot improve what you cannot identify and measure. While this seems obvious, many attempts to improve clinical and finan-

Types of Business Benefits That Can Accrue From CDS Programs

- Reduced resource waste due to redundant and inefficient activities to support clinicians' decision making
- Reduced costs of care (e.g., via more appropriate testing, cheaper and more appropriately utilized medications and therapies, reduced staff rework and better care delivery coordination
- Reduced costs associated with medical errors (e.g., from legal liability and averted safety problems, and additional work, tests, therapies to remediate them)
- Reduced liability insurance premiums based on demonstrably improved safety
- Increased revenue (e.g., from pay-for-performance incentives)
- Increased market share (e.g., from more engaged and satisfied patients and demonstration of high-quality process and outcomes)
- Improved staff retention (e.g., by providing a high-quality professional knowledge management and decision support environment)
- Improved staff utilization (e.g., redeploy QA nurse from chart reviews to CDS implementation)
- Enhanced leverage to improve outcomes from investments (and data) in CIS
- Enhanced quality of healthcare professional education provided by the organization
- Improved health services research capabilities and ability to attract grants

Source: Osheroff JA, et al: Improving Outcomes with Clinical Decision Support: An Implementer's Guide. Chicago: HIMSS, 2005. Used by permission.

cial performance fail for lack of a solid understanding of the problem, including quantifiable metrics. Healthcare organizations should develop a consolidated and carefully developed working list of their clinical performance improvement targets and parse each into more specific and measurable clinical goals and objectives.

For example, a strategic patient safety organizational goal might be to decrease ADEs. Performance targets would include decreasing severe drug interactions, as well as the costs of associated complications. However, without solid, quantifiable numbers, success in hitting those targets remains a subjective measure.

Data such as medical claims and encounters, market intelligence, demographics and financial information are all critical to pinpointing the underlying causes of an organization's quality problems and related financial implications. Understanding what is happening is not enough; an organization must also understand why a problem occurs to address it most effectively.

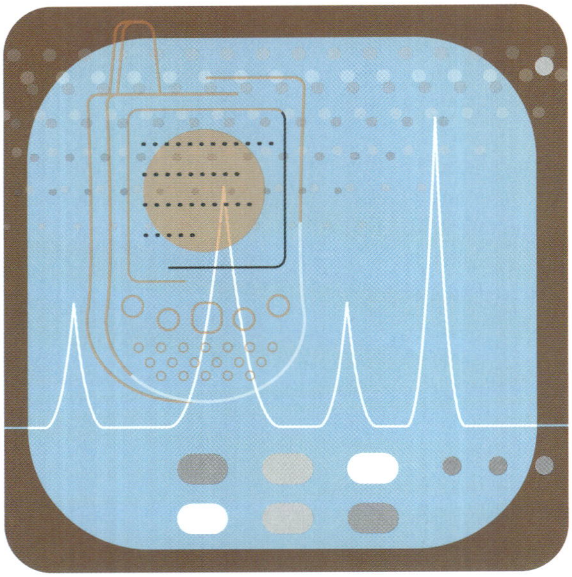

Step 2: Measure

Once an organization articulates measurable clinical objectives, business decision support tools can help determine performance against defined benchmarks, identify where breakdowns are occurring, help track progress and document where there is value and where opportunities remain.

These tools include financial analysis, utilization analysis and measurement, quality and clinical performance measurement, action lists, risk adjustment and episode methodologies. In the ADE example preceding, root cause analysis tools driven by anonymous ADE reporting can pinpoint exactly where severe drug interactions are occurring most often.

Performance measurement reports can compare the total number of patients with a complication of care for a certain disease class or ADE and the cost of care for that patient population against national or regional averages. Cost savings or opportunity costs (e.g., relative to readmissions, extended length of stay, denied Medicare claims, underpayments, capacity and productivity issues) illustrate the potential financial impact of identifying and eliminating quality deficiencies.

Similarly, sophisticated performance measurement and analytic tools can provide accessible and actionable information to drive vital strategic and tactical business decisions related to growth planning, marketing, reimbursement, costs, return on investment and other financial performance metrics.

Step 3: Empower

After an organization has clearly defined and measured performance issues, CDS embedded appropriately throughout clinical workflow can be a powerful corrective force. Broadly defined, CDS is providing clinicians or patients with clinical knowledge and patient-related information to enhance patient care. It includes a variety of approaches, ranging from alerts and reminders about potential commission or omission errors, to organizing and presenting key clinical data about individuals or populations.

For example, Partners Healthcare in Boston recently took a step forward in helping its staff address clinical questions at the point of care by providing patient- and context-specific medication and patient education information at the click of a button. Doctors, nurses and pharmacists can query the EMR application to get consistent, on-demand, point-of-care prescribing guidelines and other recommendations. Statistics from initial deployment indicate Partner Healthcare's clinicians are answering clinical questions more frequently and accurately with access to the right content, in the right format and at the right point in time. Current deployment reports demonstrate more than 400 lookups occurring daily without any employee training.

On the other hand, clinical information systems without carefully selected and implemented CDS are limited in their effectiveness. For example, a study at the VA Hospital in Salt Lake City showed continued high rates of ADEs after implementing a CPOE system lacking CDS specifically focused on drug selection, dosing and monitoring.[14]

To achieve desired outcomes from CDS, it is essential to select CDS interventions appropriate for particular objectives and deliver them through the right channel, in the proper format, to an appropriate individual at a point in workflow where the information will be most useful. CPOE is a powerful tool for performance improvement, but as the VA study emphasizes, these implementation factors must be carefully addressed. When properly deployed, CDS integrated into clinical information systems can support a variety of strategic goals such as ensuring that clinicians are aware of and are appropriately implementing evidence-based best practices for promoting health and managing disease, reducing dangerous medication errors and empowering patients to participate effectively in their care.

An approach for incorporating medical evidence into healthcare on a national basis is likely to be studied in 2006 under a contract the Office of the National Coordinator for Healthcare Information Technology is planning.[15]

Step 4: Improve

Building upon the knowledge gained from measurement and intervention, organizations can adopt process, workflow and culture changes that make performance improvement an automatic outcome of daily operations and clinician workflow.

Implementation services that include intervention testing, staff training and communication about enhanced CDS-enabled practices can help ensure the new approaches fully achieve their targeted improvements. In addition, expert consultation from business decision support providers can help organizations understand the performance data gathered during the improvement cycle and use it in a manner that yields ongoing optimal returns.

Building upon the knowledge gained from measurement and intervention, organizations can adopt process, workflow and culture changes that make performance improvement an automatic outcome of daily operations and clinician workflow.

Quality: A Clinical and Business Imperative

Healthcare customers are increasingly demanding demonstrable value from care providers. Rising to this challenge in the complex healthcare business is difficult, but robust clinical and business decision support tools, augmented by sophisticated clinical information systems, can be of substantial help.

However, achieving these goals requires a systematic approach that simultaneously addresses both clinical and business performance management, and judiciously applies information technology to achieve targeted objectives. Such an approach offers the best opportunity for health systems to remain financially strong while meeting the ever-growing expectations of healthcare's purchasers and consumers for safer, cost-effective, high quality care. ■

Endnotes

1. *Kaiser Family Foundation / Agency for Healthcare Research and Quality/Harvard School of Public Health National Survey on Consumers' Experiences with Patient Safety and Quality Information, November 2004 (Conducted July 7 - Sept. 5, 2004).*
2. *Yang S., Nationwide survey of medical groups defines high and low performers. UC Berkeley press release. www.berkeley.edu/news/media/releases/2005/08/25_medical-group.shtml.*
3. *Rothschild J, Landrigan C, Cronin J, Kaushal R, Lockley S, Elisabeth MS, Stone P, Lilly C, Katz J, Czeisler C, Bates D., The Critical Care Safety Study: The incidence and nature of adverse events and serious medical errors in intensive care. Critical Care Medicine. 33(8):1694-1700, Aug. 2005.*
4. *Bar Code Label Requirement for Human Drug Products and Biological Products. U.S. Environmental Protection Agency. Federal Register: Feb. 26, 2004. Volume 69, Number 38.*
5. *It's All in the Wrist: Improving Patient Safety with Bar Code Wristbands, Application White Paper, Zebra Technologies, Vernon Hills, IL, 2004.*
6. *An Economic Prescription for America. 2000. The Managed Care Institute, Samford University, Birmingham, AL. Sept., 2000: p. 9.*
7. *Zhan C, Miller M., Excess Length of Stay, Charges, and Mortality Attributable to Medical Injuries During Hospitalization. JAMA. 2003;290:1868-1874.*
8. *Leape L, Berwick D, Five Years After To Err Is Human: What Have We Learned? JAMA, May 18, 2005; 293: 2384-2390.*
9. *Enrado P., Health informatics programs provide savings, efficiency for payer. Healthcare IT News. June 9, 2005.*
10. *McGee MK. Computerized Systems Can Cause New Medical Mistakes, Study Says. InformationWeek, March 9, 2005. www.informationweek.com/story/showArticle.jhtml?articleID=159400302.*
11. *Ibid.*
12. *Gater L., CPOE Uncertainty. For The Record. May 9, 2005. Vol. 17 No. 10 P. 25. www.fortherecordmag.com/archives/ftr_050905p25.shtml*
13. *Osheroff JA, et al: Improving Outcomes with Clinical Decision Support: An Implementer's Guide. Chicago: HIMSS, 2005. Used by permission.*
14. *Nebeker J, Hoffman J, Weir C, Bennett C, Hurdle J. High Rates of Adverse Drug Events in a Highly Computerized Hospital. Arch Intern Med. 2005;165:1111-1116.*
15. *www.healthcareitnews/NewsArticleView.aspx?ContentID=3312*

weblink

Read why current pay-for performance models will not have a lasting impact in "Moving Pay-for-Performance to Pay-for-Value."

Telemedicine and Telehealth – Expanding the Continuum of Patient Care

If healthcare can be provided in the home through the use of IP technology, an individual may truly be able to age in place.

[Jan M. Sunday, M.A., SBC Communications, Inc.] [Patrick Pothier, M.B.A., SBC Communications, Inc.]

The rising cost of healthcare is a major concern to federal and state governments, companies and individuals. Along with the medical industry's key drivers to reduce medical errors and improve patient safety, one of the major initiatives being considered and undertaken by many healthcare facilities is the development and implementation of an EMR (electronic medical record) during the next 10 years.

The U.S. House of Representatives recently approved a $602 billion fiscal-year 2006 spending bill that includes $75 million for healthcare information technology-related projects, which has further increased interest in health information technology (HIT). The focus on HIT and the need to reduce healthcare costs has brought additional focus on ways that the utilization of technology can improve patient care while reducing cost.

How can we address the rising cost of healthcare for all ages, no matter one works or lives? Telemedicine has existed for many years. For example, the movie Apollo 13 showed a real-world use of telemedicine by monitoring the astronauts while on a mission, and the military has provided immediate medical assistance for soldiers wounded on the battlefield. However, telemedicine or telehealth is receiving new interest as technology offers cost-effective solutions to many issues impacting healthcare today.

Some of the reasons to consider the use of telemedicine include:

- Providing quality care for medically underserved communities whether they are in a remote, rural or inner city area.
- Extending the reach of a physician, nurse, program or facility.
- Improving care to specific populations:
  - Children;
  - Elderly;
  - Specific diseases;
  - Chronic care;
  - Military; and
  - Many other groups that will benefit from this care model.
- Responding to emergencies or disasters quickly and effectively.
- Allowing a rural community to survive and thrive through connections to remote specialists, training and medical technology.

While technology enables telemedicine, the primary issue to a successful telemedicine or telehealth program is people. Telemedicine isn't a new medical specialty; it simply offers another way to deliver existing services to people who can benefit from them no matter where they are.

There are many definitions of telemedicine and telehealth. In the Telemedicine Report to Congress documents published in 1997 and 2001, telehealth is defined as "the use of electronic information and telecommunications technologies to support long-distance clinical health care, patient and professional health-related education, public health and health administration." The definition for telemedicine is "the use of electronic communication and information technologies to provide or support clinical care at a distance."

The two basic technologies that enable telemedicine are "store and forward" and two-way interactive video. Store-and-forward technology is typically used in nonemergency situations where a diagnosis or consultation is made within 24 to 48 hours and sent back. It transfers digital images from one location to another. In the following example, a patient's primary care provider consults with a specialist at another location, but the care of the patient remains the responsibility of the patient's primary care provider. The direct care of the patient never transfers to the con-

Jan M. Sunday, M.A., is the director of healthcare and telehealth for SBC Communications, Inc. Within SBC, she assists marketing and sales to understand telehealth issues and develop solutions to address the needs of healthcare customers. **Patrick Pothier, M.B.A.,** is the director of medical marketing for SBC Communications, Inc. Within SBC, He is responsible for designing, developing and implementing the organization's medical industry-focused strategies that are based on a customer-centric model.

sulting physician, and in fact the patient may or may not even be present in real time for the consult.

Two-way interactive video is used when a face-to-face encounter is necessary. This involves real-time patient interaction. The patient and their healthcare provider (physician, nurse, dietician, therapist, etc.) are at one location connected via video link to a healthcare provider or specialist at a different location. In this case, the patient can receive treatment from the provider at the distant site, or the patient could receive care from the providers both at the remote site and the originating site.

The following scenario may help illustrate how telehealth can be woven into a community to improve access to care.

Joe lives in a rural community. The nearest hospital is a 10-bed acute care facility in a town about 15 miles away. A town about 35 miles away has a larger hospital (75 beds), but it is limited in some of the services provided. The state has a large, well-equipped hospital, but it's a three-hour drive.

To better monitor his heart condition, he will be sent home with a home health-monitoring device. The home health unit will capture blood pressure, heart rate, oxygenation, weight and other measurements as needed.

Joe hasn't been feeling well, and one day he experiences symptoms of a heart attack. Since there isn't an ambulance close, Joe's wife drives him to the hospital in the nearest town. At the emergency room, they take Joe to the exam room with an integrated exam table so they can fully evaluate his condition. The integrated table has multiple medical devices integrated into a computer that is located within the bottom drawer of the table. The table has an arm that has a monitor attached to it; otherwise it looks like other tables. Based on the readings that the emergency room personnel are reviewing from Joe's examination, they decide that a heart specialist's opinion would be beneficial to determine the best course of treatment. A relatively small, mobile medical video unit is wheeled into the room and a connection is made to the specialist at the large hospital located across the state. The specialist is sitting in his office in front of a computer where he can review all the information that has been captured in the patient's electronic patient record, as well as all of the results of the tests conducted and transmitted from the integrated exam table. The specialist can also see both Joe and the ER physician over the video connection.

Based on the analysis of all the data, the specialist and local physician determine that Joe can be treated there at the local hospital, rather than being transported to any of the other hospitals in the state for further evaluation. In addition, to better monitor his heart condition, he will be sent home with a home health-monitoring device. The home health unit will capture blood pressure, heart rate, oxygenation, weight and other measurements as needed. A video phone that works on their telephone line is also provided that includes an electronic stethoscope so the healthcare provider can listen to Joe's heart as well as view how Joe looks. By monitoring these measurements, an episode may be identified early and addressed so that a future trip to the emergency room isn't necessary. The focus is on Joe and his family, allowing them to heal while ensuring that the best care possible is being provided.

Now how can that save money? In many emergency rooms today, patients are transported to another hospital to obtain access to a specialist. While some of those trips are necessary, some are not. If the specialist can come to the patient on demand, no matter where the patient is, better healthcare is provided, the patient isn't further stressed by additional travel and the doctor doesn't lose valuable time to see other patients. In addition, if the patients can stay in their home community, their family and friends will be able to continue with their daily activities while supporting the patient. The family benefits because they can see their loved one while being able to take care of their home and daily living issues. While any hospital stay or illness is disruptive, if our healthcare system can provide quality care while allowing the patient to stay as close to home as possible, everyone wins.

A report by the Veteran's Administration concerning the outcome of its home health project was published in 2002 in *Disease Management*. The VA study found that by monitoring specific health conditions and coordinating the patient's care, it could reduce the number of emergency room visits by 40 percent, reduce hospital admissions by 63 percent and reduce the number of days in the hospital by 60 percent. It also reduced the number of nursing home admissions by 64 percent with a reduction in the number of days of care in a nursing home by 88 percent, all while seeing a significant improvement in the quality-of-life measurement. Other studies have validated these findings, and additional studies continue to validate the savings identified in the VA study.

weblink

Learn about how patients can become more active participants in their care through EHRs in the Q&A with John Lumpkin.

Telemedicine and Telehealth – Expanding the Continuum of Patient Care

In 2005, Frost & Sullivan released the report *North American Emerging Telemedicine Markets*. Not including the medical devices or the telecommunication connections, the study determined that the tele-videoconferencing systems in the United States in the base year 2004 was $52.8 million. Based on their research, Frost & Sullivan expect this market to expand at a compound annual growth rate of 10.2 percent from 2004 to 2008, resulting in a market value of $77.9 million for tele-videoconferencing systems alone.

The U.S. home telehealth market was valued at $140.8 million in 2004, the study's base year. Frost & Sullivan expects this market to expand by a compound annual growth rate of 24.2 percent from 2004 to 2008, resulting in a revenue value of $335 million in 2008. The future for telehealth technology, and the effective utilization of this technology, is based on the consumer and the medical community's support for this method of delivering medical services.

Telehealth has been utilizing some form of electronic patient record for many years. While the focus now is on integrating this data into a complete patient healthcare record, the experience of healthcare providers who have been utilizing this technology for years should be included in the evaluation. The telehealth community has been focused on improving care while containing or reducing costs through the use of technology. While this could be considered a competitive marketplace, the telehealth community has taken a different approach and has been built on sharing knowledge and expertise. According to the Institute of Medicine 2004 report and the Center for Health Transformation, the reported figures of 44,000 and 98,000 deaths that can be attributed to medical errors is costing the industry $100 billion each year. Therefore, many organizations are starting programs that focus on the improvement of care for the community at large - and telemedicine and EMR are at the forefront of those programs. Telemedicine Technical Assistance Documents - A Guide to Getting Started in Telemedicine, published in 2004 by the Office for the Advancement of Telehealth, Health Resources and Services Administration at the U.S. Department of Health and Human Services, is a perfect example. The editor, Joseph Tracy of the University of Missouri School of Medicine, provides an overview of how to build a telehealth program, followed by chapters written by the directors of leading telehealth programs in the United States on specific clinical applications or disease states, and includes information on building an electronic medical record for rural health systems. Many states have already implemented statewide networks for disaster response and healthcare support. Utilizing these networks for multiple applications will improve the cost benefit analysis and provide a better backbone for healthcare in many of our rural and underserved communities.

What can the future look like for healthcare using this delivery method? It is common knowledge that as the baby boomers retire, the U.S. healthcare system will be under great stress. In the last few years, many baby boomers have been managing the care of their parents and have a new awareness of the impacts of long-term care. This awareness has increased the interest in "aging in place," allowing an individual to continue living at home rather than enter a long-term care facility. But that is only one piece of the puzzle. If healthcare can be provided in the home through the use of IP technology, an individual may truly be able to age in place. This is an evolving area. The concept of the smart home is becoming closer to reality, where your home has some basic technology that allows for monitoring of health conditions and activities to ensure that the individual is functioning as expected. Whether that is an IP device that indicates the bathtub has run over or that the person hasn't opened and taken out their daily medication, the technology is becoming readily available to help baby boomers stay in their homes as long as possible. All of this health-related information can be captured and monitored and included in the patient's EMR, improving the information that the medical community uses to assess an individual's health status. Of course privacy, security and other issues will need to be evaluated; if the choice, however, is health monitoring that allows an individual to stay in their home versus moving to a long-term care facility, it may be an easy decision for many individuals. The cost to equip a home and provide this type of monitoring will have to be evaluated against the costs associated with long-term care facilities, both financial and personal.

If telehealth technology is readily available in the home, or if businesses offer wellness stations to their employees, what is the overall impact to our nation's healthcare costs? Utilization of telehealth technology has been limited due to policy issues that are continually being evaluated. As additional focus is placed on HIT, it is important to remember that the bottom line is not the technology itself, or even the money associated with implementing the technology – it still goes back to people. People must recognize the value an electronic patient record affords them, or how the delivery of care through telehealth services can help them stay in their home longer for this area to be fully successful. ■

The concept of the smart home is becoming closer to reality, where your home has some basic technology that allows for monitoring of health conditions and activities to ensure that the individual is functioning as expected.

Tell Us Where It Hurts

Everything you need, all from one source. In today's healthcare environment, the technology available to hospitals, clinics and insurance companies surpasses anything imagined just a decade ago. But along with the advances in technology come rising expectations from patients, medical staff and the government. To remain viable and competitive, healthcare facilities need to upgrade their communications with reliable networks and state-of-the-art managed services. But the last things you need are the headaches of finding in-house resources or coordinating multiple vendors. That's where we can help. The SBC family of companies is a one-stop, full-service communications provider. We provide the software, hardware, network technology and managed services you want now and will need in the future.

From the operating room to the medical records room, your efforts with IT impact the lives of patients and those who care for them. An integrated SBC solution, voice, video and data network can help make the most of your resources to address your challenges.

SBC recognizes the importance of the medical industry. We developed a vertical marketing and sales organization, with over 600 employees in our 13-state footprint, focused on identifying and meeting the needs and issues impacting hospitals and medical service providers today. This organization includes individuals who can assist your facilities in identifying areas where improved operational and administrative efficiency, and access to medical network, software, hardware and application solution expertise can have a positive impact on your bottom line. Our team will work with you and your organization to develop individual solutions that support your goals to improve access to medical services and expertise throughout your hospital system.

SBC can be a single source of comprehensive communications products and services that will fully satisfy your operational and administrative needs. Our powerful network products and services assist healthcare organizations of every size and location to boost communications efficiency by gaining broader, quicker access to administrative information, patient data bases, medical expertise, clinical data, research and much more.

We have partnerships with select best-in-class market leaders to assist us in meeting your business plan goals and objectives, by providing the capability to offer end-to-end design, support, installation and maintenance for medical applications including medical devices, video services, digital services, network infrastructure, software and equipment.

Through our partnerships we can help physicians and healthcare specialists with selecting videoscopic instruments for telemedicine applications and remote consultations, including endoscopes, otoscopes and digital stethoscopes, all supported by leading manufacturer's technical teams. Our goal is to provide an end-to-end solution including network systems, products and services to help optimize the functionality and efficiency of your medical facility and outreach programs.

Telemedicine: The Marriage Between Video and Medical Technology

Call it the magic behind the medical miracles, brought about by collaboration. Telemedicine describes the use of interactive video and medical technology to connect healthcare professionals, patients, educators and administrators in different places to expand service capabilities, save time and control costs.

Telemedicine is the new standard in modern healthcare. In cases requiring fast medical response time and specialty care, telemedicine availability could mean the difference between life and death.

We work closely with healthcare providers to identify and deploy the most appropriate and cost-effective telemedicine equipment to meet specific requirements.

Other Benefits

Improved Staff Responsiveness - In emergent cases requiring fast medical response time and specialty care, telemedicine availability could literally mean the difference between life and death.

Knowledge Exchange - IT can assist in attracting and retaining quality staff by facilitating collaborative efforts and ongoing training with other healthcare professionals around the world.

Global Accessibility - Hospitals and clinics in remote rural areas or under-

America's Most Admired Telecommunications Company, Fortune Magazine (1996–1998, 2000–2004)

SBC Communications has captured the No. 1 spot in the telecommunications industry for eight of the past 10 years. America's most admired honor is based on surveys by 10,000 executives, directors and securities analysts who rate companies in their own industries by using the following eight criteria: (1) quality of management, (2) quality of products and services, (3) innovation, (4) long-term investment value, (5) financial soundness, (6) employee talent, (7) social responsibility and (8) use of corporate assets.

Top 50 Companies for Diversity and Hall of Fame, DiversityInc (2001–2005)

In 2005, DiversityInc named SBC Communications to its Hall of Fame as a result of making the Top 50 list since the inception of this ranking. For the fifth consecutive year, DiversityInc has recognized SBC's dedication to improving diversity in its workforce, marketing, supplier diversity and communications.

Rank	Company	Score
01	SBC Communications Inc.	7.04
02	BellSouth	6.80
03	Verizon Communications	6.69
04	AT&T	6.12
05	AT&T Wireless	6.03
06	Sprint	5.96
07	Nextel Communications	5.95
08	Comcast	5.93
09	Alltel	5.88
10	Qwest Communications	4.64

Figure 1 America's Most Admired Telecommunications Companies

served urban areas can access broadcasts featuring medical procedures by experts in the field.

Service Extends Beyond the Server Room - Partnerships with select market leaders provides end-to-end design and support for medical applications including:

- Medical devices such as endoscopes, otoscopes and digital stethoscopes;
- Video services;
- Digital services;
- Network infrastructure; and
- CPE equipment.

SBC Solutions

- SBC Telemedicine Application Solutions for patient, doctors and hospitals

Infrastructure: Laying the Foundation for Any Initiative

Considering today's IT demands, network reliability is directly proportional to the quality of infrastructure. If your network handles clinical and patient information, you need a well-struck balance of performance and security.

Your network reliability is only as good as the media through which all your mission-critical information flows. With decades of experience in installing and maintaining telecommunications cable and wire systems, your network couldn't be in better hands. And if it's bandwidth you're looking for, count on us. We can provide the bandwidth you need without having to deal with another vendor. After we design and deliver your structured cabling solution we can monitor your network and make sure things run smoothly for years to come. It's modern technology designed with your hospital's future in mind.

Your Challenges

Building up bandwidth: Simply put, if the existing pipeline can't handle the flow, build a bigger pipeline. From initial design to implementation to ongoing management, bolster your capacity - and reliability along with it.

Streamline network support: People, process and systems - impact the success of each with network convergence. Access a network that protects the mission-critical traffic of millions of businesses with a built-in safety net of path diversity and backup.

SBC Solutions

- SBC PremierSERV Structured Cabling Solutions
- SBC PremierSERV Network Management

Network Performance and Security: Designed and Managed to Work Wonders

Sometimes a challenge extends beyond the bounds of your knowledge. Look to us for the most cost-efficient technology and know-how to help reduce medical errors, improve patient care and retain staff. And most importantly, become completely compliant with the latest security and privacy requirements.

Architecture framework design: Look to a variety of networking and security infrastructure solutions that focus on the development of architectural frameworks for technology and organizational enhancements.

Network management: From concept through implementation and management, make the most of the growing network investments.

Optimum network performance: Call on a staff of experts to assess your network performance, consult with your IT team or streamline design to address your challenges today. Or those of tomorrow.

Privacy: Keep data secure, yet easily available to doctors and administrators. Meet the requirements of the Health Insurance Portability and Accountability Act.

Security: Covering every angle from identifying vulnerabilities to policy development and continuity planning; seeking guidance to greatly reducing the threat of unwanted guests.

SBC Solutions

- SBC PremierSERV Consulting Services
- SBC PremierSERV Security Services

Wireless Freedom and Mobility: Connecting Staff With Much More Than Pagers

Get fully connected with a wireless solution. Mobile technology can help healthcare professionals communicate more efficiently with their patients and their colleagues.

Communication is at the very heart of the technology you use. And the evolution of wireless technology has led to even greater flexibility and the development of networks that can better serve the operational needs of medical and administrative staff.

With decades of experience in installing and maintaining telecommunications cable and wire systems, your network couldn't be in better hands.

We can offer your organization consulting, staging and installation to provide a wireless network that supplies:

- Instant wireless access to your server on a wireless LAN with connection speeds of up to 11 Mbps in the 2.4 GHz band;
- The ability to transmit to and from notebook computers or PDAs with full freedom of movement and maximum flexibility;
- Wireless phone coverage throughout your campus that works in conjunction with your existing PBX or Centrex phone system through the technology of SpectraLink™ NetLink Wireless telephones; and
- Truly portable telephones that staff can use for internal calls without incurring per-minute charges. Plus complete control over everything from server access privileges to long-distance calls.

SBC Solutions

- SBC PremierSERV Wireless LAN

We understand your needs, wants and requirements from a business plan perspective; therefore, we are focused on continuing to identify the application solutions that meet and exceed those requirements today and in the future.

We know that data services expenditures are expected to see the highest growth rates over the next three years. Growth will likely be driven by the increased adoption of broadband and dial-up Internet access, as well as the increasing adoption of new classes of value-added services, which include broadband, IP-based services and managed network-based services - like VPN and managed security. At SBC we are driven to integrate our network-based services along with the software applications that you are looking for. For those reasons we have established a series of strategies that are based on what you told us:

Be proactive and **offer data networks** that move voice communications from the traditional voice network to a data network - before the competition becomes positioned **(VoIP)**.

Continue to enhance and offer **managed services** as part of every medical **application solution**.

Continue to focus on **application solutions** that are based on the needs, wants and requirements of the healthcare client. Focus on applications like wireless mobility, security, telemedicine, IPVS, RFID and IP-TV.

Mobility solutions for enhanced patient and staff safety, improved employee productivity, increased patient and employee satisfaction and cost benefit. Integrate wireline and wireless networks.

Continue to focus on **security** in regard to patient privacy - in both a wireline and wireless environment with a focus on perimeter security, network security, intrusion detection, identity security and managed services.

Continue to focus on **telemedicine** applications - incorporating SBC consulting, video CPE, medical device CPE and managed services to meet the customer needs regarding a reduction in medical errors, and patient and employee satisfaction.

IP video surveillance - enhanced security, patient and staff safety, biochemical monitoring, temperature monitoring, moisture monitoring, reduced crime, cost benefit, protecting critical infrastructure and assets, and homeland security.

Implement a fully integrated **RFID solution** that is focused on the tracking of resources, including hospital products and services, equipment, prescriptions, employees and patients.

Implement a fully integrated **IP-TV solution** that not only is focused on "entertainment," but also incorporates an educational and informational element customized to the specific condition and treatment plan for each specific patient.

Leveraging, bundling and promotion of **Cingular Wireless** applications.

Public and private coordination of wireline and wireless networks.

All Backed by the Best in the Industry

The SBC family of companies has been designing, delivering and managing data networks and communications for decades. SBC engineers have earned more than 4,300 advanced certifications from the industry's leading equipment makers. Our engineers apply their abilities to maintain the SBC network, and we can make that same experience and knowledge available to you. We're with you every step of the way, offering technical networking expertise and the flexibility to accommodate your unique healthcare needs.

Contact us at www.sbc.com/medical. ■

SBC

SBC Companies places a priority on delivering customized communications solutions to meet the needs of the medical industry.

Edward E. Whitacre Jr.
Chairman of the Board and
Chief Executive Officer

Randall L. Stephenson
Chief Operating Officer

Rick Lindner
Senior Vice President and
Chief Financial Officer

Mark Keiffer
Senior Vice President
Business Marketing

SBC Communications
175 East Houston St.
San Antonio, TX 78205
www.sbc.com

Business Contact
Patrick D. Pothier
Director of Medical Marketing
Patrick.Pothier@sbc.com
Phone 805.583.6688

3

Using EHRs To Reduce Practice Variation

The impending necessity for physicians to interact with the EHR of their patients affords provider organizations the opportunity to translate medical knowledge into consistent action.

[Manuel Lowenhaupt, M.D., Accenture] [Lawrence M. Hanrahan, M.D., Accenture] [Scott J. Cullen, M.D., Accenture]

As health systems design the processes and information systems through which their physicians view, add to and modify EHR, they are able to structure the interaction in a way that encourages physician compliance with accepted practices - where appropriate - without diminishing the role of the practitioner's professional judgment.

Most physicians accept the premise that reducing practice variation is a good idea - that it results in better patient outcomes, more efficient use of resources and improved reimbursement statistics. However, strategies to encourage physician compliance with best practices must:

- Collaboratively seek their advice and consent regarding what those practices will be;
- Provide credible, reliable data as evidence that the new practices or treatments provide better patient outcomes than the prior ones;
- Support the new practices with information systems that make it easy for them to interact with EHR and to order the "right" medical interventions for their patients; and
- Provide feedback so that practitioners can see how their treatment choices compare with those of their colleagues.

You Can't Tell the Players Without a Scorecard

In a paper-based environment, it is very difficult to determine whether or not significant practice variations exist. Any kind of retrospective review of paper records is immensely tedious and requires enormous resources, only available to providers practicing in academic medical centers. Agencies and organizations that conduct sample-driven chart reviews are usually looking for answers to specific, narrowly focused questions. Chart reviews aimed at determining whether physicians are generally aligning their practices with prescribed protocols or Center for Medicare & Medicaid Services Core Measures that potentially drive reimbursements, are onerous to conduct in a non-electronic environment. Since managing any sort of process requires measurement of appropriate parameters, reducing practice variation depends first on electronic records.

Integrating EHR with a CPOE (computerized physician order entry) system gives all associated physicians access to the comprehensive, current patient information they need, and provides the hospital with essential monitoring and measuring tools to determine which practitioners are choosing - consciously or unconsciously - to vary from established practices. Only a process-driven IT infrastructure can easily track the degree to which physicians are complying with practices and protocols they previously adopted as best practices. An electronic environment makes analyzing practice compliance easier. It can be done routinely in a background mode, presenting the medical director with a daily report of doctors who have complied and who have not complied with use of pre-established order sets, and the extent to which they have deviated from the pathway. Importantly, data gathered during this process can also shed light on why there has been deviation, if it was appropriate and, if not, what steps can be taken to ensure the probability of future deviation is decreased.

This Is Not a Technology Journey

Hospitals and healthcare systems must realize from the beginning, and throughout the implementation process, that EHR is a

Manuel Lowenhaupt, M.D., is a partner with Accenture and the national practice leader for clinical transformation. He is internationally noted for his work in clinical effectiveness, care management and clinical informatics, with experience in organizations in the United States, Canada, Europe and the Far East. **Lawrence M. Hanrahan, M.D.,** is a senior manager with Accenture and a national resource for physician adoption strategies and clinical transformation. **Scott J. Cullen, M.D.,** is a manager in Accenture's Provider, Health & Life Sciences practice and has more than 15 years' experience in the healthcare industry, both as a practicing clinician and software developer. His areas of focus at Accenture include health package implementation, clinical transformation, business intelligence and health exchange development.

tool for change, not the driver. The real benefits of EHR come from redesigning clinical processes, aligning the tool to support best practices and providing appropriate incentives to encourage those practices. Implementing EHR within the hospital is a process redesign - not a technology - journey.

Share a Common Vision

A certain amount of practice variation reflects the diverse nature of a hospital's patient population and is appropriate, even desirable. Use of EHR to monitor and measure practitioner compliance should not be construed as limiting a physician's treatment options in situations that warrant varying from usual practices. Physicians who participate in the design and implementation of EHR understand that reducing inappropriate practice variations is a desirable outcome. All physicians who practice in the hospital also must come to that understanding. So before implementing the technology that supports EHR and the collection and reporting of compliance data, hospitals must:

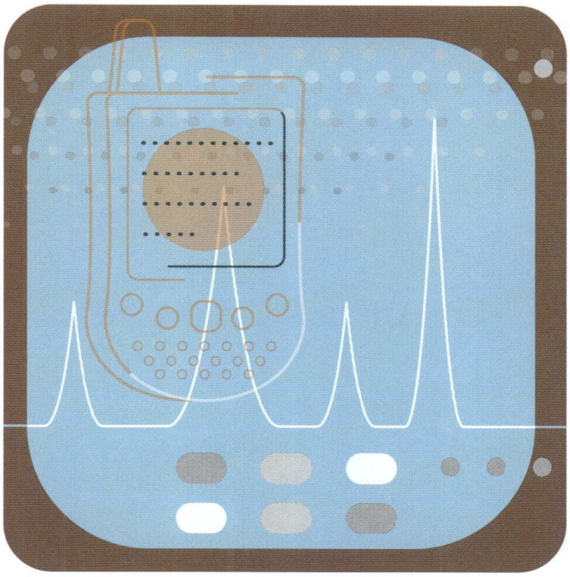

- Communicate a clear vision to all practitioners that reducing inappropriate practice variations is a desirable outcome that benefits them personally.
- Establish a systematic decision-making model, which requires both an infrastructure and a process, so that decisions regarding best practices can be made and compliance with the practices monitored.

If, for instance, in following a coordinated process of physician involvement and consultation, the hospital decides that Product X is the preferred antibiotic for prophylaxis, does the hospital have the infrastructure that can make that decision stick? Or is the situation more like "1,000 points of veto," where each doctor feels free to make an independent clinical decision, with no higher authority to consider, no accountability outside their conscience?

Vision sharing is an organizational challenge, not a technological one.

Make It Easy to Do the Right Thing

As a hospital designs the interfaces, menus and data-entry screens by which physicians and other clinicians – and sometimes patients – interact with the EHR, it also structures the processes by which best practices can be prescribed and compliance with them measured. Consequently the design process provides a vehicle for steering the physician toward best practices by making the compliant path easier to negotiate than the noncompliant path. A powerful way to encourage compliance, when appropriate, is to construct order sets in such a way that choosing treatment that complies with established care guidelines can be accomplished with a minimum number of mouse clicks, whereas varying from the established treatment requires a more laborious pathway through various menus, confirmation boxes, authorization screens and so on. The idea is to create an ease-of-use-path that makes it easier to comply with the aligned care model than to order noncompliant treatment. Most records are well-suited to presenting protocols that organize data and present them in structured ways, so that the user selecting a compliant path can enter a large amount of information with a single keystroke. The system must also permit the user to change the protocol and edit the choices on the screen, but less conveniently than ordering the "standard package." This "convenience lever" is a powerful tool that EHR can bring to the challenge of reducing inappropriate practice variation. Tools such as automatic reminders and protocols simply make it easier for physicians to do the right thing.

Use the Scientific Method

Physicians are scientists and, like all good scientists, good physicians respond well to good data. They enjoy drawing diagnostic conclusions from good data. In delivering care to patients, physicians are empowered by temperament and training to make important decisions based on the medical data in front of them. Physicians will almost always respond well to complete, accurate and comprehensive data, whether about the supply chain and the use of different medical supplies and devices, preferred drugs or different treatment options. If the hospital links good data with what they feel is an appropriate, clinically relevant outcome and a practice that supportably delivers that outcome, physicians will embrace the new practice. They welcome accurate, comprehensive and regular displays of data about how they practice relative to their colleagues. Often doctors are actually searching for a sign to make sure they are applying the right therapeutic intervention or utilizing the right medical device. The ability of physicians to quickly access accurate, comprehensive data through

Using EHRs to Reduce Practice Variation

EHR enables the hospital to share best-practice information and data about each physician's treatment choices compared with that of colleagues. Doctors will change their behaviors if they're convinced the new practice is significantly better than the old way of doing things.

However, doctors are wary of case studies, group studies with too few cases to be clinically relevant or inferior data based on ad hoc chart audits or surrogates like claims data to get at how doctors are practicing. When confronted with bad or unreliable data, doctors usually reject it and go back to their original practices.

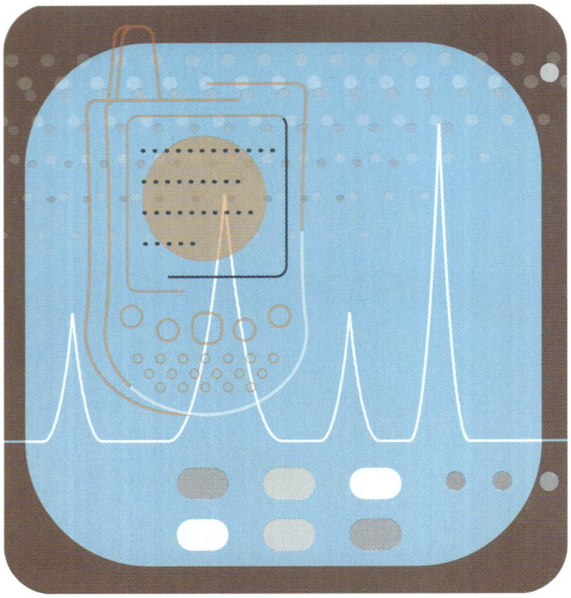

ment with prescribed practices, but it may also have the undesired result of discouraging the higher-performing doctors from varying from prescribed practices when situations warrant.

Summary

Often, we know, or think we know, the right treatment options for a patient, but our actions aren't always consistent with our knowledge. Failure to comply is almost never due to bad intent, but to the complexity of the real world of care delivery. For example, we analyzed the treatment practices of a large group of orthopedic surgeons to determine whether or not they routinely administered anticoagulants to their patients after surgery, a protocol they had all previously agreed upon. Compliance with the accepted protocol was little better than 50 percent, usually because of process delays. This was a failure of execution, not knowledge. EHR can help create a different environment where knowledge is translated into consistent, appropriate action. The power of a clinician's insight added to the foundation of a computer's ability to offer consistent and up-to-date knowledge creates the environment for world-class care. ■

Often we know, or think we know, the right treatment options for a patient, but our actions aren't always consistent with our knowledge. Failure to comply is almost never due to bad intent, but to the complexity of the real world of care delivery.

Be Careful What You Ask for

Experience has shown that physicians like knowing how their treatment choices compare with those of their peers. Their performance improves. However, experience also shows that posting these data the wrong way can have unintended and undesired consequences. Doctors are not immune to peer pressure, and so there are helpful and unhelpful ways to share compliance information. Portraying compliance as an unqualified virtue may bring the lower-performing physicians into better alignment with prescribed practices, but it may also have the undesired result of discouraging the higher-performing doctors from varying from prescribed practices when situations warrant.

ChartLogic: Leaders in Electronic Medical Office Solutions for Physicians

ChartLogic's electronic medical office solutions, featuring ChartLogic's own Precision Voice™ recognition electronic medical record, provide complete front-to-back medical office automation to physicians from scheduling, billing, charting and document management to patient education.

Moving beyond the simple framework of electronic medical records, electronic billing and scheduling systems, ChartLogic systems provide a paperless medical office environment where total workflow is managed and the standard of medical care is elevated. Through its innovative design, ChartLogic's portfolio of technology helps physicians enjoy increased free time, reduced overhead costs and increased revenues. In addition, ChartLogic's systems increasingly provide seamless electronic connectivity to other health care entities such as reference laboratories, referring physicians, pharmacies, diagnostic centers and formularies.

The flagship product, ChartLogic™, was launched in July 1999 and continues to be the only electronic medical records system that is completely voice-driven with a Precision Voice™ technology unique to ChartLogic™. Physicians have enthusiastically adopted voice-driven systems because they are already well versed in dictation and prefer using it to the keyboard and mouse.

The ChartLogic system is designed to be customized to a physician's practice and is well supported by local technical support. When thoroughly integrated into an office setting, the system saves a physician time by creating complete medical charts in a fraction of the time. Chart pulls, which typically consume 20 percent of a staff's time, are eliminated. Dictation and transcription costs are eliminated, resulting in significant cost savings. Down coding is eliminated, and increased physician time allows for increased revenues. Finally, drastically expanded medical records - the natural outcome of a simple-to-use voice-driven system - provide increased peace of mind with regard to the ever-present threat of litigation.

ChartLogic continues to acquire outside technology to complement its innovative technology. With its practice management system, an all-in-one online solution that promotes a paperless office by capturing patient information from first encounter through billing, physicians are able to remain only one click away from their schedules, messages, labs and exams.

With its acquisition of industry leader DynoMed Inc., developer of patient education software and medical multimedia programs, ChartLogic offers a patient educator series, which includes educational videos and animation for surgeons to use in their offices to help their patients visualize and understand their conditions and the appropriately recommended care.

Designed by physicians for physicians, ChartLogic's electronic medical office systems are rapidly transforming physician practices to a comprehensive automated system and allowing physicians to focus on what they do best - practice medicine. ■

Through its innovative design, ChartLogic's portfolio of technology helps physicians enjoy increased free time, reduced overhead costs and increased revenues.

ChartLogic™

ChartLogic's electronic medical office solutions, featuring voice-recognition, provide complete office automation to physicians from scheduling, billing, charting, to patient education.

Jack Savage
Chief Executive Officer

Brad Melis
Co-Founder and
Executive Vice President

James W. Strickland, M.D.
Medical Director

Bruce D. Jorgenson, M.D.
Co-Founder

Craig Hinton
Chief Operating Officer

ChartLogic, Inc.
3995 South 700 East, Suite 200
Salt Lake City, Utah 84107
Phone 801.365.1800
Toll-Free 888.337.4441
Fax 248.473.7543
www.ChartLogic.com
info@ChartLogic.com

Business Contact
Rita Schaefer
Finance & Investor Relations
Phone 801.365.1833
RitaSchaefer@ChartLogic.com

Patient Safety

Timely, accurate and complete health information, implemented through a nationwide EHR system, will improve the safety of care.

[Brian F. Shea, Pharm. D., Accenture]

Timely Access to Complete Patient Information

Today a fragmented and pluralistic healthcare delivery system processes information for the hundreds of millions of physician, clinic and hospital visits made annually in the United States. The patient records produced are either on paper or in separate computer systems that typically have limited, if any, ability to exchange data electronically, except for purposes of reimbursement. In all those files of paper and streams of data, no one has a bigger stake in the information (from a specific clinical encounter) than the patient. And in nearly all circumstances, no one in the system can know more about the patient's life than that patient.

In few other settings is it more important to provide the "right information to the right people at the right time in the right format." Yet health professionals currently have no way of accessing, compiling or managing all of the important information about their patients' medical conditions and histories. The fragmented nature of medical information systems and the difficulty of providing timely access to complete patient information are the primary obstacles to enhancing the overall safety of our patients. Better dissemination of medical information is imperative to accelerate and enhance patient care.

The electronic health record (EHR) is an essential tool for integrating the delivery of healthcare and putting patients at the center of their care. It can support the shift from episodic and acute care toward improved and continuous healing relationships with healthcare professionals. It represents a transition from a patient record that is often physician- or institutionally centered, retrospective and incomplete to one that is patient-centered, concurrent, prospective as well as retrospective, interactive and complete. The EHR can play an important role in enhancing the safety of patient care in many contexts, from monitoring and appropriately disseminating product recall information at the patient level to enhancing our ability as the U.S. health system to better "hardwire" national best practices that are shown to enhance outcomes and quality of life.

Adoption of Technological Standards

A lack of interoperable systems and data standards is a key barrier to EHR adoption. The healthcare industry has too many standards in place for disparate systems to convey patient data reliably. Healthcare professionals across a variety of settings experience difficulty in finding an EHR solution that is not fragmented over several vendors or IT platforms.

This has created a source of confusion for caregivers who believe that almost everything can be interfaced, because in the past we have been able to interface very basic clinical and administrative information about our patients. In fact, there is an implicit belief that interfaces and integration are the same terms: The logical thought is that if we build ways for systems to talk with each other through interfaces, these systems will send and receive all patient data just as if all the data were housed in one clinical system.

But the data being used by the systems today are much more complex and are coded in so many various and dissimilar ways that the path toward truly integrating our view of the patient now makes the decision to attempt interfacing disparate clinical systems an unsure, risky and sometimes impossible path to take. The safety, quality and efficiency of patient care will only be achieved if such systems are interoperable, integrated applications are seamless and electronic connectivity is accomplished, providing clinicians with key information when and where it is needed: at the point of care.

An example: One vendor may utilize its own coding system to classify patients' allergies, while another vendor employs an entirely separate classification method. When it is found that these systems cannot reliably exchange information between each other, two separate silos of (partial) truth about a patient's aller-

Brian F. Shea, Pharm. D., is a senior manager with Accenture's Health & Life Sciences practice and a former member of the Harvard Adverse Drug Event Prevention Study Group. He is a noted speaker and author in the area of patient safety and technology, and holds academic appointments, and lectures at the Massachusetts College of Pharmacy and the Northeastern University College of Pharmacy.

gies and hypersensitivities are created. As a caregiver, this raises serious process issues related to trying to understand which system may be correct, and for patients this creates a safety risk if a new allergy is entered into one system, but not the other.

Benefits of the Longitudinal Record

Patient-centric IT enables proactive improvements that are difficult or impossible to achieve through an interfaced network of specialized systems. True collaboration among multiple health providers and their patients requires a centralized, longitudinal record, as well as common systems to put the data to use. The completeness of the record, both historically as well as for each patient encounter, is critical. Instead of focusing on each encounter, a longitudinal record gathers information from both inpatient and outpatient encounters. The value of having a complete ambulatory record integrated with the acute care record allows for migration across time as well as across multiple areas of care.

The longitudinal record is exemplary for monitoring the use of medication. One example is the use of chemotherapy agents such as anthracyclines where exceeding certain lifetime maximum dosages is associated with a high risk for irreversible heart failure. Another example is for documenting vaccinations which could occur anywhere in the physician office, clinic, workplace, community, hospital, rehabilitation and long-term care settings. A longitudinal record captures information across every encounter, allowing the relevant healthcare providers access to a broad spectrum of data across care environments and administrative functions.

Missing Links Between Ambulatory and Acute Care

Even as we begin to address the integration of the record across acute care settings, we are most often missing enormous amounts of information in the outpatient setting. For example, the healthcare industry does not know how many patients are on a specific medication at any one time: When a new, significant adverse event is reported to a pharmaceutical company or the FDA, it represents one more number in the numerator - but there is no idea as to how large the denominator really is. Because patients now can fill and refill their prescriptions at too many points of access (e.g., local pharmacy vs. mail order), there are even more opportunities for drug interactions and allergy issues to occur than when patients once used a primary pharmacy (and often, pharmacist) for all their medication needs. Each healthcare entity, public and private, gathers and holds its own information, most often in paper form, in other types of "silos of (partial) truth." Only a fraction of their data is accessed and transferred digitally; the vast majority of healthcare transactions are still conducted by phone, fax or mail.

As a result, critical information is not available when and where it is necessary to support both clinical decision making and patient care as patients navigate a complicated healthcare system. If a patient enters an emergency care facility, alone and unconscious with a high fever, clinicians are often forced to deliver often lifesaving care with incomplete information about the circumstances behind the patient's condition. Caregivers still rely far too much on patients and their families to carry medical records and reports across the boundaries of a fragmented health system. Since many patients see different doctors for different medical conditions, physicians never have access to all of the information collected over the course of all those visits. The absence of readily available, comprehensive and patient-centric health information negatively affects healthcare at every level and puts the patient at greater risk.

Raising the Bar for Patient Safety

For the EHR to heighten the levels of patient safety, records must be easily accessed by patients' caregivers, contain extensive medical histories that encompass all medical encounters and share a standardized format for the storage and exchange of data so that caregivers do not need to know or access multiple sources of information. Only a common framework can support improved health information exchange nationwide while protecting patient privacy. The new health information environment should be based on open, nonproprietary standards and methods for their adoption, connectivity built on the Internet and other network types and uniform policies that protect privacy and assure security.

We are already behind in addressing these safety issues while we are soon to be facing the next horizon of clinical information, such as genomics. For example, today we understand that some chemotherapy regimens can be curative in some patients and not work at all in others, but why this is occurring may be due to variations on a genetic level that would be vitally important to characterize and capture so that clinicians can make far more meaningful decisions about what agents to use and how to use them to enhance their therapeutic affects and minimize toxicities. Genetic information such as this, paired with clinical data, will be integral in making care decisions, and customized care can be developed through the application of data mining, pattern recognition and clinical decision tools to EHR. The scrutiny of patients' medical histories, genetic composites and health risks, combined with access to the most current data available on breakthrough treatments and genomic research, can result in better treatments and faster recoveries. The ideal infrastructure is one that links EHR with clinical, genetic and other research data from all healthcare institutions.

Conclusion

The most compelling reason to implement the EHR is that it allows healthcare providers to offer safer and more consistent care to all patients. All relevant information needs to be available and legible whenever and wherever patients are seen – in acute settings, clinics, examining rooms, nursing stations and offices. All components of a patient's medical record – including progress notes, test results, images and medications, advance directives, future appointments and demographic data – need to be readily accessible at the point of care. ■

Maximizing Hospital Efficiency Using Palm® Mobile Devices to Automate Patient Flow

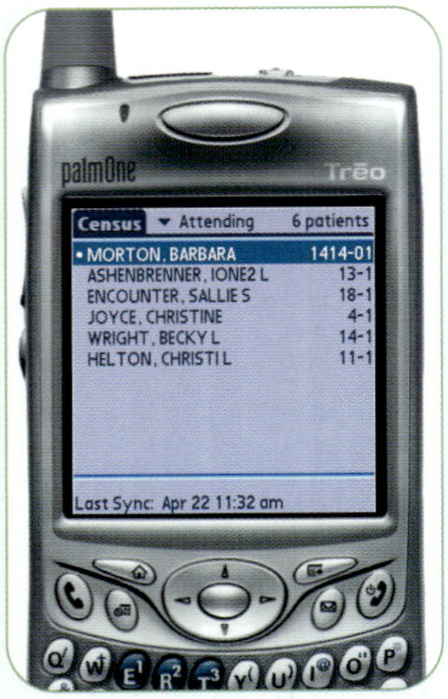

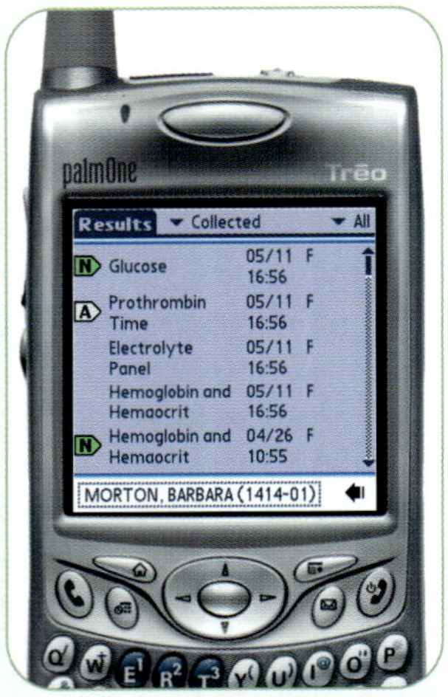

McKESSON
Empowering Healthcare

Challenge

St. Luke's Episcopal Health System is one of Houston's largest hospitals – it provides care to 22,155 inpatients and 101,861 outpatients every year. The hospital has more than 1,800 credentialed staff with 949 licensed beds and an occupancy rate of 95 percent.

Physicians and administrators wanted the ability to access patient data from the hospital's clinical information systems on mobile devices with the goal of developing a more efficient rounding system.

Solution

St. Luke's responded to these needs by deploying McKesson's Horizon MobileCare™ Rounding software to 42 Palm® users – 19 on Treo™ smartphones and 23 on Palm handhelds of total 80 deployed. The solution offers more portable and more ubiquitous access to patient results, which means greater flexibility for the physicians.

Benefits

Efficiency

In general, physicians have 20 to 35 patients on their rounding list and it takes approximately eight hours to see those patients in a hospital. McKesson's Horizon MobileCare™ Rounding software on Treo smartphones and Palm handhelds has, for many of the patients, cut their rounding time in half. Physicians benefit from the ability of seeing patient vital signs and statistics before visiting patients so they are well prepared prior to the consultation and they can better prioritize their visits rather than just working their way from the top to the bottom of the hospital.

Time

Patients benefit from physicians not being interrupted during consultations – physicians can stay with their patients without leaving the room to check results. By eliminating time-consuming tasks, physicians spend more time with patients and deliver enhanced levels of care. Having all the information in hand makes them more efficient.

Safety

In addition, the use of mobile devices cuts down on possible communication snafus – instead of asking nurses or technicians what a value is on a lab result or x-ray the physician can read the value for themselves.

Ease of Use

Physicians also enjoy the devices' ease of use. Synchronizing the smartphones and handhelds with the hospital clinical information systems ensures that physicians have the most recent data available. They can transfer data from the hospital system a number of ways: cradle sync, infared beaming or WiFi (802.11b wireless network) for their handhelds, or over cellular networks for their Treo smartphones.

In terms of adoption, for physicians who already had Palm® devices, there was virtually no training involved. Physicians learned about the Horizon MobileCare™ Rounding features and how to back up their devices and they were ready to use the solution on their rounds. "About 20 of the physicians had never touched a smartphone or handheld and most of them thought that it was easy to get on board."

"I've heard comments that a couple of doctors have shown patients the data that is on their devices and that puts the patient at ease. Patients also feel more comfortable knowing that they are at a "state-of-the-art" hospital. It makes patients feel like they are getting world-class, cutting-edge care because their doctors are connected and wired to the hospital."

— **Curtis Burkhart**
Lead System Analyst
St. Luke's Episcopal Health System

ST. LUKE'S®
Episcopal
Health System

Enhancing Patient Care With Palm® Mobile Solutions

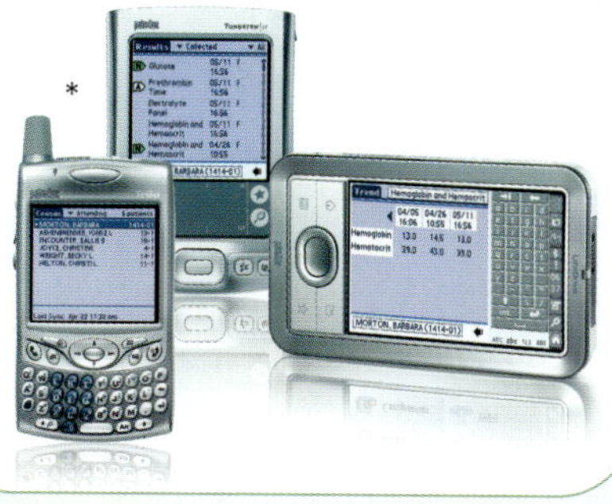

Palm® helps healthcare professionals enrich patient care by developing mobile solutions that improve efficiencies, reduce costs, improve the quality of care and reduce medical errors.

Healthcare professionals are mobile – on the go, often seeing patient after patient with little time between visits. These providers depend on the mobility of Palm handhelds and smartphones. Instant access to critical information is crucial. Handhelds and smartphones from Palm, together with software from leading healthcare solution providers, offer clinicians a powerful tool to more easily:

- Access vital patient data;
- Communicate and collaborate with patients, colleagues and pharmacies;
- Reference important drug, disease and diagnostic information;
- Manage their practices and schedules;
- Ensure accurate charge capture; and
- Increase physician, nurse and staff efficiencies.

Solutions That Deliver — At the Point of Care

Applications from Palm partners – like patient management, drug reference, e-prescribing and charge capture – provide healthcare professionals with critical information when they need it most. New solutions are being developed every day, including:

Patient Management

- McKesson – www.mckesson.com
- MercuryMD – www.mercurymd.com
- PatientKeeper – www.patientkeeper.com

Drug and Clinical Reference

- Epocrates – www.epocrates.com
- Skyscape – www.skyscape.com
- Unbound Medicine – www.unboundmedicine.com

E-prescribing

- DrFirst – www.drfirst.com
- iScribe – www.iscribe.com

Security

All Palm OS® handhelds and smartphones include a built-in security application featuring power-on password protection and auto-locking. This simple yet effective application has no back doors and uses the MD5 hashing algorithm to encrypt the password.

HIPAA

If your organization handles protected health information, then the Health Insurance Portability and Accountability Act may apply to your usage of handhelds and smartphones. Palm mobile solutions can be made HIPAA-compliant by taking a few simple steps to defend stored and transmitted data.

Featured Products

Treo Smartphone – The Potential Is As Great as Your Dedication

The Treo™ smartphone takes mobility a step further for healthcare professionals. The Treo makes it easier than ever for physicians, nurses and clinicians to stay connected in every way, every day. It simplifies your life by combining a compact mobile phone with email, an organizer, messaging and Web access plus many valuable healthcare applications. The ultimate tool, be it for a physician at a large hospital or running a private practice.

LifeDrive Mobile Manager – Practice From Where You're Standing

Palm introduces the LifeDrive™ mobile manager. With a 4-gigabyte hard drive and built-in Wi-Fi® and Bluetooth® support, you can easily carry patient files from office or desktop computer, 2.5 hours of video, 1,000 photos/images and more. And see it all on the large, color-rich display in landscape and portrait views. Includes support for POP, IMAP and Exchange email accounts, plus onboard voice recorder. The ultimate tool, be it for a physician at a large hospital or running a private practice. ■

Palm, Inc. is a leader in mobile computing and strives to put the power of computing in people's hands so they can access their most important information.

Ed Colligan
President and CEO

Ken Wirt
Senior Vice President, Worldwide Marketing

John Hartnett
Senior Vice President, Americas Sales and Customer Support

Palm, Inc.
950 W. Maude Avenue
Sunnyvale, CA 94085-2801

Sales Contact
Dexter N. Siglin III
Enterprise Solution Sales
Phone 1.888.548.9394
dexter.siglin@palm.com

Marketing Contact
Gail Moody-Byrd
Director, Healthcare and Professional Services Marketing
Phone 408.617.7518
gail.moody@palm.com

* Application software sold separately

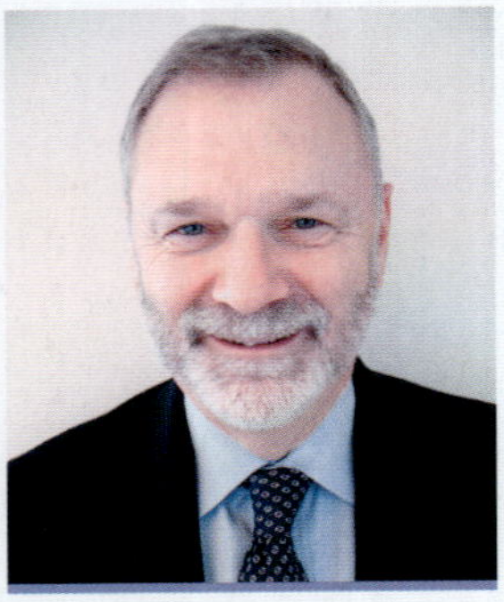

Donald W. Simborg, M.D.

Donald W. Simborg, M.D., was the co-founder of HL7 and founding member of AMIA's College of Medical Informatics. He founded and is the former CEO of two EHR companies and the author of over 100 articles and book chapters on a wide range of medical informatics topics.

Q&A With Dr. Donald W. Simborg

The key developer of HL7 predicts what standards are on the horizon in healthcare.

Healthcare Technology: *You developed the interchange protocol that became the first version of Health Level 7 (HL7), which today is the most widely used data interchange protocol in healthcare. In addition to HL7, what other standards do you see on the horizon?*

Donald Simborg: In addition to HL7, there are not only other standards on the horizon, but many other standards already in place. HL7 is an important standard for data interchange, but there are other important standards in use. These include healthcare-specific standards like LOINC, which is the laboratory standard, and DICOM, which is the image standard. In addition, we have non-healthcare-specific standards that are very important in healthcare – the Internet (TCP/IP) being the most important. XML has become a very important message transfer type standard that is being incorporated into HL7. So fortunately, in healthcare we don't always reinvent wheels, but we do benefit and use standards that are more general.

Getting to your answer of what is on the horizon, I think the major standard that is emerging has to do with the data content of clinical records and clinical care. The main standard there today, and I think emerging for the future, is SNOMED CT. I see that becoming much more widely used, and it's very necessary. HL7 primarily deals with the messages, what kinds of messages and what things need to be in messages, but it doesn't go down to the level of how you code all the various concepts that are used in healthcare records and healthcare communications. SNOMED CT takes it that next step. Another entirely new area of standards development in healthcare relates to interoperability in the emerging National Health Information Network and its component sub-networks.

HCT: *How do EHRs apply to physician input systems?*

DS: EHRs must deal with physician input – you don't get anything into the record that comes from a physician unless the physician puts it in there directly or indirectly. Obviously everything in a health record doesn't come from a physician; it comes from other professionals and it comes from laboratories and other places. A substantial part of what is in a health record, however, comes from a physician. There must be facile ways for physicians to enter their encounter notes and orders into an electronic format that can be understood by not only computers but also obviously communicated to other people in the healthcare system. So it's essential that we have physician input systems. This has been the largest barrier to date to the adoption of EHRs.

HCT: *What are some of the types of information captured?*

DS: The main areas are ones I just mentioned: the encounter note itself; that is, the note that a physician records in a record during and after seeing a patient at a patient visit. That usually includes components defined by the acronym SOAP: subjective, objective, assessment and plan. Subjective is the history information – what the patient tells you about himself or herself. The objective part of a note contains the things that the physician observes or things that are determined by testing procedures. The assessment, which is a critical part of the input from a physician, is what the physician thinks about all this, what's the physician's impression of the patient's problem and how bad the problem is – the severity of the problem. The fourth component, the P or the plan part, is what the physician is going to suggest or recommend. It contains the diagnostic and/or therapeutic next steps, which would include the orders, such as the prescriptions or orders for procedures.

HCT: *What are some of the benefits and risks of electronic record capture, storage and transmission?*

DS: Well, being someone who's been working most of his career trying to get physicians and others to use electronic records – I have a strong bias that the benefits far outweigh the risks. But there are risks, so let me start on the risk side. I'd say the primary risk is the potential for loss of privacy or confidentiality of records and the potential for abuse of that information. So I would say that's the biggest risk we need to guard against, and make sure there are appropriate safeguards to reduce that kind of a problem. On the benefit side, it's a long list, a huge list, and they fall into two main categories: clinical benefits and financial benefits. Clinical benefits are almost self-explanatory. The fact that a physician or other health professional can have access to legible records is one main benefit. To have access to information virtually anywhere, any time, without having to find a chart is just an enormous clinical benefit. In addition to just the availability of the information, the more modern systems all engage in what people call decision support. These are methodologies that are available in computerized systems that will help alter or improve the decisions that are actually made by the physician. All physicians make errors – they can't be expected to be perfect. In addition to reducing errors, decision support systems can suggest better ways to do things according to the latest published evidence. So decision support is a huge benefit of these systems.

Just having access to information widely between physicians, which isn't available today, will prevent unnecessary care and unnecessary duplication in care.

On the financial side, there's just no question that these systems are going to be important in reducing the costs, particularly the rising costs, of healthcare. These decision support components have already been shown to reduce errors. Errors, in addition to being bad medicine, are also very costly. Someone has to take care of the complications from these errors that are made. Just having access to information widely between physicians, which isn't available today, will prevent unnecessary care and unnecessary duplication in care. So there are many ways that these systems are going to reduce costs in addition to improving clinical care. The benefits are enormous. There are risks, though, and we can't let the concern or the threat of the risks impede the benefits that we're going to get. We just have to deal with the risks.

HCT: *Do you think there will be widespread adoption?*

DS: You know, I have a saying: "paper records are dangerous to your health." They really are.

HCT: *Do you think there will be widespread adoption in five years?*

DS: I think we're on a rising part of the curve, largely because of a lot of the stimulus going on at the federal level now, with things Dr. Brailer is doing and the things going through Congress now. So I think we're going to have a lot of stimulus, a lot more adoption. Widespread in five years? It depends on what you mean by that. I'd say if we're at about 5 to 10 percent adoption now, we'll be in, perhaps, the 30 to 50 percent range in five years. I'd say that's widespread compared to today. Not anywhere near 100 percent. The key will be changing the economic model, particularly with regard to the financial incentives to physicians to adopt these technologies. If Congress passes legislation requiring Medicare to provide the proper financial incentives, we will get much higher adoption in five years.

HCT: *You're way ahead of your time.*

DS: Well, I am working on it. ■

The Logical First Step for EHR: E-Prescribing

With more than 3 billion prescriptions written every year, medication prescribing has become one of the nation's most paper-based, inefficient processes – one prone to life-threatening errors.

[Jodie Thellin Skyberg, Accenture]

While the variability of technology and solutions for overall electronic health record (EHR) may intimidate physicians and cause reluctance to adopt this approach to better healthcare, e-prescribing provides a safe introduction into the process for the ambulatory arena. A properly deployed e-prescribing system creates a win/win solution for all stakeholders and a pathway for future deployment of EHR and related applications. With a fully connected e-prescribing solution, payers and providers can begin to communicate in real time and in a relevant and efficient manner. It can establish the electronic highway that enables a more robust and relevant dialogue between payers and providers as well as establish an infrastructure on which to build.

By connecting to the payer environment, physicians enjoy immediate operational efficiencies and can comply with pharmacy and pay-for-performance programs. The operational efficiencies can be significant for a physician office. A majority of patients leave a physician visit with at least one prescription, and in today's manual paper environment, that translates to a large number of pharmacy calls for prescription verification, modifications and renewals. With each of those calls, a physician's office encounters a series of manual steps to address the question or correct the prescription, which in turn wastes valuable physician, nurse and office staff time.

For payers, the benefits of electronic prescribing come through improvements in formulary compliance, generic utilization and in establishing relevant and timely connectivity with physicians that can be leveraged to the benefit of both parties.

The benefit to the patient should also not be overlooked. Beyond the apparent patient safety benefits, there is ability for physicians to actually assess patient medication compliance. In today's manual environment, physicians may only know what prescription they wrote for a patient but they do not have a way to view if that prescription was ever dispensed. E-prescribing provides physicians with dispensed medication history, thereby giving physicians a view of what was actually dispensed which can lead to patient-physician discussions around compliance issues where they exist. The hassle factor is also removed for the patient, no longer needing to wait at the pharmacy counter as the pharmacist calls the physician office to verify or modify a prescription.

We would also be remiss if we did not address the value to the retail pharmacies. Studies have shown that the paper-based process adds a significant amount of administrative manual work to pharmacists' jobs, impacting productivity and taking them away from their primary clinical role.

Everyone – especially the patient – derives benefits from enhanced information access and greater safety. E-Prescribing creates an infrastructure that benefits all stakeholders and provides a platform from which to expand into future applications.

Incentives for Implementation

Over the last year a number of forces have come together to make e-prescribing adoption more probable. One significant force is the current political environment that encourages and supports e-prescribing and EHR. The Medicare Modernization Act (MMA) solidly promotes the use of e-prescribing technology and the development of standards. While MMA does not mandate the use of e-prescribing, it does encourage differential payments for physicians who participate in Medicare Advantage Prescription Drug plans and who e-prescribe.

The federal government has also expedited the development of standards around e-prescribing, issued the foundational standards in 2005 and is expediting the development and testing of addi-

Jodie Thellin Skyberg is a senior manager with Accenture's Health & Life Sciences practice. She has extensive experience working across the payer-provider healthcare continuum including e-prescribing and EHR initiatives. Ms. Skyberg is a founding member of Café Rx, an alliance of companies and organizations working together with a common mission to facilitate the use of end-to-end electronic prescribing, and an active member of NCPDP, HL7 and eHI.

tional standard elements. All providers using e-prescribing will need to adhere to these standards, so, logically, payers must be able to accept and operate with them as well. The federal government encourages payers to create incentives that drive e-prescribing forward in the provider environment. As a primary payer, the federal government will probably follow suit with its own incentives as MMA implementation progresses.

Standard-setting organizations have also come together to help propel the movement forward. Organizations like NCPDP and HL7 for the first time have collaborated on mapping their standards to enable the sharing of information between inpatient and ambulatory environments. They have been joined by organizations such as RxHub, SureScripts and a number of private vendors to make this a reality.

Numerous foundations and private companies have also provided funding and leadership to move adoption of technology forward in healthcare. Health plans and employers are structuring incentives to encourage the use of technology by providers in their network. The incentives can and have taken several forms. One approach is pay-for-performance incentives that reward physicians for using an e-prescribing or an EHR application.

While this provides the carrot for adoption, it may not be enough to get some physicians over the hurdle of the initial investment. This is particularly true for physicians in small- to medium-sized practices. As such, some employers and health plans are considering sharing the cost of the initial investment; an approach that helps reduce the initial cost barrier to entry.

The Centers for Medicare & Medicaid Services is also exploring pay-for-performance demonstration projects and the federal government has targeted $50 million in funding in 2006 for e-prescribing programs for ambulatory physician practices. These practices serve as the keystone for regional and national health infrastructures, and e-prescribing starts the process by creating infrastructure building blocks. The government has taken the approach of funding demonstration projects and allowing final models to evolve as various infrastructures prove their viability.

E-Prescribing Captures Information

Full e-prescribing encompasses a broad spectrum of information and capabilities, including:

Eligibility status at the patient level for pharmacy coverage. Eligibility information reflects current status, provided the primary systems adjudicating claims remain current, which they tend to do since their business depends on real-time processing and payment of pharmacy claims.

Details about patient-level pharmacy benefit coverage. The information reflects individual details instead of aggregate group-level data, and integrates benefit coverage with formulary and preferred medication lists.

Formulary and preferred medication lists. This interactive listing of medications, coupled with the specifics of a patient's benefit plan, transcends static listings of medications.

An ambulatory history of dispensed medications. Each physician or prescriber can access this electronic record of prescriptions (this information can be shared across physicians if the patient has provided consent). This history, which crosses prescribers and payer plans, includes active and past medications.

An ambulatory history of written medications. Each physician or prescriber can access this electronic record of prescriptions. (This information can be shared across physicians in the same practice if the patient has provided consent.)

The ability to assess written versus dispensed medications for a patient and identify medication therapy noncompliance.

The ability to integrate clinical messaging and rules. This capability integrates tools such as prior authorization, quantity-level limits, step therapy rules, disease management triggers, care management messages and evidence-based care guidelines.

When integrated with an EHR, e-prescribing information can be coupled with a patient problem list, tests (lab, radiology) and results.

> Existing technology can accommodate a variety of physician office and workflow requirements and support different business models that can make adoption more feasible for the smaller practices.

Implementation — Today

Today's technological environment enables a relatively smooth implementation of e-prescribing. Existing technology can accommodate a variety of physician office and workflow requirements and support different business models that can make adoption more feasible for the smaller practices.

In addition, vendors and strategic alliances can provide turnkey solutions today that make it possible to migrate tomorrow to EHR. A group of companies, for example, each with vast experience in strategically applying technology to the needs of the healthcare industry, has come together to create an e-prescribing solution for the ambulatory market. They have combined best-in-class software, hardware, consulting and support services to connect physicians and clinicians directly with pharmacies for instant e-prescribing capabilities. This solution incorporates all components of the e-prescribing process, including interfaces to major practice management systems and the ability to load patient demographic and scheduling information directly into the application.

The single largest challenge to adoption of e-prescribing clearly is not technological – reluctance to adopt in the ambulatory market presents the most significant obstacle. Fragmentation of the ambulatory market in small and single practices further complicates the situation. These practices face considerable financial and other challenges if they wish to adopt and integrate new approaches and maintain them for the long term.

To encourage ambulatory providers to adopt e-prescribing, sponsors, payers and vendors must deploy a hands-on, high-touch model and work with providers to educate, train and navigate through the learning curve. Behavior modification in a busy environment takes time for office staff and physicians.

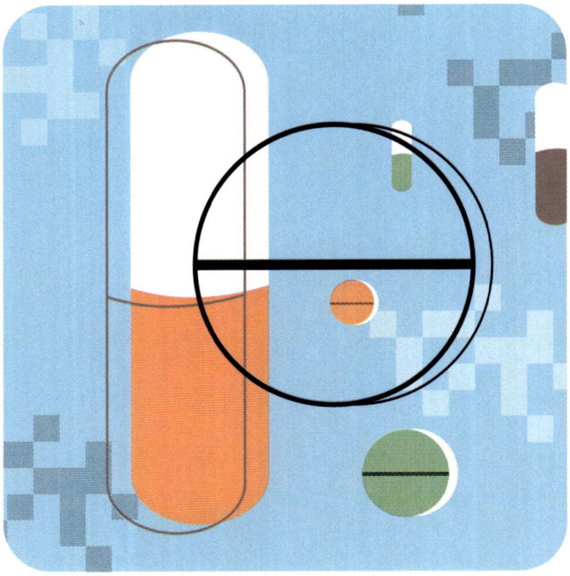

As e-prescribing becomes more mainstream – the standard for payers and providers to do business – adoption rates will increase. Payers (including the federal government and large commercial health plans) can encourage this evolution by incorporating incentives into their contracts, such as reimbursement strategies tailored to e-prescribing or pay-for-performance rewards. Economics often serves as the major driver for behavior change. Because payers tend to benefit from e-prescribing more quickly and to a larger degree, accruing about 75 to 80 percent of the initial benefits, they need to share these benefits through co-funding strategies to lower the initial barrier to entry for ambulatory physicians.

With the federal government standing solidly behind e-prescribing and EHR, the ambulatory market enjoys an incredible opportunity for making these changes. Realizing improvements through reduced medical errors and fewer deaths from adverse drug events will fuel further action.

The Risks and Benefits

One of the major risks facing implementation of e-prescribing is that not enough health plans or payers will get behind the effort and encourage standardization of technology and business processes. If the federal government, as the single largest payer in the U.S., does not provide meaningful funding incentives, the effort will lose steam. Walking the talk is critical.

In addition, if enough of the large-group-practice e-prescribing/EHR systems remain isolated from payer systems, we may see one model for large providers and another for the ambulatory segment. How will large payers react to this market? At this stage, some large e-prescribing/EHR vendors have moved forward to gain access to ambulatory information, but the risk remains that this effort will not move forward quickly enough to gain momentum.

An additional risk is with stand-alone e-prescribing vendors that do not have an EHR platform/application. These vendors need to position their offering to allow integration with EHR systems. Physicians may take e-prescribing as a single application but they will eventually want and need to move to a full EHR application that includes e-prescribing. The challenges may include both the ability of the e-prescribing vendor and the willingness of the EHR vendor.

By and large, the benefits of implementing e-prescribing far outweigh the risks. The e-prescribing component of EHR is the easiest to implement and serves as a leading-practice model for all other pieces of the care continuum. The process can build on well-established pharmacy and interim technology standards, making it much more likely that the industry will reach MMA goals for full e-prescribing by 2009.

Where Is Deployment Today?

In the past couple of years, studies have indicated that somewhere between 5 to 15 percent of physicians use some version of e-prescribing applications. However, in the past year, with the alignment of various forces, e-prescribing seems to be taking off. According to RxHub, the last six months have seen double-digit growth in eligibility transaction volume (a core transaction for e-prescribing) month over month. This indicates large deployments and use of e-prescribing technology.

Some large payers, such as WellPoint, have made efforts to move their physician network forward in the use of technology in the ambulatory setting. WellPoint's initiative focused on reducing the cost barrier of entry for physicians, and illustrates a payer's understanding of the value that they as well as physicians derive when technology such as e-prescribing is deployed and used in the ambulatory setting. Other examples of large-scale efforts include RxConnect, a collaborative effort between Blue Cross Blue Shield Massachusetts and Tufts University, and a Blue Cross Blue Shield project in Michigan with employers such as GM, Ford and DaimlerChrysler.

In addition, standards development organizations have stepped up efforts to promote e-prescribing standards. This includes the key project between the National Council for Prescription Drug Programs (NCPDP) and HL7 to map their respective standards to allow pharmacy transactions across the inpatient and outpatient/ambulatory settings. This begins to break down the silos of information that exist between inpatient and outpatient environments with pharmacy leading the way for a more patient-centric view of information. It also includes recommendations for e-prescribing standards by the National Committee on Vital and Health Statistics (NCVHS) Subcommittee on Standards and Security. NCVHS has already recommended a subset of transactions to be foundational standards for e-prescribing based on the fact that these transactions are already widely used in the market. Additional transactions related to e-prescribing such as the medication history transaction are in the process of certification via ANSI-accredited organizations such as NCPDP.

E-prescribing applications have existed for more than 10 years and the maturation of technology and applications makes it truly deployable in the ambulatory market. Likewise, maturation of associated business models has made e-prescribing more affordable, especially as payers serve as catalysts for deployment and enter into collaboration with physicians/providers where they share in some of the cost as well as the benefits. As payers continue to look for new ways to collaborate with providers, the likelihood of success increases. Ambulatory physicians hesitate to invest in vendor-dependent systems that may lose relevancy and remain confused by the offerings of the many vendors currently in the market. They need true partners to help them cut through the crowd to the solutions that fit their practice needs.

Integration of ambulatory practice systems with inpatient systems will further encourage deployment of e-prescribing. Inpatient systems are much more developed and implemented (even though the level of use and deployment remains suboptimal). Ambulatory systems remain fragmented between large-group practice systems and small- to medium-sized practice systems. The large group practices can more ably interface with inpatient environments, provided they operate on the same systems, while small to medium practices typically have no connection with inpatient environments and run on completely different systems.

By creating specific capabilities that provide value for both, e-prescribing systems can overcome this fragmentation and link inpatient information with ambulatory care. For example, the HL7-NCPDP mapping project has created the ability to access a patient's ambulatory medication history in an inpatient setting (such as in the emergency department). It has also provided the capability for discharging physicians to access patient ambulatory benefit coverage, write a prescription per that coverage and route it to a retail pharmacy.

... maturation of associated business models has made e-prescribing more affordable, especially as payers serve as catalysts for deployment and enter into collaboration with physicians/providers where they share in some of the cost as well as the benefits.

The Time Has Arrived

Today, e-prescribing continues to grow rapidly because of increased pressure on the healthcare industry to improve quality, safety and efficiency. The MMA and its requirements for reasonably short-term deployment fuel this acceleration, as does increased payer emphasis on collaborating with providers and members to promote this beneficial tool.

A significant percentage of large group practices already have some level of EHR/e-prescribing (although not usually connected to ambulatory prescription data) in place and the rate of adoption is expected to increase over the next few years. Smaller groups and solo practices must keep pace to remain viable and competitive. E-prescribing – a relatively low-cost, easy-to-implement solution – is the logical starting point toward full-scale EHR implementation for all ambulatory practices. ■

Driving Care Management Home: EHR and Patient Self-Monitoring

When patients and providers have real-time access to data about chronic diseases, they can become aware of and respond to early indicators.

[Kimberly O'Keefe, Accenture] [Wendy L. Wilson, M.D., Accenture]

Health plans have begun to use biometric devices to assist in managing chronic diseases such as diabetes, asthma and chronic heart failure. These devices include glucometers, electronic scales, spirometers and sphygmomanometers. They generate data that, when analyzed through a clinical rules engine, share early indicators with providers and patients. Studies indicate that this approach improves self-care by patients. Despite implementation challenges associated with cost, configuring technology for the home setting and integrating the process with EHR, some benefit plan designs and reimbursement programs use biometric devices to drive better outcomes.

Why Use Biometric Devices?

Biometric devices educate and empower the patient, increasing awareness, accountability and responsiveness. When integrated with EHR, these devices extend benefits beyond the patient's immediate realm. Information also reaches physicians and healthcare professionals in real time, enabling proactive treatment.

Every health plan contains a group of people under case management for chronic diseases. Of those with conditions such as chronic heart failure, diabetes or asthma, the most severely affected account for an overwhelmingly high percentage of total treatment costs. They also tend to reap the benefits of EHR with biometric device integration and therefore tend to participate meaningfully when this approach is launched.

Clinical rules engines drive the true value of integrating biometric devices with EHR. These rules engines do not simply generate values with date and time stamps, they generate knowledge (based on objective algorithms) about trends and other key diagnostic issues related to those data.

The Glucometer

The glucometer checks blood sugar levels for diabetic patients. A 2003 study of veterans revealed that self-monitored blood glucose testing drives clinically important and sustained results. [1] When integrated into EHR, the device helps physicians ensure that their patients follow directions, and it tracks the results.

Jane, a 43-year-old female with a 26-year history of diabetes, has had trouble controlling her blood sugar. Her physician has instructed her to check her blood sugar four times a day. Midway through the day, she tests her blood sugar with her electronic glucometer. The device transmits an elevated reading of 600 mg/dL via the EHR and her customized rules engine generates an instant message to "take 15 units of regular insulin and go immediately to the emergency room as directed by your physician." Jane prepares to follow these instructions while the EHR sends a message to her physician and her health coach, who immediately calls Jane's cell phone to check on her.

The Sphygmomanometer

The sphygmomanometer, which measures blood pressure, is typically used by patients with chronic heart failure or diabetes with elevated blood pressure. A three-month study showed significant

Kimberly O'Keefe is a partner with Accenture's Health & Life Sciences practice, concentrating in strategy and transformation for health payers as well as leading large, complex Web-application development and package implementation engagements. She has worked in the managed care industry for over 14 years and has focused in several areas, including medical management, provider network development and product development. **Wendy L. Wilson, M.D.,** is a senior manager with Accenture's Health & Life Sciences practice. She has over 20 years' experience in healthcare. Her work as a consultant has been diverse and has extended both across payers and providers, most recently including clinical intelligence, outcomes, care management and payer-provider collaboration.

improvement in nurse-managed telemonitoring of patients with chronic heart failure when EHR incorporated these devices. [2] The strategy reduces hospitalizations related to chronic heart failure, myocardial infarction and stroke.

Jack, a 54-year-old man with a history of heart failure related to his longstanding hypertension and two previous myocardial infarctions, has started a new medication to treat his heart failure and elevated blood pressure. His physician has asked him to check his blood pressure twice daily, since mild elevations in his blood pressure cause decompensation of his heart failure. When Jack checks his blood pressure, the 144/94 reading creates an instant message from the rules engine based upon his customized instructions. The device instructs him to take an extra dose of his medication and call his physician the following morning. At the same time, his physician and health coach receive a nonurgent message apprising them of the situation. The following morning, Jack's health coach calls him to remind him about salt intake.

The Electronic Scale

Generally used by patients with chronic heart failure, the electronic scale measures body weight. Mortality rates are significantly reduced for patients using technology-based daily-weight and symptom-monitoring systems. [3] In addition, inpatient visits decrease by an average of 57 percent and related delivery costs drop about 55 percent per patient per year. [4]

Jack has achieved good control of his blood pressure and, per his physician's instructions and health coach's prodding, checks his weight every day via his electronic scale. On this particular day, Jack feels normal but his scale indicates an increase in two pounds since the day before. He instantly receives a message customized by his physician to decrease his fluid intake, watch his salt intake, take his medication and weigh again the next morning. Jack then logs on to his health plan's website and notices that his weight occasionally fluctuates one or two pounds. (He can track this because his electronic scale populates his personal health record on this site.

The Spirometer

The spirometer helps asthmatic patients measure peak respiratory flow on expiration. Spirometer studies have demonstrated significant improvement in mean "quality of life" scores after 12 months. [5] These studies also show that implementing a comprehensive disease management system increased expenditure on asthma drugs by 45 percent, but reduced hospitalization costs for asthma by 146 percent, total costs by 21 percent and total direct healthcare costs by 22 percent.

Don is a 27-year-old with a nine-year history of asthma whose physician recently changed his medication. During this period of transition, his physician has instructed him to check his peak flow using the electronic spirometer twice daily. On this particular spring afternoon, the pollen counts are high and, when Don checks his peak flow, the indicator shows he has crossed from the "green zone" into the "yellow zone." He receives an instant message to use his rescue inhaler and check his peak flow again in 30 minutes. He does so, and returns to the "green zone." Don's health coach calls him to check on his status and suggests that, in accordance with his physician's wishes, he electronically submit his peak-flow results for the past week to his physician via the health plan's website.

The Benefits, Risks and Challenges

For patients, linking self-monitoring devices to EHR provides many significant benefits. This approach increases proactive self-management and enhances communication with physicians and other healthcare providers for improved outcomes and better quality of life.

Improved communication with patients means physicians can track compliance with instructions more meaningfully, versus use of patient-generated and usually incomplete paper calendars. Access to fundamental real-time clinical information leads to more timely and useful interventions between office visits.

Health plans see improved participation in chronic disease management programs, with consequent reductions in cost. Integrating biometric devices with EHR also makes it possible for health plans to collaborate with pharmaceutical organizations, academic medical centers and other entities. Finally, by having the same view of the same data, health plans and physicians can integrate their care plans and reinforce each other's activities.

The major risk of integrating biometric devices with EHR is inefficiency or wasted activities due to false positives or device use by someone other than the patient. Proper tools and processes for identification can overcome this obstacle.

The primary challenge to implementing EHR/biometric device integration relates to behavior change on the part of patients and providers.

Although it would seem fundamental that patients would modify their behaviors to improve their quality of life, incentives tend to accelerate compliance. For example, health plans can improve glucometer compliance rates by waiving one month of co-payments for insulin or providing a 10-percent-off coupon for use at the pharmacy. Studies have shown that such approaches work well, especially for economically disadvantaged patients.

From the physician's perspective, changing processes means new and different ways of working with patients and a consequent increase in activities such as checking Web summaries or receiving pager notifications of patient trends. Health plans generally use two models to encourage physicians to accept these changes. They either pay a fee per member per year or enable billing for "technology consults," such as patient communications via email. (These incentives must include timely requirements for reacting to information generated by biometric devices to manage liability concerns.)

Costs and technology challenges associated with integrating biometric devices can be considerable. Volume dictates the cost of technology, so projects must involve a significant population of patients and physicians to be cost-effective. Patients must receive devices costing from $100 to $200 and, in many cases, "e-calendars" ranging in cost from $400 to $500. This does not include ordering, packaging and shipping of equipment to each patient. Decision makers must determine whether to use wireless, telephony or some combination of both technologies. Rules engines must be developed and configured. Portals must be developed for physicians, patients and health coaches. Training and other support also comes into play.

Where Does It Stand?

Although some health plans have begun to integrate biometric devices into EHR as part of disease management programs, activities have not progressed much beyond that level. As success stories spread, however, the true value of this approach will become better known and appreciated. Having access to a continuum of data based on proactive information from real-time testing will prove too compelling to ignore. ■

Health plans can improve glucometer compliance rates by waiving one month of co-payments for insulin or providing a 10-percent-off coupon for use at the pharmacy.

Endnotes

1. *Diabetes Outcomes in Veterans Study [DOVES],* Diabetes Care, *June 2003.*
2. American Journal of Hypertension, *2003 and* Heart Lung®, 2001.
3. American Heart Journal, *October 2003.*
4. Disease Management, *2003.*
5. American Journal of Respiratory and Critical Care Medicine, *International Conference of the American Thoracic Society, Toronto, Canada.*

Connecting Healthcare To the Digital World

CaduceuX

The CaduceuX software solutions enable healthcare teams to schedule and assign appropriate individuals into the most relevant events and ensure equitable distribution of scheduling events. Our mission is to bring value to our customers, employees, stakeholders and the healthcare community by delivering advanced technology solutions that enable our clients and trading partners to operate, interoperate and compete more effectively.

Our flagship product A.S.A.P. (Advanced Scheduling & Administrative Program) is a state-of-the-art scheduling system designed and developed in-house. We have pioneered the use of Web technologies in developing best-of-breed processes to satisfy the unique requirements of scheduling healthcare personnel. From our corporate headquarters in Denver we provide our clients with services in healthcare, billing, staff augmentation, network support, remote administration, software, hardware, maintenance and hosting services.

Story

The solutions developed by CaduceuX help our customers simplify, streamline and automate business processes. Caduceux was founded on the development of a state-of-the-art scheduling system that optimizes information flow among existing applications, data, schedulers, physicians and facilities. Standardizing and having complete visibility of these processes creates better and more consistent information across all channels to better service providers and patients.

CaduceuX provides solutions that streamline the ability to schedule a case, check for availability, forecast time off and significantly reduce billing cycles. These solutions provide a foundation for additional CaduceuX systems to increase operational efficiency, improve customer service and enhance provider relations.

CaduceuX's industry expertise minimizes project risk while maximizing the benefits of process improvements and the bottom line to the stakeholders. Seasoned industry professionals design, build and deliver every CaduceuX implementation into a pre-built package that can then be customized to an organization's unique processes. Our goal is to significantly improve our customer's major business processes in order to increase their enterprise's value across a multitude of areas. Key customer rewards include, but are not limited to, increased employee satisfaction, decreased turnover, enhanced patient service and experience, improved administrative costs, managed medical costs and the maintenance regulatory compliance.

A.S.A.P. was designed and developed in the real world, to address all of the scheduling requirements of a healthcare provider group practice. A.S.A.P. is an interactive, cost-effective, high-quality scheduling system that provides flexible front-to-back office process management. Web-based access protocols provide for virtually unlimited accessibility.

Key features include a customized resource assignment algorithm, continually updated CPT codes, auto routing and error resolution, embedded reports, instant messaging, auto-distribution, personal time-off calendars, revolving on-call, block time assignments, billing system integration and much, much more.

CaduceuX is committed to delivering high-value group management software that enables our customers to successfully execute, monitor and measure against expected outcomes. By implementing published standards, CaduceuX applications provide an advanced, flexible technology platform to enable our systems to function in a client-specific environment and allow them to be easy to implement. Additionally, continued commitments to new product development, advanced software research and healthcare technology ensures our ability to be proactive within the industry and flexible to our customers' requests. ■

weblink

Read how healthcare leaders can implement EHRs in an integrated manner in "Navigating the Maze."

CaduceuX offers the provider practice an affordable and practical back-office staff scheduling software solution. Our software dramatically improves back-office efficiencies by allowing for the automation of credentials, preferences, personal time off, distribution, case acceptance and on-call details as well as a plethora of other staff scheduling intricacies.

Odell Isaac
President and CEO
oisaac@caduceux.com

Dr. Vincent Muscat
COO
vmuscat@caduceux.com

Jon Wisda
CTO
jwisda@caduceux.com

Stevenson Sommer
VP Network Solutions
ssommer@caduceux.com

CaduceuX, LLC
4600 S Ulster St., Ste. 700
Denver, CO 80237
Phone 303.740.6772
Fax 303.740.6774
www.caduceux.com

Business Contact
Odell Isaac
oisaac@caduceux.com

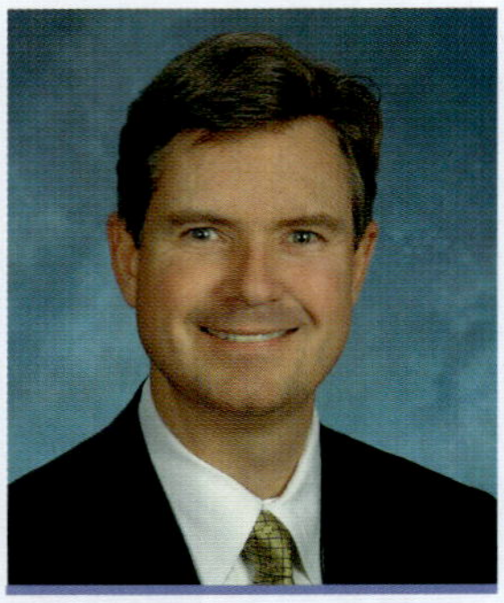

Scott Whyte
Vice President, IT
Catholic Healthcare West

Scott Whyte is a vice president of clinical systems at Catholic Healthcare West (CHW). Prior to his role at CHW, he was vice president and CIO at Phoenix Children's Hospital and has spent over 17 years consulting with Capgemini, Siemens Medical Solutions and Ernst & Young to hospitals, health insurers and life sciences companies.

Q&A With Scott Whyte

A VP of IT at Catholic Healthcare West explains the impact that clinical genomics could have on electronic records.

Healthcare Technology: *You are a leader in the clinical genomics space. Can you tell us a little bit about your work with genomics?*

Scott Whyte: A few years ago, I became interested in the topic of genomics and its ultimate impact on clinical information systems (CIS). I had heard one of the leading researchers with the National Institute of Health, Jeffrey Trent, comment that one of the biggest challenges was the exchange of genomic information. Independent researchers would work on sequence and profiling information but it was difficult to share that information electronically with others without human intervention to reconfigure the information before it got loaded into another database. He said that, to a certain degree, this slowed down research collaboration and progress.

Although I'm not a researcher, I predicted we would have a more significant problem when it ultimately came to patient care. We are now moving from bench research to translational research, where researchers are looking at specific drug therapies or diagnostic techniques; some of which are in place and being used by doctors and hospitals.

Today the volume of these therapies is relatively low, but as the volume builds, we need to be able to exchange genomic information from one machine to another without having a human intervene. I have a background on solving these types of problems, so I volunteered with Health Level 7 (HL7), which is an international standards organization. They had not yet begun work in genomics, so I helped form the team, and I'm currently a co-chair of the Special Interest Group on Clinical Genomics.

HCT: *Can you explain the connection between EMRs and clinical genomics?*

SW: Today most of the genomic-related information is not stored in an electronic medical record (EMR) at all, and if it is stored, it's stored in a text-based note. There aren't discrete data fields that can be sorted and queried or reported upon.

So if you think about a routine lab test, a blood chemistry, for example, those values come back from a lab instrument into a laboratory information system and then through an interface over to the main EMR. When the results get to the EMR, they're stored in very discrete values – there are numeric measurements for the glucose, calcium, electrolytes, etc. Each of those is stored as a value in a little bucket within the EMR. As a result, you can graph that information and trend it, and you can sort across patients and do all kinds of work it information. Quantitative information is much more valuable to the clinician. Since the genomic information now currently comes in as text, you can't do any searching, graphing or comparison between patients or for a given patient over time.

There's very little use of genomic information within the EMR today. There are very few exceptions where more leading-edge institutions are building discrete attributes in which to store genomic information. The Mayo Clinic is one, for instance. The Marshfield Clinic in Wisconsin is also doing this. So there are some institutions that are starting to integrate genomic information into the EMR.

HCT: *What are some of the security and privacy concerns.? What kind of barriers are we encountering?*

SW: Well, the security and privacy concerns are essentially the same areas of concern for all other healthcare information. Federal regulations, such as HIPAA, are mandating privacy and security standards and compliance with those standards. However, the genomic area is of particular concern because of the predictive nature of the information. You can predict that there's a higher likelihood for a particular disease to occur prior to it occurring. And a patient may have the concern that if an insurer knew future likelihood of disease based upon genomic information that the insurer might make his/her policy either more expensive or effectively make them uninsurable. You can start to extrapolate other implications there as well; for example, relating to employability. The areas of concern are the same for all health information. The degree of the concern, and sensitivity related to privacy is just much higher for genomic information.

I personally think that we will overcome the security and privacy issues. We have exposures today that are still of great concern that we are addressing with technology, laws and prosecution. I also think there's a certain scientific humility as we learn more about the genomics. We learn about the value of genomics and also learn more about the limits of the meaning of the genomic information. For instance, certain gene markers tell us disease likelihood, but there absolutely are behavioral and environmental factors that affect the disease. So while you may have a particular single nucleotide polymorphisms (SNPs), it is not a foregone conclusion that you're going to get breast cancer or some other disease.

The value of genomics in medicine will outweigh privacy concerns. Today breast cancer and the BRCA1 and BRCA2 genes are talked about the most. In addition, there's work with other cancers, diabetes, heart disease and obesity; there are many other research and development efforts related to predisposition. But much of the work goes beyond predispositions to evaluating which particular therapy is effective on the person. There's significant work being done on pharmacogenomics, which doesn't predict your ability to acquire the disease but assists in the development and predicts the effectiveness of a particular drug.

HCT: *What's on the horizon for EMRs and clinical genomics in the next five to seven years?*

SW: I would say within a year or two we will see a number of pilots of genomic information in EMRs. There's will still be an early adopter phase, maybe in three to five years. Ultimately I do see that the information will be more routinely stored in the EMR. And there's a question about what that means. Initially only very small fragments of information about a person's genome will be stored – only the fragments that result from testing for specific conditions. Those test results, identifying the presence of a particular SNP or mutation for example, will be placed in the EMR. Your whole genome sequence will not be in the EMR – at least not initially. I think that'll be a long way off. As the volume of information increases, security and storage issues become much more significant.

We still wrestle with the issue that there is not a common vocabulary in the clinical setting and I think that's really the biggest barrier. We need a common vocabulary to describe the whole topic of clinical genomics and all the various pieces and parts. There aren't universally accepted terms for genomic components and how they interact with each other from a care delivery perspective. Until that common vocabulary is better defined, it's going to be harder for widespread adoption to occur. So it's really more of a clinical issue or medical terminology issue than it is a computer issue. Right now the advances are so rapid, there are billions of dollars being invested worldwide by government entities and by pharmaceutical companies. The knowledge is growing at an incredible pace. The method to categorize and agree on the meaning of those findings is not keeping pace with the progress. There is no shortage of challenges and opportunities to including genomic information in the EMR. ■

> Until that common vocabulary is better defined, I think it's going to be harder for widespread adoption to occur. So it's really more of a clinical issue or medical terminology issue than it is a computer issue.

weblink

An electronic medical record (EMR) is a computer-based patient medical record. A patient medical record contains information related to specific visits to a health provider (e.g., hospitals, doctors offices). In contrast, an electronic health record (EHR) includes the information in an EMR but adds general health-related information that is not necessarily related to a disease or visit (e.g., diet, exercise, weight, nonprescription medications).

Laboratory Services: A Key Island of Information for EHR

In the grand scheme of patient care, laboratories do far more than just receive orders and return results. They aggregate and provide fundamental information upon which clinicians base critical decisions.

[Jeff Hawley, Accenture] [Ashif Jiwani, Accenture]

Throughout the care continuum, laboratory services provide test results and interpretations that drive and affect medical decisions as well as billing and other business matters. In a world of centralized and decentralized laboratory models, many and disparate pieces of information about the same patient reside in different systems and different places. Additionally, this information is not uniform from system to system.

How does one integrate these systems with EHR so that all information – from the most basic blood chemistry results to the most complicated biopsy interpretations – can be aggregated, accessed and consumed by clinicians and other decision makers in a meaningful way? And how can EHR extend the functionality of laboratory systems as a broker of information between organizations and individuals?

What Do Labs Do?

Laboratory systems provide test results for patient samples. The scope of the typical laboratory includes clinical and anatomic pathology. Consequently, laboratory systems capture information such as patient demographics and order information. They also generate a broad range of result data including numeric, textual and derived or calculated data. Interpretations of clinical data by laboratory clinicians are a subset of this information. In the laboratory setting, information crosses all of the care venues (primary care, acute care, post-acute care, home care, the emergency department and ambulatory settings) and may include clinical trial environments. Information is received and transmitted in various ways, from automated, integrated systems to standalone systems with no electronic interface.

Labs receive primary information about patient demographics from client registries, provider registries and master patient indexes. The lab system must rationalize information complexities and correct information disparities to ensure it performs the right test for, and routes results about, the right patient to the right individuals and organizations. For example, multiple physicians (including the primary care physician) must be able to receive results when conditions dictate. Further complicating matters, the laboratory must track how to route results to the various recipients.

Laboratory information systems capture test orders, such as:

- Test codes and descriptions;
- The date and time a test should be performed or samples collected;
- Test conditions;
- Provider(s) involved;
- Result instructions; and
- Test status (whether routine or immediate, for example).

Essentially this equates to what to do, when and how to do it and who needs the results. Many labs do not standardize the codes for describing test codes beyond the common procedure terminology (CPT) convention. Nomenclature for test codes and descriptions varies, even when translated over a standardized HL7 data stream. This complicates the ability to share laboratory data in a way that enables a cumulative view of the data (when result codes are not uniform). A clinician wishing to view a patient's hemoglobin, for example, may have difficulty rationalizing the result if three different labs describe and code that test as "HGB," "Hemoglobin," and the hemoglobin component of an "H&H."

Jeff Hawley is a manager with Accenture, responsible for managing selections, implementations and strategy planning for laboratory and clinical systems both nationally and internationally. He developed the methodology to select vendors to provide multiple healthcare information system applications to health districts within the province of Saskatchewan. **Ashif Jiwani**, a senior manager with Accenture, focuses on building sustainable business solutions in healthcare, most recently on Microsoft platforms. He has developed solutions in such areas as enterprise application integration, clinical mobile tools and clinical portal frameworks, and has implemented one of the first Web services.

Results information encompasses the actual test result, including the method used and associated reference ranges, and the specimen type and parameters for its collection. The LOINC nomenclature (Logical Observations Identifiers Names and Codes) has attempted to rationalize and standardize ordering and results nomenclature. While this method is highly effective for a broad range of laboratory testing, deficiencies exist in areas such as microbiology, anatomic pathology and cytology.

Laboratory systems also contain derived data from accumulating results over time. As with orders, internal and idiosyncratic nomenclature makes it difficult to pool and exchange results.

Benefits and Risks of Transcending Paper

EHR integration offers multiple benefits over paper for record capture, storage and transmission. It permits multiple viewers to obtain multiple views of data, building collaboration between and among organizations and individuals.

Folding laboratories into the EHR system permits rapid inquiry into the status of orders and results. It also enables linkages to decision support engines so that laboratory data drive actions and interventions. For example, the system can incorporate alerts based on any lab value outside of acceptable ranges or to indicate potential contraindications of a medication order for a patient based on a specific result of a laboratory procedure for that patient.

Another benefit of EHR is the aggregation of data, representing a centralized and rational approach, thus reducing unnecessary testing, with a concomitant reduction in costs. It improves storage and tracking of specimens, reducing the incidence of repeat testing, which is costly and often incurs patient inconvenience or discomfort.

Finally, EHR presents significant opportunities for standardization of nomenclature and processes. Creating an electronic perspective naturally fuels agreement on standards for naming and describing tests and results.

On the downside, the EHR approach includes some risks for laboratories and their "customers," such as loss of data or lack of accessibility at critical times if electronic systems fail. This concern can be mitigated with appropriate technology, ensuring near fault tolerance. Additionally implementation depends on all pertinent organizations and users accepting and adopting the technology, including standard data and approaches. In a time when idiosyncrasies are still the norm, this presents certain political and organizational challenges.

Fully electronic approaches also require a different view of security. Access to paper records is inherently difficult and insecure, whereas electronic systems ease access but can be vulnerable to inappropriate disclosure. Systems containing patient health information must incorporate appropriate technology to ensure security and limit access to appropriate members of the healthcare delivery team. The ability to restrict and audit access down to the data element level is becoming required.

Where Things Stand

From an organizational perspective, laboratories tend to be progressive in terms of data integration and systems change, so they offer a natural place to start. The kind of data common to this environment, for the most part, accommodates standardization and interoperability.

Fundamental development in this area has focused on creating a clinical data repository (CDR) standard that will allow cohesive and coherent description and storage of results. Many organizations already hold data and interpretations in a precursor of the CDR, but the end result must accommodate clinical documentation and multiple viewer access from the "vaults" of information.

The diagnostic services industry is a competitive one, with a variety of companies trying to differentiate themselves in the marketplace in order to maintain and grow their customer bases. Laboratory results rank as among the top two or three pieces of information that caregivers demand in order to make appropriate decisions regarding their patient care. One popular strategy by diagnostic companies focuses on providing physicians with tools and systems. In the hospital setting, providers with existing infrastructures want to extend their value by doing more testing and competing with stand alone diagnostic services. (For the most part, both have focused on results delivery, although some have created Web-based order entry.)

Web portals hold great promise, but fragmentation poses considerable challenges.

All of these strategies will have an ongoing impact on the kinds of systems and technologies adopted for EHR. Hospital providers, for example, have become creative with third-party vendors, using Web portals to deliver results to physician office computers, pagers and other equipment. Naturally this technology must be balanced with the potential overload of information that could result from laboratory results.

Use of Web portals will continue to grow as trends change from viewing relationships as technical to seeing them as service-based. Laboratories will extend the value of existing systems and become important partners with clinicians by using upcoming technologies to provide remote specimen tracking; proactive, profile-based data reporting; and other customer relationship management features.

Web portals hold great promise, but fragmentation poses considerable challenges. Various organizations and their departments hold separate silos of data. In order to access this information, several methods can be leveraged. One option involves consuming all data and placing them in a master database, then providing access to the database through the Web. Another places an umbrella of Web-based technology over all systems, allowing physicians to consume data in a standard format through controlled access, as and when it is needed.

Challenges to Implementation

Creating standards for messaging, common terminology and results must occur in order to meaningfully integrate laboratory systems with EHR.

The HL7 standard continues to be a "moving target," with continual version updates that incorporate more capabilities and require retooling of interfaces. In addition, different interface engines can format and inject information into the HL7 data stream, making it relatively easy to modify data to fit specific systems. Although most laboratories use HL7 to send their results, most currently identify tests with their own codes. As a result, receiving systems cannot recognize and file results unless they adopt the same codes, an impractical solution for those using multiple laboratories, or match each laboratory's code with their own codes, a costly and time-consuming process. Using the LOINC (universal identifiers for laboratory and other clinical observations) solves some of this problem but has limitations with free-text reporting, such as commentary that has an impact on interpreting results.

Creating common terminology presents the same kind of challenges, and not just with test codes. Reference ranges vary from method to method, lab to lab and region to region. Results differ depending on source such as primarily numeric values for chemistry, alpha-numeric for hematology and microbiology and text-based for anatomic pathology. EHR must accept and properly interpret all of these diverse data.

Modifying results in a real-time environment adds further complexity. When technical difficulties occur, EHR must be able to accept the modified results (while maintaining the original results) and produce modified results that explain the differences in values.

Progress is being made in creating systems that can communicate or receive results in diverse environments and interface with decision support engines, so that clinicians can mine data, for example. However, the ability to define federated data or rationalize laboratory testing over the continuum from diverse entities is still a challenge.

Where It's Working: A Case Study

PACLAB Network Laboratories, based in Bellevue, Washington, has implemented a Web-based portal to improve its position in this competitive business.

PACLAB serves physicians, clinics and large hospitals throughout Washington state (about 30 percent of all outpatient medical laboratory services in the western part of the state, including the Seattle metropolitan area). Its solution provides a consolidated and comprehensive view of a patient's lab results and medical records to participating physicians and hospitals within their own organizations or from Pathology Associates Medical Laboratories, the primary esoteric lab for, and managing partner of, the PACLAB network.

Previously, hospitals and physicians participating in the PACLAB network experienced difficulties receiving lab reports and an inability to know for certain whether or when patients had tests performed in other healthcare facilities. They also incurred unnecessary costs associated with overlapping or redundant testing.

PACLAB sought an integrated system that would provide real-time access to clinical inpatient and outpatient lab records across multiple organizations. It chose a Microsoft .NET-connected solution called LabsNow, which uses Web services to query systems for lab results and present them in a unified way. Physicians can access the portal through a secure website, or hospitals or clinics can integrate the solution into their own systems to provide their physicians with an in-house portal.

This approach overcame the inherent problem of delays in receiving paper-based lab reports, which increase the risks of misdiagnosis or mistreatment, exacerbate inefficient reimbursement processes and create duplicate testing and added costs. Physicians now go through one channel to build a real-time view of all tests from disparate systems, including mainframes, desktop computers and other systems.

LabsNow also removed concerns about loss of control over patient data. Hospitals, clinics and physicians maintain control over their own data but provide full access to those data when needed elsewhere. The LabsNow solution also allows participating organizations to leverage the resources of others, so that they can offer and charge for additional services without developing their own capabilities. The solution also provides secure methods for transmitting information and is HIPAA compliant. Participating members own their data and choose which information to share.

The Bottom Line

Implementing EHR in the laboratory setting leads to improved access to lab results by caregivers, providing greater efficiency, safety and higher quality of patient care. This leads to cost savings for greater profitability and competitive advantages for improving business position. ■

4

Securing Physician Buy-In

In order for physicians to adopt a change in clinical process and technology, they must believe that it will enable them to provide better care for their patients as well as improve their work flow. Once a system is implemented, continuous improvement is necessary to keep physicians using the system. Management needs to understand what the organizational culture is willing to accept in terms of clinical transformation and tailor their expectations accordingly.

Securing Physician Adaptation And Adoption of EHR

If it addresses their concerns and helps them provide better care, physicians will adopt a change in clinical processes.

[Manuel Lowenhaupt, M.D., Accenture] [Lawrence M. Hanrahan, M.D., Accenture] [Scott J. Cullen, M.D., Accenture]

As hospitals contemplate implementation of EHRs, they need to be realistic about what physicians are willing to adopt. Importantly, designers must monitor and understand how willing their medical staff will be to adapt their clinical processes to a new electronic environment. The goal is to create a clinical information system and an electronic environment that physicians will want to use, both in the beginning and increasingly over time. The ability to interact productively with an integrated clinical information system providing access to a global and comprehensive EHR and providing computerized physician order entry is rapidly becoming a vital part of every physician's medical practice. But physicians are diverse in their aptitudes and appreciation of these technology tools. To lead their physicians gracefully (i.e., not kicking and screaming) to a necessary electronic environment, hospitals must disabuse themselves of two prevailing myths, each pointing to an opposite but equally unhelpful implementation strategy:

Myth 1: If You Build It, They Will Come

Adopting an electronic environment for the long term means providing benefits that are worth the effort of learning the system and the perceived time it takes to use it. In order to gain physician acceptance, any new technology must have a positive and convincing answer to the question, "How's this going to help me and my patients?" There must be personal and professional gain, because physicians, although they're slowly beginning to accept some organizational values, are typically still autonomous and individual in their values and culture. To date, IT vendors have had limited success gaining physician acceptance of computerized clinical systems.

Myth 2: Physicians Are Averse to Technology

In fact, physicians see themselves as scientists, believe in evidence-based medicine and routinely take the time to learn technology they perceive as useful. Physicians in general embrace technology as soon as they are confident it can help them provide better care to patients.

Attractors: What's in It for Me?

As caregivers and as gatekeepers to various and occasionally costly medical interventions, physicians have had their motivations closely examined. Money? Power? Largesse from pharmaceutical companies? The consistent answer in surveys and questionnaires, and as evidenced by physician behavior is – cynics beware! – the desire to give quality care to patients. The real reason a physician gets out of bed at 3 a.m. to care for a patient having a serious episode in the ER is a professional commitment to quality health care. In implementing EHR and its processes and technology, there is no stronger motivator for physician support than a clear demonstration that the system will help them take better care of their patients.

Increased safety for patients – and the resulting mitigation of risks such as malpractice – also motivate physicians. If the hospital can show them – all other things being equal – that EHR and its accompanying electronic environment can give an alert when the physician prescribes a drug to which the patient is allergic, or issue a reminder when a diagnostic test is overdue or tap into its evidence-based treatment protocols at 3 a.m. when the physician perhaps isn't thinking all that clearly, they would see those benefits of EHR as powerful motivation for change.

Manuel Lowenhaupt, M.D., is a partner with Accenture and the national practice leader for clinical transformation. He is internationally noted for his work in clinical effectiveness, care management and clinical informatics, with experience in organizations in the United States, Canada, Europe, and the Far East. **Lawrence M. Hanrahan, M.D.,** is a senior manager with Accenture and a national resource for physician adoption strategies and clinical transformation. **Scott J. Cullen, M.D.,** is a manager in Accenture's Provider, Health & Life Sciences practice and has more than 15 years' experience in the healthcare industry, both as a practicing clinician and software developer. His areas of focus at Accenture include health package implementation, clinical transformation, business intelligence and health exchange development.

Any system that integrates electronic health records (EHRs) into an electronic, interactive environment will include an order management tool. Ample data demonstrate that where such tools are in place, the time between the physician prescribing a drug and the patient experiencing the therapeutic effects of the drug is dramatically reduced compared with a paper-based process that involves prescription pads, several handoffs, inboxes, fax machines and other manual processes.

Owning the system and its processes is another important attractor for the physicians who will use the clinical information system. Physicians – or any other users of such a ubiquitous system – tend to be more forgiving of the system's imperfections and the bit of extra time it may take to use it if they were involved in its design and implementation from the beginning. As owners and sponsors, they tend to expend effort remedying the inevitable "bumps in the road" rather than blaming those who shoved a pre-ordained set of policies and practices down their throats.

easily accomplished in an electronic environment. Physicians perceive this aspect of the electronic environment as a strong benefit.

Documentation control, such as inputting treatment notes and updating medical histories, can be time-neutral or burdensome, largely dependent on the physician's typing abilities. This aspect of interacting with EHR can be agonizing for a physician who is a hunt-and-peck non-typist.

Viewed narrowly – i.e., how long does the interaction take me versus how long does it take between the time I order an intervention and when the intervention happens – order entry takes 10 to 20 percent longer in an electronic environment, especially for a novice or inexperienced computer user.

Experience has shown that the real challenge in gaining physician acceptance of a clinical information system is in reducing the perceived time to conduct a transaction. Typical issues include:

- Placement of terminals; and
- Complexity of logging in.

Physicians must share the hospital's vision of why a computerized information system is worth their time and trouble and must take a pivotal role in deciding how the system will be implemented.

The issue of physician ownership must be addressed early and often. Physicians must share the hospital's vision of why a computerized information system is worth their time and trouble and must take a pivotal role in deciding how the system will be implemented. Whatever costs are involved in developing the appropriate organizational structure, resource infrastructure, education and increasing cycle time for physician involvement will be returned tenfold in the hospital's ability to achieve a successful system implementation.

Barriers to Implementation: How Much of My Time Will It Cost Me?

Solution vendors like to claim that an integrated information solution around EHR is time-neutral or perhaps a slight time saver. Realistically, from the physician's perspective, interacting with EHR takes a little more time than handling pieces of paper, although it reduces the clerical functions of other clinical staff. Physicians have three kinds of interaction with a clinical information system:

- Access to results;
- Electronic documentation; and
- Order entry.

There's no question that access to results such as lab tests, radiology images and other diagnostic procedures is most quickly and

There's often a discrepancy between the number of terminals clinicians think they need and the number administrators are willing to buy. Practitioners who see a resident, a physical therapist and a social worker queued up at computer terminal are not going to wait in that line to place an order. Many hospital architects still like providing bedside terminals, even though doctors and nurses both are saying that's not an access point they want to utilize. Hospitals need to bring more sophistication – such as dynamic queuing modeling familiar to supermarkets and fast-food restaurants – to planning terminal usage. The food may be fast, but if the line is slow, the customer opportunity may be lost. The same is true with physicians' access to terminals. The cost benefit looking at the number of terminals and/or hand held tablets or PDAs must be completed with the end goal of maximizing physician use and minimizing physician time.

The complexity of logging in to a clinical information system can present another barrier to physician usage. A client hospital

weblink

Learn about the challenges of qualifying patients for Medicaid in "Utilizing Credit Scoring to Predict Patient Outcomes" in this book and on the Web.

with an investment of many tens of millions of dollars in a clinical information system discovered that only 20 percent of its medical staff were logging in to use the system. An investigation revealed that their system was so secure that no one could use it. Logging in involved two levels of security, each requiring tedious data entry, a password that expired every 60 days and other measures. The designers reasoned that compliance with HIPAA necessitated such onerous security measures. However, they also neglected the fact that a clerical or administrative user logs in only a few times per day and interacts with the system for hours at a time, while a physician must log in to the system dozens of times per day for only short periods. In the end, a much-simplified system used each physician's proximity ID card – the same one used to gain access to the physician parking lot – to identify each physician, and a simple biometric fingerprint scanner that used each physician's index finger as a password, to take physicians directly to the application they use 80 percent of the time. Log-in time decreased from nearly two minutes to a few seconds. With these improvements, 80 percent of the hospital's physicians now actively use the system.

Early Adopters – 10%	Progressive, computer-savvy physicians eager to embrace information technology; leading the way toward EHR and other information initiatives.
Majority – 60%	Physicians who want to contribute, and trust their colleagues who are leading the way, but are wary and will use EHR and other information initiatives only when they're confident they will work and cost them a minimum of inconvenience.
Occasional Users – 20%	Senior physicians and/or infrequent users more comfortable with paper-based clinical methods.
Active Resisters – 10%	Older, experienced physicians who will resist any information initiative unless their perspectives are recognized and respected; can become engaged and help to implement IT, but won't use it themselves; likely to need an interim parallel or "workaround" process to interact with EHR.

Champion Spectrum: To Whom Are We Talking? Physicians are a diverse group of highly motivated, fiercely independent professionals with varying aptitudes and attitudes toward information technology.

Continuous Improvement: Recognizing This Is a Journey, Not a Sprint

Physician adoption of the capability to interact with EHR through a clinical information system is not a one-time project; it is a never-ending process (or at least a 10-year hyper-marathon). Continuous improvement of the system is required to retain physicians previously recruited. For one thing, expectations change over time – often dramatically. In one example, a client with a clinical information system in place for seven years initially had 60 to 70 percent of its physicians agreeing that the system brought value to them personally. In two years' time, that percentage of physicians viewing the system favorably fell to 40 percent, largely due to changing expectations. In the beginning, the ability to retrieve results of current lab tests represented satisfactory performance. Now physicians want to see retrospective results, such as a patient's glycohemoglobin levels for the last 20 instances. If the system is clumsy in its ability to access that depth of retrospective data, physicians feel disappointed. As expectations change, cutting-edge capabilities become baseline functions almost immediately. Functions that weren't even on the physicians' radar screen in the beginning become essential capabilities.

Hospitals need to realize that the original planning of their EHR system deployment – everything from application design to placement of workstations throughout the hospital – must be constantly re-evaluated in the light of changing expectations and evolving needs. The key to retaining physician usage is disciplined, structured, two-way communication between system users and system implementers. Hospitals with EHR implementations that have been most successful at not just recruiting but retaining clinical users have built disciplined and formal communication models around the experience of using the tools. One hospital's IT department sponsors free pizza lunches to keep an ongoing dialogue with the house staff using their system. They ask for and receive feedback on how the system is working and how it is keeping up with escalating expectations, what new features and functionality are desired and other relevant issues.

System implementers must avoid surprising system users with enhancements that alter the ways they interact with the information they need. Physicians with busy schedules and/or waiting patients who need to get at their patient records quickly, and who log on to discover that the system has changed and they can't readily find the information they're looking for, get angry and frustrated. When changes occur, physicians must have simple, one-step access to a "super user" or other real person to help them.

Pay Your Respects: Design Alternative Pathways Before Users Do It for You

In any system implementation, users fall into four broad categories: the technophiles or early adopters who like computers; the majority who aren't especially interested in using computers except when it can benefit them personally; the occasional users who will use the system only infrequently; and the active resisters, the vocal minority who oppose changing the paper-based "natural order of things." Most system implementations focus on providing a satisfactory experience for the majority of users, and although that's the right group on which to invest the most time and effort, the other groups deserve a fair share of consideration.

The technophiles will appreciate being able to bypass some of the menu-driven pathways to frequently accessed functions and information. Treating them as "power users" and letting them go below and beyond the user-friendly interfaces lets them save time and better tailor their interactions to their individual needs.

Many doctors nearing retirement are reluctant to invest in learning new processes and practices. They're hoping to just ride out the computer revolution. In the case of private hospitals, where practitioners have shown great loyalty over many years, establishing a "take it or leave us" attitude toward computerized access and data entry would be disrespectful, and many hospitals have built a transition pathway with a clear end date. Though investing in this parallel pathway puts some burden on the hospital's operations staff, the good news is that many senior and influential physicians, given the extra time to get acquainted with the tools, eventually develop a comfort level using them and become proponents of the electronic environment.

The hospital that neglects to respect its technophobic physicians sometimes sadly discovers that the resisting physicians, who tend to be senior, influential practitioners, have more clout than the hospital thought – these physicians conspire with their colleagues to bring the whole electronic initiative to a dead halt. Showing respect for these active resisters is an effective strategy, even though there are costs involved in providing a parallel pathway. The parallel pathway should not be so attractive as to cause defections from the groups adopting the new tools, but hospitals that fail to provide a workaround for resisting practitioners often learn that the physicians have built them themselves, usually at higher cost and greater inconvenience to support personnel than if the hospital had provided the option. Typical workarounds include asking nurses or ward secretaries to work with the resistant doctors to print out lab tests and patient records, and to type in orders, treatment notes and other data from the physician's handwritten notes.

The hospital that neglects to respect its technophobic physicians sometimes sadly discovers that the resisting physicians, who tend to be senior, influential practitioners, have more clout than the hospital thought ...

Summary

Obtaining physician adoption of a realistic and workable electronic environment requires careful examination – and a persuasive response – to the following issues:

- What are the attractors that would compel physician acceptance of an electronic environment?
- What barriers keep them from adopting such a system?
- Once implemented, what methods of continuous improvement will be necessary to keep physicians using the system?

Physicians will adopt a change in clinical processes and technology if they believe it will help them provide better care for their patients, that their interests and concerns are adequately addressed and that their professionalism is respected. ■

Automated Discharge Summary Delivers Value to Physicians and Patients

The standardized and rapid communication of patient care details between healthcare institutions and referring providers is central to the improvement of healthcare delivery.

[Beth Sample, D.O., DINMAR]

Challenges for HIT vendors are universal: a highly competitive market, software functionality issues, unrealistic visions and customer dissatisfaction. At the 11th annual Oacis Users' Group Conference, I discovered some impressive customer success stories. One in particular describes how success can be achieved incrementally. The story is told by Oacis users from South Australia and it revolves around the deployment of an EHR system to eight hospitals and associated clinics in the state of South Australia. Though originally slated for the renal service only, the benefits realized were so immediate that the department of health decided to expand functionality and continue the implementation to include hospitals and clinics throughout the state (see Figure 1).

One of the most impressive achievements is the separation or discharge summary, a brief snapshot of the health of a patient at a particular point in time. By achieving standardized and rapid communication of patient care details between healthcare institutions and referring providers, the South Australia experience is an exemplar both on that continent and for North America as interoperability standards become central to the improvement of healthcare delivery. In fact, South Australia's discharge summary is well-aligned with the continuity of care record standard being published by ASTM International, one of the largest voluntary standards development organizations in the world. It allows a primary care provider timely access to useful and potentially life-saving information from the patient's previous episode of care, so that care can continue uninterrupted when the primary provider resumes responsibility. In the United States today, patient information remains locked in silos available only to providers practicing in the same facility; referring and community providers typically do not have ready access to information about their patients' care in those facilities.

In South Australia, the facilities across metropolitan Adelaide may have different clinical care systems (laboratory, radiology, therapies, etc.) but because of the robustness of the EHR's data repository, information captured in those systems is immediately available to all providers in each facility. This means the data is also instantly available for automating the compilation of intelligent discharge summaries. This benefits the referring or primary provider because pertinent patient data is available in hours rather than days. As a physician, I see a vast improvement in this model since I could have potentially life saving information in my hands prior to the next patient encounter – rather than having to hunt down that information when the patient appears in my office.

Typically the discharge summary is a document that a physician writes post-discharge that captures a variety of data intended to inform the primary or referring provider of the highlights of the patient care episode. This information could be but is not limited to patient allergies, current medications, consultations, procedures, test results, operative report, admitting and discharge diagnoses and description of the course of the patient's hospital stay or encounter. Having been the recipient of many discharge summaries, I have concluded that the differences between a good summary and a bad one are profoundly important. A good summary provides concise and accurate information and helps ensure continuity of care of the patient. A haphazard summary is an unnecessary obstacle and may even be dangerous. A bad or incomplete summary forces the reader to take the time to go through the body of the chart to glean the information that is not readily available in the summary – assuming the reader even has access to the patient chart. The discharge summary implemented in South Australia leverages the power of the EHR's data repository to automatically update and pull forward information on the patient throughout the encounter or hospitalization, thereby ensuring consistency and completeness in the final summary report.

Beth Sample, D.O., is a family practitioner and the director of medical informatics at DINMAR. She attended UHS-COM, completed her residency in St. Louis and practiced medicine in southern Illinois. Prior to medical school, Dr. Sample was a registered nurse. She is licensed in Virginia and is a member of AAFP, ACPE, AMIA, HIMSS and VAFP.

A high degree of physician acceptance of the South Australian discharge summary is reported, perhaps because a wide range of information is automatically populated into the draft summary for the physician to consider. The specific information presented can be customized by each facility or provider, and is typically organized into logical sections:

- Patient demographics;
- Allergies;
- Current medications;
- Problem list or diagnosis;
- Procedures or surgeries;
- Clinical synopsis;
- Test results;
- Discharge plan;
- Hospital details;
- Nurse and ancillary notes;
- Encounter included in summary; and
- Future appointments.

In addition to automatically populating fields with online data from the current episode, the discharge summary can be integrated with voice recognition software to speed completion of comment fields.

The practical patient safety benefits of a timely and well-written discharge summary can be illustrated by a simple example. Assume Susan arrives at the emergency room with an acute case of appendicitis. Thankfully she is already in the facility's EHR system, and the ER staff note her allergy to penicillin. Susan is taken to surgery and prepped with Betadine, which leads to a severe skin reaction and wound infection that delays her discharge. Upon completing the discharge summary, the care team includes the updated allergy information on the summary and transmits it via secure email to Susan's primary care provider. Susan's doctor is now immediately informed of this important new information and can monitor her condition carefully in follow-up care. Timely access to such critical data for the provider can also translate into appropriate patient education in the primary care setting, since Susan may not have remembered the Betadine allergy in the confusion of the ER admission. This example is mirrored in the South Australian model, where allergies and medications are updated and carried forward from the Oacis EHR to the discharge summary automatically.

In my clinical practice, I would see a patient in my office for routine follow-up after the patient had previously been seen by clinicians at another facility. My staff would spend at least an hour questioning the patient and telephoning other facilities to determine the most recent test results, current medications and recent therapies performed. Access to a current discharge summary would save my staff, me and the patient a significant amount of time. Since I practiced in a rural environment, I often referred patients for care to a larger facility 100 miles away. My patients often had diagnostic tests performed and new medications initiated, then presented to me for care before I ever received correspondence from the consultant detailing the patient's care. Given the application used in South Australia, I would have had immediate

Oacis is being deployed across eight Adelaide metropolitan public hospitals, enabling real-time sharing of clinical information. In addition, selected community and mental health facilities have been enabled to facilitate patient movement and to deliver patient services.

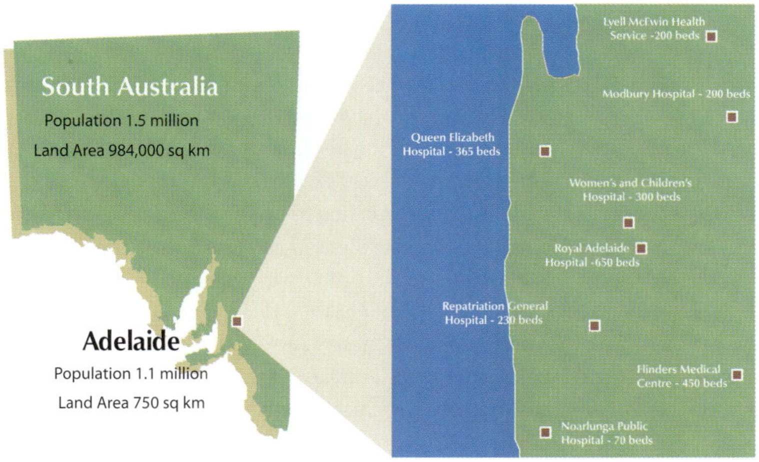

Source: South Australia Department of Health

Demographic	
Metropolitan Adelaide (DHS Annual Report 2003-04)	
Average daily available beds	2,667
Accident & emergency attendances	312,841
Outpatient visits	1,312,337
Inpatient separations	267,465

Usage Statistics	
As of May 31, 2005	
Clinical users trained	22,845
Active users	4,673
Hours usage	108,825
Average hours of usage per clinician	23.29
Clinical units enabled	400+

Figure 1 Program Scope

access to all pertinent patient information without being an attending physician associated with the testing facility.

What about the cost savings to the patient? The cost benefit would be evident if a patient went to a consulting physician who decided to start the patient on a new medication that required liver function tests. On her next visit to her primary care physician, she reports the new medication but does not recall that liver function tests were performed. If her primary physician has a timely and thorough discharge summary, the patient avoids the costs of duplicate testing and also the discomfort and inconvenience associated with another trip to the lab – especially important for patients living in rural areas. Potentially this could improve patient compliance since redundancy could be virtually eliminated. Physicians do not want to order duplicate tests, and if the patient is unaware of tests that were previously performed and there is no record available for the physician to view, this can easily occur, and quite often does. The South Australia EHR helps eliminate duplicate testing in just this way, where benefits accrue both to the patient and the state health system. Deployed in the U.S., fewer unnecessary testing equates to less claims processing and review for insurers and health care professionals and ultimately reduction in patient anxiety.

Even a cursory review of the literature reveals compelling data regarding the importance of timely discharge summaries. One article written by Dr. van Walraven showed that discharge summaries were available only 15 percent of the time and that 27 percent of patients discharged from a hospital were urgently readmitted. Another article discussed the trend toward decreased readmission if the primary provider had access to a discharge summary but concluded that further study was needed to quantify that trend. As a physician, I do not need further study to acknowledge that access to a good discharge summary would help prevent the readmission of any one of my congestive heart failure patients. An accurate discharge summary available at the first follow-up visit is worth more than words can express to the patient and the provider.

Supporting Technology

At the core of the South Australia clinical information system is the Oacis EHR, a comprehensive, longitudinal, patient-centered repository that delivers real-time clinical information whenever and wherever it is needed. The South Australian Oacis repository contains approximately 260 million service records, over 12,500 trained clinical users from over 400 clinical units, and nearly 50 HL7 interfaces into the repository. The system is run in a high-availability environment and currently stores 1.2 terabytes of data, growing at the rate of approximately 1 gigabyte per week and processing an average of 80,000 transactions per day.

Relevance to Interoperability Movement in the U.S.

I enjoyed reading the statement from HIMSS in June 2005 about interoperability. We seem to find different buzzwords every few months without having a solid understanding of how it pertains to HIT until a few months later, when another word is found and the cycle starts again. The six key characteristics of interoperability made in this statement were: uniform movement of data, uniform presentation of data, uniform user controls, uniform safeguarding data security and integrity, uniform protection of patient confidentiality, and uniform assurance of a common degree of system service quality. Upon reviewing the South Australians' discharge summary implementation, I found consistent parallels regarding this statement and the system used by our friends in Australia. The uniform movement of data was easily seen in the discharge summary distribution (via email, fax or postal service). Security and patient confidentiality is addressed at each facility and within the system itself. Uniform presentation of data was seen on each of the discharge summaries but allowed for each facility to decide what information was to be included on a patient-by-patient basis.

The South Australia Oacis EHR delivers both out-of-the-box functionality and a toolset that allows the end user to tailor the system in support of their workflow. I think that this end user functionality leads to increased end user support and satisfaction. Each facility was able to include in its discharge summary those important pieces of data that they deemed necessary for a complete document. Further increasing end user satisfaction is the ability for users to decide what particular vital signs and laboratory or radiology reports are needed to make this a complete and succinct document; and retrieving all that information automatically from the EHR reduces the time required for clinicians to complete the summary.

In summary, the South Australia state government set out to "improve the quality and safety of services, to strengthen and re-orient services toward prevention and primary healthcare, to develop service integration and cooperation. ..." This paper has discussed the coordinated efforts of the hospitals and clinics in South Australia based on their deployment of a patient-centric interoperable EHR.

The discharge summary is key to continuity of care for the patient and for the primary care provider. The discharge summary can alleviate the need for the patient to repeat allergies and medications to every facility and clinician providing patient care. The automated version implemented in South Australia can augment the process of dissemination of these important discharge summaries to the primary care provider or to another facility or physician who might treat this patient.

A system that automatically adds data to the discharge summary and updates it can decrease the amount of time a provider has to document, while making it easier for the provider to complete that final piece of critical patient information.

Those in the U.S. who are extolling the virtues of interoperability and RHIOs should take a closer look at what Australia has accomplished as a model to incorporate into our vision of the future. ■

Healthcare IT Solutions Focused On the Way Healthcare Really Works

DINMAR
dealing with the REALITIES of HEALTHCARE

Through a highly experienced team of professionals, DINMAR effectively assists its healthcare customers in all aspects of technological change, from establishing new business objectives and strategies through designing and implementing the complex information systems and processes that support them. The company's expertise includes:

- Management consulting;
- Customized systems development;
- Data center services/ASP;
- Systems integration services;
- Implementation services; and
- Support and helpdesk services.

When DINMAR opened its doors in 1992, the company's vision was grounded in a realistic grasp of healthcare and the information systems that support it. The belief that IT could drastically improve care quality and reduce costs prevailed companywide, but the pragmatic management team knew better than to propose pie-in-the-sky approaches. For DINMAR, it was about understanding the strategic needs of the customer's organization and devising *realistic* IT solutions to address those needs.

In a matter of years, the customer base, as well as the entire company, had grown significantly. And while headed down the right track, fully realizing the vision in the absence of reasonably priced, well-designed EHR solutions was difficult at best.

Many healthcare IT suppliers had not delivered on promises of improved patient care and reduced operating costs. In fact, costs for electronic health record systems had skyrocketed, patient safety incidents were at an all-time high and the road to "technology paradise" was littered with failed endeavors.

Fortunately DINMAR had discovered an innovative, interoperable EHR called **Oacis.** After spending several years as a certified installation expert, the company felt so strongly that Oacis was the solution that could complete the vision, that DINMAR bought it outright. Since 2001, Oacis has been the centerpiece of DINMAR's portfolio of products and services. ■

The belief that IT could drastically improve care quality and reduce costs prevailed companywide, but the pragmatic management team knew better than to propose pie-in-the-sky approaches.

Relevant Expertise

Delivery of high-quality care demands a multidisciplinary, team-based approach.

Likewise, DINMAR applies a similar strategy to the challenges of healthcare IT, so both patients and providers can benefit. The company's diverse skills help organizations adjust effectively to new information systems while fostering a better understanding of how technology enhances clinicians' productivity.

To every engagement DINMAR experts bring extensive real-world experience in clinical practice, strategic planning, IT deployment and product development. Moreover, the company offers a world-class training and professional development program to keep pace with evolutions in healthcare, technology and management.

In addition to DINMAR's broad array of skills and services, the company also offers the industry renowned *Oacis EHR* – electronic health record system.

DINMAR is a leading North American healthcare information technology solutions provider. The company's Oacis EHR product was instrumental in launching the "open systems" revolution, which spawned many innovative technologies and clinical interoperability standards in commercial use today.

Mark Groper
President and Chief Executive Officer

Dinis Cabral
Senior Vice President

Ian Robinson
Chief Operating Officer

DINMAR
755 Baywood Drive, Ste. 190
Petaluma, CA 94954
Phone 707.658.5110
Fax 707.658.5155
www.dinmar.com

Business Contact
Jason Huckaby
Director of Oacis Sales
marketing@dinmar.com

Oacis EHR
A DINMAR SOLUTION

EHR Usage: A Compendium of Recent Studies Performed by KLAS

Product capability versus market penetration by product use suggests old habits are today's principal roadblocks for EHR adoption and use.

[Karen Ondo, KLAS Enterprises] [Kent Gale, KLAS Enterprises]

Old habits, not technology, are today's roadblocks for EHR adoption and use. Physicians traditionally handwrite orders or tell someone else what to order. Clerical personnel typically transcribe orders into the system and maybe a nurse validates the order. When physicians need a test result they ask a nurse or clerk to print it. Today everything can be done online but it is tough to train and move the professionals who are impacted by this new technology to adopt a new way of doing business. This, coupled with the fact that incentives and downstream benefits are not aligned to support this automation (costs, reimbursement, lack of standards, Stark Law), makes today's environment one that has so far been defined by the early adopters.

As clinician awareness of the benefits of using an integrated medical record increases, there is an increasing belief that EHRs will soon become a standard of good practice for both ambulatory and hospital-based care. Computerized physician order entry (CPOE) plays a pivotal role in this discussion and many care delivery organizations are talking about CPOE as a component of a more comprehensive patient safety strategy. Medication-related activities are, in particular, receiving a lot of attention, including e-prescribing.

By way of introduction, KLAS, a market research and intelligence firm specializing in healthcare IT performance monitoring, gathers HIT vendor performance data from provider organizations, and offers research and consulting services based upon that data. They do this by first collecting product evaluations and then performing in-depth, confidential interviews with the IT executives and department directors who complete questionnaires. They gather valuable insight into specific strengths, weaknesses and future expectations for products.

CPOE

The 2005 CPOE Digest is the third successive annual report from KLAS regarding CPOE usage and its vendors and systems. The objective of each study was to survey every live North American CPOE site that was using a commercially available product, where there was a linkage and/or a relationship between the inpatient and ambulatory environment and a potential need to affect or be responsible for patient care treatment across these boundaries. The 2005 survey participants reported using the following products (listed alphabetically): American HealthNet, Cerner Millennium, CliniComp, Dairyland, Eclipsys (SCM, TDS and Emtek), Epic EpicCare, GE Centricity, IDX (LastWord, Carecast), McKesson Horizon Expert Orders, Meditech (C/S, Magic), Misys CPR, QuadraMed, Siemens (Invision, Soarian) and VisualMED.

The software objective of CPOE is for physicians to electronically enter virtually all clinical orders that they previously ordered via paper. In one user's estimate, the focus on the software represents only about 15 percent of what the installation is about. Today users describe a CPOE project as a journey that never ends. CPOE is not a project; it is a paradigm shift in the delivery of care.

The challenge with CPOE is that while measurable progress is being made, much is left to be accomplished. CPOE is in use at less than 5 percent of U.S. hospitals and is in active use (physicians entering over 50 percent of patient orders) at 2.5 percent of hospitals measured. The really good news is that the progress this year has been primarily from non-teaching facilities. To the industry, this may be the most important finding of this year's report. This is the first real evidence of CPOE adoption outside of the teaching environment. Non-teaching sites represent the hurdle that CPOE must overcome and usage in this environment provides an indication that adoption by privileged, non-employed physicians is possible.

Karen Ondo is the executive vice president of KLAS Enterprises and has 30 years of healthcare experience. She is on the HIMSS board of directors and the DocuSys Advisory Board. **Kent Gale,** president and managing partner of KLAS Enterprises, has 30 years of healthcare experience as a vendor, provider and consultant. He formed KLAS to improve the delivery of HIT software and services by monitoring vendor and product performance in the healthcare market.

The 2005 verifiable live sites totaled 245 versus last year's total estimate of live sites at 199 (with 159 verifiable and 40 reported but not verified), an increase of 23 to 54 percent depending on which figure is used. Given CPOE's small numbers, however, we are still at the early adopter stage and while progress is encouraging, critical mass has not yet been accomplished; but today's results may very well represent the groundswell everyone is looking for. Sites that are live speak across the board to the benefits of efficiency, reducing errors and enhancing patient safety.

There are more "100 percent" users. CPOE usage is multi-dimensional and there is an indication of more "100 percent" use based on the three ways it is measured: (1) the percentage of physicians doing CPOE as compared to the number possible, (2) the percentage of orders a physician enters as it relates to all patients orders, and (3) the percentage of medication orders that are electronic.

CPOE Advice for Others

The commentary regarding benefits realized is more detailed in 2005 – providing greater insights into operational benefits spanning a wide range of activities, from clinical to financial. The benefit most often stated as being realized is efficiency and streamlines processes (46 percent), reduce transcription errors was second (40 percent) and reduce errors/enhance patient safety was third (38 percent). Workflow changes (36 percent) and physician acceptance (34 percent) top the list of surprises encountered or hurdles overcome.

At a macro level, users speak to CPOE being harder than envisioned and the general underestimating of the effect of CPOE on the whole order process, through the ancillaries and back to delivery of the results/medications. The advice for others spans a wide range of suggestions; at the top of the list were suggestions involving physician buy-in/involvement (38 percent) and the need for physician/nurse champions (22 percent). Mandating CPOE is at the bottom of the list (2 percent). Commentary at a more micro level with some not-so-obvious detail involves:

- **Physicians:** The fact is, CPOE does take longer than paper and our physicians all know that now. They are realizing they cannot have the exact same workflows they used to have. Training is a large component and the different doctors need specialized strategies to engage and properly train. The physicians themselves were surprised at the amount of training necessary for CPOE. We underestimated the hand-holding the physicians needed. Start with a control group such as orthopedics, anesthesia or OB/GYN, where standing order sets are well-accepted and controlled before moving to other departments. Physicians who do not use the system on a regular basis really struggle. The real value is in the mining of complex data for the physician. Rules help to push this data where the physician can use it most. The biggest surprise is good news: Now that it works the doctors want more usability.
- **Nursing:** In-depth and aggressive training of physicians, nurses and pharmacists is more important than you will think. While we knew from the beginning CPOE would be a challenge for the physicians, we underestimated the impact CPOE would have on nursing. Moving from paper processes to an electronic method is challenging. In the past, nurses were not required to be adept computer users. Nowadays, it is important for nurses to perform the key online clinical data documentation of vitals and other key daily data for the knowledge/rules CPOE needs to be effective. We have had difficulty implementing CPOE without having nursing online. Do everything else first: observations, nursing flow sheets, nursing documentation and ancillary system interfaces. The combination of CPOE and eMAR (electronic medication administration record) is a winner.
- **Management:** Make sure you understand what the organizational culture is willing to accept in terms of real clinical transformation and tailor the expectations accordingly. Be aware of how fast the organization can adopt change. After five years it is hard for the leadership not to be distracted. Obtain and maintain executive ownership, not just involvement. Get board, executive and medical leadership buy-in up front. The project must be a hospitalwide initiative, not an IT project. Keep patient safety as your focus. Prepare for wholesale organizational changes. Do not underestimate the culture change. It will cost twice as much as people think it will, and take twice as long to implement.

Be aware of how fast the organization can adopt change. After five years it is hard for the leadership not to be distracted. Obtain and maintain executive ownership, not just involvement. Get board, executive and medical leadership buy-in up front.

- **Process:** You cannot cookie cutter your approach in multiple organizations. We were surprised that over 7,000 abbreviations (some with multiple meanings) were used across our enterprise. Supporting workflow in high intensity areas and critical care units is more difficult. I was surprised at how inconsistent we were with processes across the organization. Every hospital has workarounds for processes that are broken and CPOE tends to uncover them. You cannot rely on the computer system to resolve all your procedural problems and changing a process is a much bigger deal. Procedural issues are often viewed as system issues. We underestimated how much the role of the unit secretary would be revamped. It has been a constant discovery process regarding how broken our old paper ordering process was before.
- **Implementation:** The secret in CPOE is setting the expectations. There is not a single formula to make this work. It takes a lot of time to build useful and effective order sets – this is the key to making it all work. We converted two years of detail clinical data and 10 years of visit history; we should have been more careful in making sure we expired the MD relationship on the converted data. We only occasionally make the fancy parts work well. Put your "A" team on the project. It is less than ideal to use resources that will not be around after implementation. It takes a lot more effort and attention than we ever guessed. Do not underestimate the importance and impact of workflow redesign. We provided elbow-to-elbow support and training. I recommend that all trainers be clinicians in order to add credibility to the understanding of the process. Many workflows are missed during implementation and then result in negative feedback during installs. The issue for us is preparing for all the contingencies downstream once the order is entered. We are wearing thin on having enough people to get this implementation done and keep the business running. Do not automate an existing bad process. Spend a lot of time up front getting the workflow right.
- **Technology and Ongoing Support:** The mix between keyboard and mouse is not clean. Some things can only be done by keyboard, some only by mouse and they often both exist when performing the same task, impacting both task efficiency and hardware choices/usability. We were not prepared for the large amount of click errors the staff made. We were shocked at the level of user dissatisfaction that can be caused related to system response time and uptime: We found we needed to deploy more equipment. We have not been able to develop a system for effective communication and notification of changes to CPOE users once it is live. The help desk for major clinical applications required restructuring. CPOE would not be possible without wireless carts or mobile devices.
- **Interfacing/Integration:** Interfaces are still a challenge. All vendors claimed that their CPOE solutions were fully integrated, while only three mentioned that in some cases there is interfacing to other relevant clinical systems. Although these integrated systems may exist, providers reported that much of the data getting into the CPOE system (laboratory, pharmacy, etc.) is interfaced. Integration of pharmacy and CPOE from same system vendor(s) was less than expected. The majority of vendors reported that their pharmacy system and CPOE system were integrated, however, all vendors had some sites that had to re-enter orders in the pharmacy system except for IDX and Epic. Thirty-one percent of all pharmacy orders entered with CPOE are re-entered in the pharmacy and this represents a 35 percent improvement overall (since 2003) and a 14 percent improvement from last year's reported 36 percent re-entry. Additional challenges with CPOE and pharmacy are observed from state laws. A foreign ADT system creates challenges. Radiology tells us that 75 to 80 percent of the orders are wrong and that they do not have the ability to change or communicate back.

Alerting

Alerts are ignored if they occur too frequently. The results on alerting are mixed: 1) There are more complex active alerts (in the magnitude of thousands), 2) Those who are doing alerting are doing more (complex alerting), but 3) With the increase in CPOE sites reported there is an increase in the number of sites doing no alerting. Commentary does speak to alerting challenges, alert fatigue and alerts being turned off. Some users have established low- and high-level alerts. The low-level alerts are seen but can be ignored versus high-level alerts that "require action steps." The challenge appears to be in the development of "high precision rules," ones that eliminate the firing both of false positives and false negatives.

Commentary does speak to alerting challenges, alert fatigue and alerts being turned off. Some users have established low- and high-level alerts. The low-level alerts are seen but can be ignored versus high-level alerts that 'require action steps.'

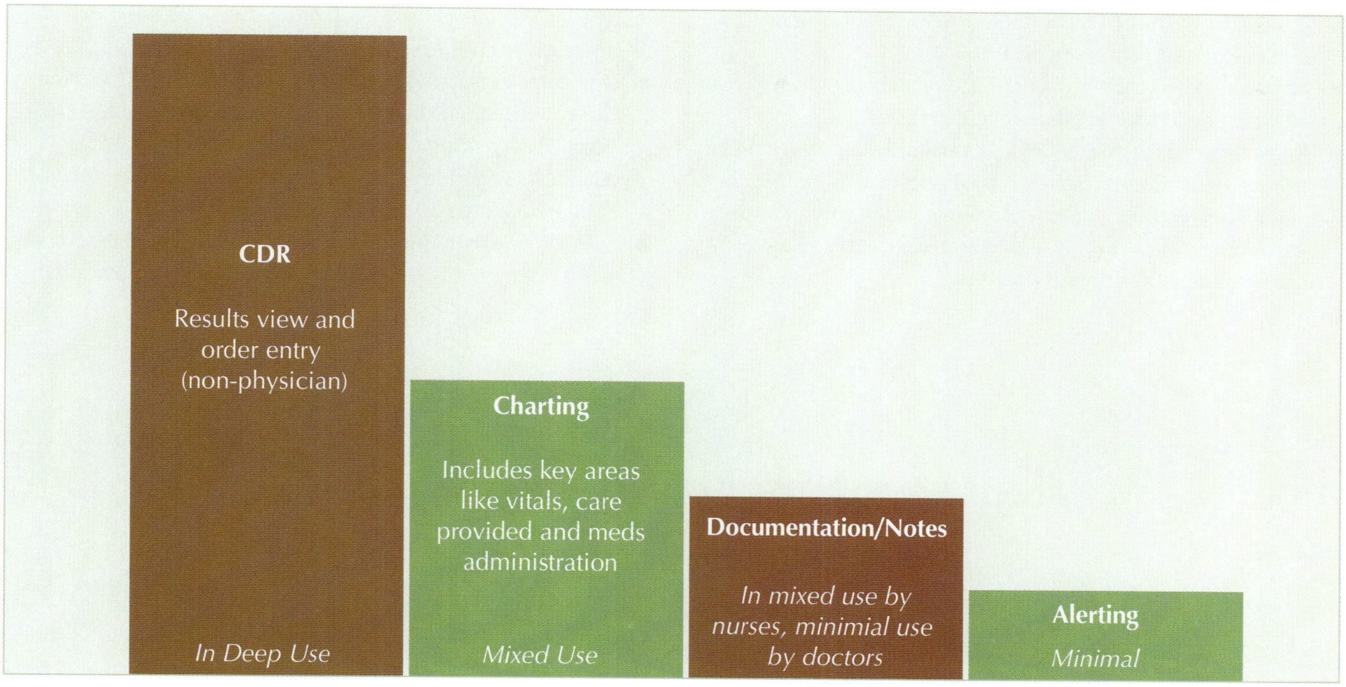

Figure 1 Usage of Healthcare Technologies

Medication Management

(Source: Medication Administration Study, September 2004) Systems and technology surrounding the area of medication management are a growing market due to the focus both of regulatory agencies and consumer groups calling for patient safety initiatives, specifically in the area of medication administration. In addition, bar code medication management (52 percent) was the No. 1-cited response by healthcare industry professionals as the most important computer application in the next two years (15th Annual HIMSS Leadership Survey sponsored by Superior Consulting).

The foundation elements to accomplish the goal of closed-loop medication ordering, alerting, administration and tracking are offered and put to use. The ability for physicians to enter all medication orders and to be notified of alerts from decision logic at the time of the medication order is generally, but not always, available. Making this environment more complex is the fact that nearly a third (31 percent) of all pharmacy orders are re-entered by the pharmacy. Access to medical or knowledge content during the ordering process, an online MAR (medication administration record) complete with all medications dispensed and positive patient ID at the time of medication administration is somewhat vendor/product-related.

Bar code technology is emerging as a solution in support of closed loop medication administration and the "Five Rights" (the right patient receiving the right medication at the right time by the right route in the right dose), laboratory specimen identification and blood verification – are based upon positive patient identification at the time the activity is conducted.

Today's performance suggests the emergence of a strong product market as the three capable of being measured scored strongly (Bridge Medical MedPoint, Siemens Med Administration Check [MAC], and McKesson Admin-Rx) and 14 others are in various stages of development and deployment (AMTSystems PatientSafe, Baxter Patient Care System, Cardinal Health, Care Fusion wCareMed, Cerner Power POC Care Mobile, Eclipsys Knowledge-Based Medication Administration, GE Centricity Admin in Motion, IntelliDOT, MDG Medical Corporation, MEDITECH BMV, Mediware, Misys CPR, Omnicell SafetyMed and QuadraMed PC Affinity Med Charting).

With the industry looking for systems and technology to increase patient safety, reduce medical errors, improve communication between pharmacy and nursing, as well as meet intense pressure for these solutions from regulatory and consumer groups, the market share is expected to grow and seriously increase as seen with the 17 vendors cited in this report. Information at a more detailed level involves:

- ICU (31 percent) and Labor & Delivery (31 percent) were the two most common areas where survey participants indicated difficulty in implementing this technology (due to the immediacy of drugs needed in both of these medical specialty areas).
- Survey participants indicated that the barrier to the ease with which nurses use the medication administration system was related to the comfort level of the user regarding PC use, not the application itself.

- The average length of medication administration system implementation was seven months.
- An organization's ADT and pharmacy vendors are chosen most often for medication administration products.
- Regarding quantifiable benefits, the majority of respondents (89 percent) indicated that increased patient safety is the "top" quantifiable benefit. Improved communication with pharmacy and nursing was a distant second at (18 percent) and better documentation was third (14 percent).

Studies indicate that physician offices are not interested in stand-alone e-prescribing systems, but are seeking an integrated EMR solution that includes one integrated database and e-prescribing functionality, including drug-to-drug and drug-to-allergy interaction checking.

Ambulatory EMR

(Source: Ambulatory EMR Report, March 2005) As expected, there has been tremendous growth in the ambulatory EMR market with hundreds of EMR vendors currently offering products to physician practices. Moving forward, we expect to see continued growth in this sector with increased competition, vendor solutions or strategies that support a wide range of physician office practice sizes (solo practitioners to large group practices), mergers and acquisitions.

As clinician awareness of the benefits of using computers (as a tool to reduce medical errors) increases, more physician offices are looking at an e-prescribing/ambulatory EMR strategy. The ambulatory EMR marketplace offers many choices to physician offices. Each vendor offers unique benefits and challenges, but success in this space will require systems to be easy to use, adaptable both to physician workflow and specialty care areas. Ambulatory EMR systems do offer a wide variety of functionality and may include storage and retrieval of patient electronic charts, histories, schedules, claims and insurance records; capture of coding data at the point of care; workflow management to streamline and eliminate redundant data collection; prescription management, including contraindications; paper document scanning; referral management; electronic orders and results-reporting capabilities; health maintenance reminders and patient education; voice and handwriting recognition capabilities; standardized clinical vocabulary; and wireless point-of-care devices (PDAs or PC tablets).

Vendors in the ambulatory market are capable of meeting the high demands of clinicians and there is evidence of adoption that exceeds that seen in the inpatient environment. Today the ambulatory EMR vendors and products being measured are in relation to physician practice size:

- Over 25 physicians (A4 HealthMatics EMR, Allscripts TouchWorks, Cerner Millennium PowerChart Office, Epic EpicCare EMR, GE Centricity Physician Office EMR, InteGreat IC Chart, LSS [Meditech] EMR, McKesson Horizon Ambulatory Care, Misys EMR and NextGen EMR);
- 6-25 physicians (A4 HealthMatics EMR, Allscripts TouchWorks, Amicore Penchart, CHARTCARE EMR, GE Centricity Physician Office EMR, Greenway PrimeSuite Chart, Misys EMR, NextGen EMR, PMSI Practice Partner EMR and WebMD Intergy EHR & OmniChart);
- 1-5 physicians (A4 HealthMatics EMR, Companion EMR, eClinicalWorks EMR, GE Centricity Physician Office EMR, Greenway PrimeSuite Chart, JMJ EncounterPRO, MediNotes Charting Plus, Misys EMR, NextGen EMR, PMSI Practice Partner EMR, VitalWorks Intuition EMR and WebMD Intergy EHR).

E-Prescribing

Studies indicate that physician offices are not interested in stand-alone e-prescribing systems, but are seeking an integrated EMR solution that includes one integrated database and e-prescribing functionality, including drug-to-drug and drug-to-allergy interaction checking (Source: E-Prescribing/Ambulatory EMR Perception Study, March 2005). In a recent study, 60 percent of survey respondents have already chosen an e-prescribing/ ambulatory EMR strategy and decision points of feature/function and sole source were the key drivers in choosing the system. Of the 40 percent of respondents who had no e-prescribing/ ambulatory EMR strategy, 43 percent indicated that 2005 will be the year to determine their strategy. The top eight e-prescribing vendors most often considered by survey respondents were: A4, Epic, GE, IDX, McKesson, Misys, NextGen and WebMD. Large physician practices are more likely to have an e-prescribing/ ambulatory EMR strategy than smaller practices. Based upon survey results, the e-prescribing/ambulatory EMR market is healthy, is growing and vendors are ready to provide systems to meet physicians' needs. ■

Accelerate the Positive Transformation Of Your Healthcare Organization

NEC

NEC Solutions America

Imagine getting more out of your technology and staff investments. Imagine an environment where physicians and clinicians are able to focus their efforts on improving care delivery. Imagine your costs reduced and under control, patient flow and physician loyalty increased. Recent studies are validating that investments in technology and workflow improvement are measurably improving patient outcomes and are leading to higher levels of performance. Higher contracted rates and increased patient throughput are a few benefits being realized by hospital systems leveraging advanced technology. NEC's Healthcare Solutions Division is integrating technology with workflow in new and innovative ways to help healthcare organizations achieve performance benefits.

NEC's healthcare solutions are designed specifically for the dynamic demands of the healthcare environment. Enterprisewide security, performance and workflow improvement drive cost reduction, increase organizational efficiency and help improve patient safety. These are some of the tangible results NEC Healthcare solutions delivers.

Improved Caregiver Efficiency

Physicians are inundated with different passwords for the myriad of software applications running today's healthcare facilities. Passwords can secure sensitive patient information, but unfortunately the frustration of password management impedes the caregiver and often ties up valuable IT resources. NEC can solve this problem, empower the caregiver and decrease IT expenditures with TouchPass – Secure Single Sign-On.

Physician adoption of new technology can make a huge difference in quality of care and workflow. Caregivers need to access patient information as quickly and accurately as possible. TouchPass enables users to use a single log-on, either by password or finger biometrics, to gain access to all enabled applications.

Coupled with TouchPass Context Management, users not only gain the benefit of single sign-on but also save time through context management. TouchPass Context Management allows applications to share information so that they appear to behave as a single system, allowing information in separate healthcare applications to be synchronized so that each individual application refers to the same patient, encounter or user. This means that when a clinician signs on to one application and selects a patient, that user's sign-on is simultaneously executed on all other applications that have been enabled, and the same patient is automatically selected in all of the applications, saving clinicians time and improving efficiency. TouchPass delivers the highest physician adoption rate.

Physician adoption of new technology can make a huge difference in quality of care and workflow.

If your organization is interested in improving performance, NEC can help you explore your options and accelerate achievement of optimum results. NEC's solutions and workflow innovations focus on key performance issues such as staff efficiencies. Examples include:

- **PersonalPass** – Automated patient ID and admissions (ADT solutions fully integrated with clinical applications);
- **Vocera Communications System** – Wireless hands-free communication (improved workflow, i.e., 15 minutes per nurse per shift time savings);
- **Disaster Recovery Fault Tolerant Solution** - Servers, recovery software and services for 100 percent run time; and
- **Performance Improvement and Process Redesign Consulting Services** (i.e., patient safety audits).

NEC understands the value of IT in healthcare. We understand the need to improve staff utilization and reduce costs. We understand the value gained from leveraging your existing IT investments. Contact us. Together we can make a positive difference. ■

NEC Solutions America, Inc. is a premier provider of integrated healthcare solutions for the connected enterprise in North America.

Tadao Kondo
President and CEO

Phil Scarfo
Senior Vice President, Public Sector and Health Care Solutions Divisions

Lauryn Jones
General Manager, Health Care Division

Yuji Ichimura
Vice President, Corporate Planning & Marketing

NEC Solutions America
2890 Scott Blvd.
Santa Clara, CA 95050
Phone 408.844.1119
Fax 408.844.1497
www.necsam.com/healthcare

Business Contact
Greg Sarrail
Director of Sales & Marketing
Healthcare Solutions Division
greg.sarrail@necsam.com

Shelly Greenhalgh
Director, Marketing Communications
Solutions Platform Group
shelly.greenhalgh@necsam.com

Technology Devices for Healthcare

In the evolving world of electronic healthcare record keeping, technology devices are the key to getting the right information to the right people at the right time.

[Sarah Danielson, Accenture] [Charles Colander, Northwestern Memorial Hospital]

Many Choices, Real Benefits

Desktops, tablet PCs, mobile laptops, computers on wheels, handheld devices – technology devices that access an EHR system provide a universe of opportunity.

Despite the real benefits these devices offer, the devil is in the details. How can a CMIO or CIO navigate the technology needs of a healthcare organization based on anticipated benefits? The challenge must be resolved between caregivers and devices. Caregivers must adapt their processes to the right devices and devices must be flexible enough to adapt to caregiver needs.

There is no "silver bullet" solution. The key to choosing appropriate devices lies in a careful assessment of the advantages and disadvantages of each device and how the devices will plug into existing systems and the greater EHR enterprise.

Improve Patient Safety

Technology devices have a role in enabling the success of critical initiatives such as clinical documentation and computerized physician order entry (CPOE). These devices can help reduce medication errors in inpatient settings and improve patient safety by adding access points to medical data, increasing the chance that clinicians will have the right patient information at their fingertips when needed.

For example, by using mobile technology devices, nurses can use the clinical system at the point of care to ensure the right medication is being administered at the right time to the right patient. Accurate recording of medication administration becomes a mere byproduct of this action. Similarly, direct CPOE provides widely cited patient safety benefits, such as immediate expert rules and other alerts for the physician to guide the ordering process in real time.

Increase Care Efficiencies

The use of technology dramatically increases care efficiencies. High-tech monitoring devices can "auto capture" information for monitoring patients. For example, critical care nurses spend most of their time monitoring the vital statistics of critically ill patients. During any one shift, they may record great quantities of patient data that are vital to their patients' well-being, a time-consuming process.

In a technology enabled healthcare environment, an IV pump can be programmed to administer medication at a certain rate. A nurse can use a handheld device to scan a bar code on the pump. The handheld is connected to the hospital's wireless network, so the handheld identifies the pump, based on the bar code, and issues a request across the network. The IV pump responds by broadcasting data back and populating a screen on the nurse's handheld device. By simply scanning the bar code on the IV pump, the caregiver instantly records a great deal of data without investing the time or encountering the potential entry errors of the manual effort.

In addition to substantial patient benefits, direct physician order entry increases efficiency because it eliminates paper and the extra steps – each with extra potential for human error – needed for medical transcription and data entry.

Increase Charge Capture

By moving to electronic charge capture, the cumbersome coding and charge entry process can be dramatically streamlined. Physicians use handheld devices to capture and wirelessly transmit professional charges from the examination area to a coding and billing support team, eliminating the paper trail. In addition, hospital technical charges can be entered into the system immedi-

Sarah Danielson is a senior manager at Accenture in the Health & Life Sciences practice. She has more than eight years of consulting experience leading large-scale and complex, multihospital clinical information system implementation projects. **Charles Colander** is the director of technology management at Northwestern Memorial Hospital and is responsible for all technical infrastructures at NMH including networking, telephony, desktop and computer services. He is currently leading significant initiatives for VoIP, wireless services and point-of-care device strategies.

ately, as a by-product of clinical documentation recorded by nurses and ancillary department technicians, reducing – if not eliminating – both the entry and payment lags.

Enhance Mobility

Handheld electronic devices enable clinical staff to carry medication reference information to the point of care. These devices are small enough to keep in pockets or on belts, leaving hands free for other duties. Information on drug indications, doses, interactions and other considerations can be downloaded to these devices for quick reference.

Many hospitals are piloting the use of handheld electronic devices linked via high-bandwidth, wireless networks to the main hospital network. As devices converge, physicians can now use a single device such as a cellular telephone, personal digital assistant or pager and an access point to the hospital network for accessing patient records. In this way, a physician could go home or on vacation and remain actively linked to hospital information.

Save Time

RFID tags, a wireless identification system, can save time in a hospital setting. By embedding them into patients' armbands when they are admitted to the hospital, the tags allow hospital and emergency personnel to track the status and exact location of patients quickly and easily. RFID, coupled with location-based services, can also be used to locate critical equipment and gear.

Ease of Use

When technology devices or processes are difficult to use, they become a barrier to the success of an overall EHR initiative. For example, physicians inputting data into a desktop workstation in patient rooms may be required to log in each time they enter a new room. Without a seamless sign-on, this step in the care-giving process becomes cumbersome, causing frustration and reversing any efficiency gains from adding the technology.

Interoperability

Interoperability among devices, applications and platforms is a huge issue, especially with the EHR initiative in its infancy. Although most applications are moving toward a Web-based infrastructure, the sheer number of applications being developed makes it difficult to link systems under a connected EHR model.

Sometimes technology devices deliver benefits but are not used by nurses or physicians due to personal preferences about how to deliver patient care.

Barriers to Success

Despite the many benefits offered by technology devices and electronic record keeping, significant barriers to success remain.

Costs

Technology devices are expensive; no hospital can afford to buy what it won't use or what will be used less than optimally. It's important to determine the devices that will clearly help physicians, nurses and other professionals. Correctly estimating the number of devices needed is also imperative. When healthcare organizations fail to accurately predict the volume of devices needed, the equipment is either underutilized or in short demand.

Ownership and Maintenance

A key decision point that influences the number of devices an institution will purchase is who owns and maintains the devices. Devices can either be owned by an individual caregiver or by a work area. When providing devices for each individual (such as a pager), responsibility falls clearly on the user. This requires the purchase of additional devices but it fully engages the caregiver in the "care and feeding" of the device. When devices are assigned to a work area, such as a nursing unit, responsibilities must be clearly outlined. Although this seems mundane, devices without owners quickly become unusable due to unreported problems, creating dissatisfaction with performance and lack of availability within the community.

For example, hospitals that embrace tablet PCs are often surprised to discover that applications that run on these devices cannot run on desktops or laptops. On the other hand, laptops and desktops are universally compatible and can share applications.

Likewise, most handheld devices require a specially coded "client" that recognizes that the limited screen size will demand a focused approach to interacting with the caregiver.

Care-Giving Preferences

Sometimes technology devices deliver benefits but are not used by nurses or physicians due to personal preferences about how to deliver patient care. For example, some clinicians do not like to be distracted by computer hardware when they are in a patient's room, as they prefer to focus attention on the person receiving their care. Alleviating the problem by moving devices to the hallway creates challenges with privacy and accuracy. Locating devices at the nursing station is next to impossible in most institutions because of the limited workspace and competing needs. The location and types of devices used must be matched to personal preferences while providing for ease of use.

Security

As more and more IT systems are converted to Web-based infrastructures, healthcare providers will continue to incur risk in exchanging health information over the Internet. Technically these problems are solvable; however, the perception of reduced security is enough to hamper the adoption of new technology devices in many organizations.

In addition, the physical location of some devices compromises the security of patient information. In some hospitals, desktop PCs are located outside patient rooms, requiring nurses to "chart" in the hallway, making it easy for patient health information to be divulged to passersby.

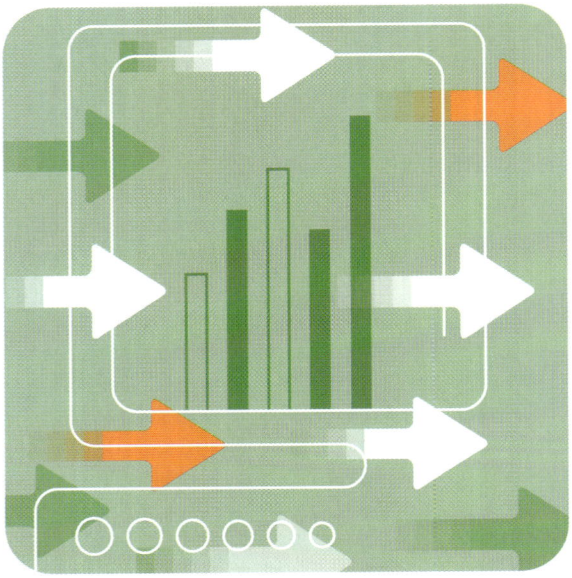

Obsolescence

Technology devices change rapidly, creating cost barriers to purchasing new equipment. The possible obsolescence of a technology device and its software should be considered as part of an organization's overall device strategy.

The Approach: Establish a Technology Device Strategy

Before investing in technology devices and software, healthcare organizations must take a conservative approach by assessing needs and creating a design for implementation. One of the most important considerations for all players must be how these devices will work in to individual EHR systems and the community EHR as a whole. Several steps and considerations are helpful for organizations that are developing a technology device strategy.

Plan for Evolving Standards

Because interoperability is a huge issue, organizations must decide which standards will be adopted as part of a technology device strategy. For example, HL7 is the leading, ANSI-accredited, international standard for data exchange among computer systems in healthcare. There are additional standards for fixed and wireless networks, operating system platforms, bar coding, security and authentication, coding and electronic health record architecture. Healthcare organizations should choose an infrastructure and devices that comply with evolving healthcare standards to minimize roadblocks and incompatibilities that might be encountered with individual EHR initiatives.

Conduct a Needs Assessment

Needs assessment is an evaluation of the functions desired from computer and networking technology or the needs the technology is expected to meet. This step helps determine exactly what devices are needed and can save hours of wasted effort and expenditures.

All players need to be considered when crafting a needs assessment. A surgical nursing unit's needs differ greatly from those of a critical care nursing unit. Likewise the billing department needs different equipment than the pharmacy. A cross-functional team of clinical professionals who will use the devices, technology specialists and EHR application specialists should form the core team for conducting the needs assessment.

After determining the types of devices needed to complement the EHR functionality, criteria should be established to guide the final decision.

Consider Usability

Consider usability when selecting devices. For example, many hospitals prefer using desktops to communicate patient information because they are relatively inexpensive and easy to use. They are, however, cumbersome in patient rooms. By developing workarounds, such as mounting the desktop on a platform affixed to the wall with an adjustable, swinging arm, nurses can access computers without adding to room clutter. In this way, hospitals make a desktop device "usable," increasing the chance it will be utilized.

Allocate for Device Footprints

Some devices are larger than others, so consider a device's footprint as part of the selection criteria. For example, many hospitals use computers on wheeled carts (COWs) to make desktop computers mobile. These devices also provide additional workspace for writing when necessary.

Address Security

Technology devices, such as laptop computers and memory chips, are valuable and are often stolen from hospitals. Some hospitals have solved this problem by chaining computer equipment to carts or workstations, but this can compromise the mobility of these devices. Healthcare organizations with expensive equipment must develop a security plan that protects technology assets without sacrificing usability.

Consider Maintenance and Upkeep Requirements

Most mobile devices use batteries so purchasing and maintaining batteries must be considered as part of a healthcare organization's workflow.

For example, if a clinic decides to equip patient rooms with mobile laptops, someone must round up all used laptop batteries at the end of a shift and ensure they are charged for the next person's use. Also many batteries have a one-year warranty, so a decision must be made up front concerning who will buy and replace them.

Support components for the devices, such as the COWs themselves, can provide just the needed fix for battery challenges and should be considered and selected together with the device. Although handy, carts take up space and a hospital must create a "corral" for its COWs so they are not left unattended and are readily available to medical staff.

Other component considerations, such as wireless capabilities integrated into the desktops or laptops, reduce the challenges of separate cards to be maintained.

Consider the Vendor

Whether purchasing desktop PCs for a nursing unit or designing applications for a laboratory, healthcare organizations should seek vendors that make these tasks easy and help choose technology equipment and software that will interoperate with the evolving EHR model.

Vendor collaboration is also a must. If physicians begin using handheld devices, they must deal with a handheld vendor and a separate company that develops handheld applications. For maximum success, both vendors must come together to help users address interoperability issues.

Finalize Selection

Once needs are assessed and criteria are established, a device fair should be scheduled to finalize the selection of specific devices. In addition to the team of experts, the user community as a whole should be invited so that usability feedback can be considered from different perspectives.

The device fair affords the opportunity to rapidly assess how a device meets needs and selection criteria. The fair should also include components such as mobile carts and adjustable, swinging arms, so devices can be assessed in the proper context.

Understanding barriers to success and addressing these concerns up front will help healthcare organizations develop the right device strategy to ensure technology helps rather than hinders practitioners.

Summary

There are many technology devices available to healthcare practitioners and the benefits they offer are real and tangible. Improved patient safety, reduced error and increased efficiency – healthcare organizations that are experimenting with new devices are achieving impressive results.

Understanding barriers to success and addressing these concerns up front will help healthcare organizations develop the right device strategy to ensure technology helps rather than hinders practitioners. In addition, the need for planning cannot be overemphasized. By assessing needs and planning for different players, evolving standards, usability, security and other factors, organizations can develop a device strategy compatible with a connected EHR.

The best strategy in device selection is to focus on functionality and results. Too many healthcare organizations become distracted by gadgetry and lose sight of the real reasons behind introducing technology – improving patient care and saving time and money. ■

Q&A With Jeff Goldsmith

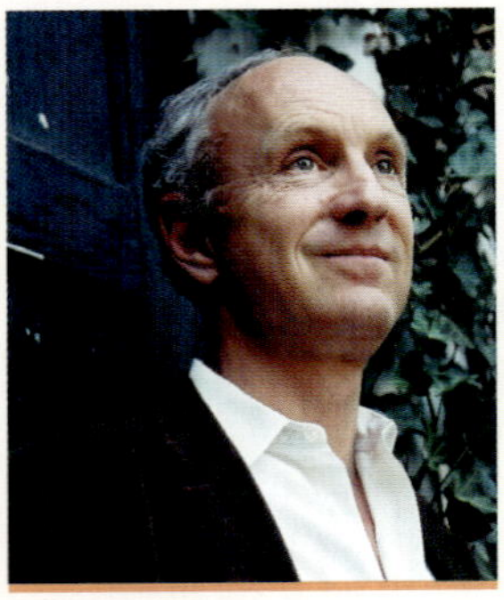

Jeff Goldsmith
President
Health Futures, Inc.

Jeff Goldsmith, Ph.D., is president of Health Futures, Inc. He lectures on healthcare technology at the Wharton School of the University of Pennsylvania. He is the author of *Digital Medicine: Implications of Healthcare Leaders* (Health Administration Press: 2003).

The author of *Digital Healthcare* describes what has not changed in healthcare in the past 30 years.

Healthcare Technology: *In your book* Digital Healthcare, *you described how the medical records were stored in the basement of the University of Chicago's hospital in 1975. What percentage of healthcare systems continue to store records like that? Do you think that in five years we'll have total adoption of EHRs?*

Jeff Goldsmith: I would say that less than 2 percent of the healthcare organizations in the U.S. of any description are paperless, if you define paperless as no paper charts and complete electronic ordering. In five years, that number may be 20 percent. I think it's going that slowly – the larger the institution, the slower it goes. It's actually a lot easier to do this from a green field than to lay an enterprise solution over dozens of poorly integrated legacy applications. The numbers that I've seen suggest that clinical information systems (CIS) spending is no more than $8.5 billion a year in the U.S., and growing at perhaps 10 percent a year. You're not going to get from that to $276 billion – which is the amount that is required – any time soon.

HCT: *Do you think we are 10 years away from total adoption of EHRs?*

JG: I think it's a lot longer than that. I understand what Dr. Brailer is doing and he's doing the right thing. It really does not make sense for the federal government to be subsidizing IT investment until the systems can talk to one another. But the reality is, it's going to cost tens of billions of dollars in federal money to get the safety net providers, the community health centers, the critical access hospitals, the large urban public hospitals and the cash-strapped primary care physicians to do this. I don't think we're anywhere close to getting this right as a society.

There's a cone of hype surrounding this effort. Inside the cone, everyone agrees on how important this is. Outside the cone, it's business as usual, and managers and clinicians are worrying about the same things they were worried about five years ago. I don't think this has penetrated very far into the consciousness of people who are actually operating healthcare institutions. I don't think this is yet the No. 1 agenda item on the minds of most health system or health claims CEOs. Twenty years looks a lot more realistic to me. It's a generation's worth of work.

HCT: *Over a year ago you published a paper in Health Affairs entitled "The Federal Health Information Policy: A Case of Arrested Development." The paper argued that federal action is needed to speed the implementation of digital CIS. How much federal action has there been, and how far along are we in the process?*

JG: Well I think the most important thing that's happening is the creation of a certification process that drives interoperability. Until you have a consensus of how you define an appropriate record system, you can't incent people to adopt it. So I think that Dr. Brailer started in the right place. The problem is, it's going to take forever to do this. And very few of the actors involved in this process really have an incentive to reach resolution quickly. To an extent, this is unavoidable. You have a $2 trillion health system that you're essentially trying to rewire while it's operating. That's the size of the entire German economy. In terms of degrees of difficulty, this is very, very difficult. So the fact that it's going to take a lot longer than ten years is as much a reflection of how vast, complicated and unwieldy our health system is as on the quality of the leadership.

HCT: *Your book discusses the roadblocks implementing a transformation, such as gaining physician support, balancing competing priorities and managing IT vendors. Which roadblock is the greatest barrier?*

JG: I would have thought it would have been physician support, but I don't think it is. I think physicians are ahead of the people running their institutions on this. If you show physicians a paperless world, a world in which they don't have to have five full-time employees in their office wrestling with medical claims, they can relate. They would really like to have the resources freed up, either to pay themselves a little more generously out of the money they're getting or to use their clinical resources for enhanced service to their patients. I think the big problem has been the inability of hospitals and health systems to allocate a sufficient amount of capital and political bandwidth to actually make this happen. I don't think this is top of mind for a significant number of CEOs. I'm not talking about the leadership at places like Kaiser or Ascension Health; these folks get it, and they're making the investments to make this happen. It's just that these places are still not the norm. I think we'll be surprised at how long it takes the investor-owned firms, who have fewer valid excuses than the nonprofits, to get there.

HCT: *Do you think that standards and privacy are two of the major barriers?*

JG: I don't think they're the big ones. I think that the generation of people running healthcare organizations is just not comfortable with information technology. I think there is still a great degree of not only skepticism but frankly fear and ignorance about the use of these tools. And I don't think CEOs really get that there's a big gap between the institutions that they're operating on a day-to-day basis and other sectors of our economy.

They ought to be embarrassed. But they're not; they're frustrated, and they blame their people, they blame their vendors, they blame Dr. Brailer, they blame the state legislature, they blame the health plans, and the health plans will blame the physicians. Blame, blame, blame. There's a lot of finger pointing going on (just like there is on patient safety). But at the root of the blaming is a fundamental failure to take ownership. It's interesting. If you look at the "big iron" companies that invested in clinical IT, such as GE and Siemens, what are they discovering? That the core businesses from which they generated capital to invest in clinical IT are actually growing significantly faster than clinical IT is. Imaging is eating IT alive. There are a lot of exciting new imaging applications – you've got the promise of molecular imaging, you're got tremendous new hardware that's coming out and for this generation of CEOs, purchasing more "big iron" is a lot easier to understand and do than buying a complex clinical IT product.

Implementing clinical IT is hard. If you do it right, everybody's cheese gets moved. It's disruptive, and yet to fundamentally improve clinical process requires disrupting existing routines and reconfiguring work flows and relationships. To do that you've got to be willing to not only understand the technology, you've got to be willing to commit yourself to working with it and working through it. And I don't think that commitment is yet there in this industry and I wish I could say otherwise.

The fundamental challenge in the book *Digital Medicine* was a call to leadership. And I'm not sure we've got that leadership yet. We need it. And it may just have to wait for a new generation of leaders that grew up with these technologies, for whom using them is as natural as breathing, before we really get that whole-hearted commitment needed. We're not making optimal use of our clinical resources. We're burning out our workforce. We're needlessly damaging patients. A lack of patience with an unsatisfactory status quo is essential to making the digital transformation happen anytime soon.

HCT: *There are some trends that could reshape the healthcare system such as consumer-directed plans and pay-for-performance. Do you think we'll continue to see more of this?*

JG: At the heart of both of those issues is changing incentives, changing the signals that are being sent to the care system, as well as to patients and their families, about what we want them to do. Here, too, I think the progress is just glacial.

At max, there are 3.5 million people right now in consumer-directed plans. In order for them to have a transformative impact on the way the healthcare system works and on the way people behave and on their own health, we need 40 million to 50 million people enrolled.

With pay-for-performance, I think it's very important to send signals that folks that adhere to clinical protocols and that listen to their patients and that are responsive to professional guidance about standards of care ought to earn more than people who don't or aren't. But if it's 2 or 3 percent, or 5 percent difference in someone's income, summed across all their payers, I don't think it's going make that much of a difference. Pay-for-performance is an area where the fragmentation of payers and the bewildering contracting maze hurts the ability to make real progress.

I think until the payment system starts saying we're not going to pay for fixing the errors, we're not going to pay for the re-admissions, we're not going to pay for the extra week that someone spent in an ICU because we gave them an infection or the wrong drugs, then the industry is not going to deal with its quality problem. I recently read an article in *JAMA* that said there has not been significant progress in reducing avoidable deaths in our hospitals in the last five years. Here, too, it's a question of ownership. Are management and boards going to own these issues? Are they actually going to take responsibility for them and change what they do on a day-to-day basis or aren't they? ■

4

The Final Centimeter: The Physician/Machine Interface

As more and more physicians get comfortable with the technology, peer pressure is providing momentum to accelerate the move to an electronic environment for technophiles and technophobes alike.

[Manuel Lowenhaupt, M.D., Accenture] [James R. Lynch, R.N., M.B.A., INTEGRIS]

Introduction

Building a clinical information system (CIS), especially as an instrument for integrating a hospital's clinical and financial functions with each patient's EHR, looms as a task for most healthcare providers. A vital consideration in implementing these costly and complex systems is how to get physicians to use them. A great deal of thought and discussion currently centers around establishing a flexible server-peer structure, a robust database architecture, and standardized communication protocols; but experience has shown that, very often, not enough thought or planning goes into providing a usable interface between the computer and the person who must use it.

The following case study of an EHR implementation was undertaken by a leading private practice health system in the Southwest. The "bumps in the road" experienced by this 13-hospital health system, and the lessons learned while traversing them, provide an instructive lesson in how to approach the physician/machine interface.

The Bumpy Journey

The project undertook implementing information system automation and clinical decision support at one of the health system's largest facilities. This major transformation project included hundreds of hours of consulting time to re-think and re-design clinical processes. The first deliverable was an online admission history and physical assessment form for deployment in inpatient nursing units. The second deliverable, 13 months later, included major transformations of processes from printed charts and reports to online documentation, including medication administration and post-discharge scanning of all remaining paper documents. Physicians were required to provide an electronic signature for all medical records. The elimination of as many paper documents as possible was established as a major system benefit. The strategic plan called for all clinical users to view clinical results online. The plan also established a direction toward computerized physician order entry (CPOE), evidence-based practice guidelines and further conversion of clinical documents to electronic records.

Bump No. 1: Lack of Physician Involvement

From the beginning, physicians were resistant to the idea of computerizing their cherished paper charts. There was little involvement of physicians in making critical decisions. Training was another challenge. Nurses are difficult to free from their responsibilities for formal training. The hospital's all-private physician staff has multiple demands on their time and a strong distaste for classroom-style instruction. Efforts to deliver personalized training to each physician were met with reactions ranging from indifference to outright avoidance. Although the hospital had established that physician training to use the electronic signature application was mandatory, only 15 percent of the active staff received training prior to the system's go-live date.

Predictably, when the system went live, physicians reacted poorly to what they saw as a worse-than-useless administrative albatross and nefarious government plot. They felt the EHR implementation was an injustice being done to them rather than

Manuel Lowenhaupt, M.D., is a partner with Accenture and the national practice leader for clinical transformation. He is internationally noted for his work in clinical effectiveness, care management and clinical informatics, with experience in organizations in the U.S., Canada, Europe and the Far East. He received his undergraduate degree, Phi Beta Kappa, from M.I.T. and his medical degree from Harvard Medical School.
James Lynch, R.N., M.B.A., is director of applications for INTEGRIS Health, Oklahoma's largest healthcare organization. Mr. Lynch and his team are responsible for the implementation and support of all clinical, business and infrastructure applications. He received his B.S. degree in nursing from the University of New Mexico, and his M.B.A. from the University of Phoenix.

a clinical tool they had a part in designing. Worse, the physicians as a group dug in their heels and refused to use the new system. The hospital had a hard time understanding their opposition, in part because there was little interaction with them as the system was being implemented. The lesson learned was that re-designing, integrating, and automating clinical processes and workflow is less a technical journey controlled by IT professionals than it is a social and cultural journey that needs strong user champions led by physicians. Decision makers quickly decided that they needed to take a step back and listen to physicians' complaints rather than continuing to enforce a solution that caused more problems than it solved.

Bump No. 2: Too Much to Learn

With support materials such as instructional mouse pads, posters and pocket guides, most physicians were able to master the basics of signing a medical document online. However, accessing and viewing clinical results online, or placing orders for tests or treatment, proved too complicated for most physicians. They complained of a too-complex user interface, a dearth of user-determined options, and too few available devices. The hospital realized that its expectations of what could be achieved with technology alone were unrealistic. The system's technical barriers were tolerated by physicians who were experienced, sophisticated computer users, but novice computer users who happened to be good doctors suddenly found the EHR implementation to be a huge impediment to caring for their patients. Those who made enough noise or complained to the right people were able to opt out of using the system altogether, going back to the paper documents with which they were comfortable.

Bump No. 3: Too Much Security

Information is never more secure than when nobody uses it. Physicians were discouraged by a time-consuming and unfriendly security environment. Users had to log in first to the network, then into individual applications. Waiting 45 seconds to get to any useful information poses a big imposition on busy doctors, especially since they typically log in for each patient interaction – perhaps dozens of times per day. Reducing the time and effort to log in to just a few seconds has helped to improve physician acceptance of the clinical information system.

Smoothing the Bumps in the Road

Physician involvement that was lacking in the original implementation – in identifying common concerns and suggesting improvements and customizations to the clinical information systems – is now the responsibility of a standing committee, whose ongoing efforts are coordinated by a soon-to-be-full-time medical informatics specialist. Changes applied to the system as a result of this committee include custom screen views, organization of information flow, and global options settings. Realizing that the EHR implementation as originally conceived was not gaining physician acceptance, the hospital decided to take a more evolutionary approach to adoption of clinical information technology. Physicians are no longer required to use laptops or workstations to access the hospital's information network. Each physician has been issued a wireless "rounding tool," a handheld PDA. Custom screen views allow physicians to access and review clinical and financial information, including a patient list, laboratory results, transcribed reports, limited nursing documentation such as vital signs and intake and output data, basic patient demographics, and insurance carrier and policy data. Physicians download the data to their personal devices wirelessly through a traditional infrared synchronization station, a wireless Ethernet connection, or their cellular-based Internet service.

The data they receive are for viewing purposes only – physicians cannot send any information or transmit an interaction back to the computer system. Even though the PDAs lack the ability to store or display large amounts of data, don't permit two-way communication and lack the broader and more sophisticated range of functions required for CPOE, they represent a first step towards an electronic clinical information system and have proved to be just what the doctors ordered. As physicians get more experience using the PDAs, they gain a better appreciation of the value of electronic clinical information. Already, physicians are requesting training on the core system, and they're beginning to show wider acceptance of the clinical information tools they were recently so eager to burn and bury.

Already, physicians are requesting training on the core system, and they're beginning to show wider acceptance of the clinical information tools they were recently so eager to burn and bury.

Design Principles

It's important to realize that enhancing physician acceptance of this hospital's EHR implementation had nothing to do with altering the basic information system itself. All the data elements, all the storage and communication processes with which the physicians happily interact on their PDAs are the same as those in the original system they reviled. The difference is in the design of the physician/machine interface – how information traverses the final centimeter between circuit and synapse.

Fundamental Attributes

Certain attributes of an electronic information environment make it fundamentally different from a paper-based information environment. In a computer, input and output are no longer coupled. Though the physician may enter data though one interface, such as a keyboard, the information may be displayed in an entirely different format, layout, sequence and structure. There's great power in decoupling input from output. Clinicians type lab tests or scan radiology results into the system, but the physician is likely to see that same information in a completely different structure or context.

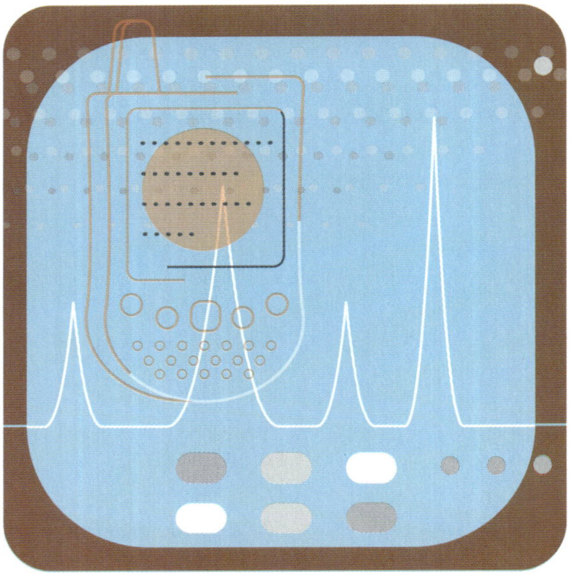

Decoupling input from output permits interface automation, the ability to customize a data display to present information in a way most useful to a person's role. For example, one of the early constructive criticisms of this hospital's interface was that physicians found that the way data were displayed – their sequence and placement on the screen – made it difficult to dictate a discharge summary. Information was awkwardly placed, and physicians had to search around for the data they needed. To solve this complaint, programmers redesigned some of the display screens so that physicians could easily dictate a discharge summary simply by scrolling down a list of data that were more conveniently displayed.

Physicians, clinicians, clerical and administrative staff, and others can access different levels of information in a variety of ways – some intuitive enough to require minimal training, others requiring significant time and effort to learn the system's more advanced functions and capabilities.

Visual Design Should be Simple, and Reflect the Importance of Displayed Functions

Good interface design makes use of color, font size and other visual differentiators to emphasize the most critical elements of information in a display. For example, abnormal lab values may be highlighted in red, high-priority messages may flash, and completed encounters are often shown in gray. Visual design is also highly dependent on the capabilities of the interface itself. For instance, a good interface for a particular process displayed on a laptop screen would be impractical or impossible to display on a PDA.

Whatever the type of display, effective use of the screen real estate is important. Screen design should be simple and elegant, showing only what is critical to the functional purpose of the current interface page. It's important to strike the right balance between completeness of data and an overwhelming list of largely unreadable data. Distractions such as superfluous design elements need to be minimized to keep the user focused on the data. Compressing a huge amount of eye-wearying data onto a single screen increases the risk that a physician will miss critical elements.

Help Users Get to the Information They Need as Fast as Possible.

A well-designed user interface displays the most-needed data at the most immediate level. If a physician uses a particular function 80 percent of the time, that physician should be taken to that screen immediately after login. The user interface is what determines whether particular data are deeply embedded, requiring numerous mouse clicks and menus to access them, or whether they are easily accessed with a few clicks or keystrokes.

Documentation by Exception

The use of templates and defaults greatly speeds up interactions with information systems. The ability to use templates in generating clinical notes and defaults in placing orders saves an enormous amount of time, especially for the mediocre typist. A busy doctor can zip through templates and defaults, quickly completing many clerical and clinical transactions. However, the programmer's good intentions in saving physician's time and typing can also set them up for trouble if they forget to read what's in the template. In documenting a medical exam, for instance, it's easy to zip down the list, checking off items that weren't actually examined. In placing orders, templates make it easy for doctors to quickly check off items in an order set and end up ordering items that are either unintended or duplicative. Tricks like adding a stopper such as "Is the patient currently breathing?" to a long list of conditions likely to have a checkmark in the "No" column annoys doctors. One suggestion that works is to move around elements of the interface every six months or so. This forces physicians to slow down enough to be more careful in their selections.

Mass Customization

Most information systems are used by multiple constituencies and so need interfaces customized for each of them. Different types of users, and users with different access privileges and levels of computer expertise, must have different ways of interacting with the system:

- User capabilities: novice vs. expert;
- User level: physician vs. R.N.; and
- User focus: primary care M.D. vs. surgeon.

Each has different needs in terms of interface design and accessibility to information.

Familiarity vs. Function

Sometimes, it's useful to design an interface to resemble what newer users are used to seeing in an older medium. Interfaces that use manila folder tabs or other design elements to resemble a paper chart can help computer novices become more at ease in the electronic medium. However, extensive or prolonged use of interfaces that mimic paper charts can diminish the power of an electronic interface by blocking its ability to use capabilities that have no paper analogue, such as menu-driven (tiered) logic or hyperlinked text, or ignore more efficient structures for data presentation. At each step in implementing a clinical information system, the design of interfaces must be driven by the needs of the clinical processes they support, not the other way around. Maintaining a legacy look and feel to interfaces often subverts this basic design principle.

Different types of users, and users with different access privileges and levels of computer expertise, must have different ways of interacting with the system.

Conclusion

No clinical information system will achieve the goals expected for it unless the physicians use it. Gaining their acceptance in this case study has been a result of designing the final centimeter – the physician/machine interface – so that the computer is perceived by physicians as an ally, not as an onerous intrusion, to their ability to provide better patient care and to get their work done.

The hospital realizes that reaping the full value of an EHR implementation and its capabilities for computerized order entry, enhanced compliance with evidence-based medical practices and other clinical and financial benefits, requires that physicians eventually transition from the PDAs to a system more like the one originally envisioned.

All physicians are now routinely using PDAs to access and review significant but limited sets of clinical and patient demographic data. For some physicians, the PDAs represent a wholly satisfactory alternative to more comprehensive and powerful electronic interactions. Getting this faction to move on from their PDAs to more sophisticated and interactive tools may prove more difficult than coming to terms with their original resistance. ■

References

Amit X, Garg, Neill K, Adhikari J, McDonald H, Rosas-Arellano M. Patricia, Deveraux PJ, Beyene J, Sam Justina, Haynes R. Brian. "Effects of Computerized Clinical Decision Support Systems on Practitioner Performance and Patient Outcomes: A Systematic Review." JAMA. *2005;293:1223-1238.*

Wears RL, Berg M. Computer Technology and Clinical Work: "Still Waiting for Godot." JAMA. *2005;293:1261-1263.*

Koppel R, Metlay Joshua P, Cohen Abigail, Abaluch Brian, Localio A. Russell, Kimmel Stephen E, Strom Brian L Role of Computerized "Physician Order Entry Systems in Facilitating Medication Errors." JAMA. *2005;293:1197-1203.*

Note: *This paper was first published in the 2005 AHIMA Convention Proceedings*

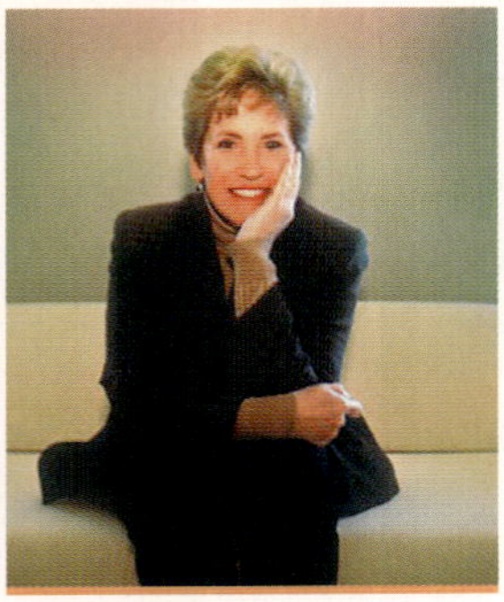

Molly Joel Coye
CEO
Health Technology Center

Molly Joel Coye, M.D., M.P.H., is the founder and CEO of the Health Technology Center (HealthTech), a not-for-profit research organization dedicated to advancing the use of beneficial technologies for healthier communities. Prior to HealthTech, she served as health director for two states, executive in health delivery system and health software development firm and advisor to investors in emerging healthcare technologies.

Q&A With Dr. Molly Joel Coye

In terms of general adoption of EHRs, providers with low margins will need help with financing the first two to three years.

Healthcare Technology: *Can you tell us a little bit about San Francisco's Health Tech?*

Molly Joel Coye: HealthTech forecasts emerging technologies in biotech, pharma, IT and medical devices; that includes the timing of market entry, the nature of the products and services that will be offered and the potential impact and consideration in strategic planning for hospital-based delivery systems and health plan and federal agencies.

HCT: *Is the lack of data standards the key obstacle to adoption?*

MJC: I think that the lack of data standards is a key obstacle, a critical obstacle. But establishing data standards is like laying railroad tracks: You also need support for the investment for physicians because it's not in the economic interest of a solo or small group practice to pay for an EHR. And you have to establish actual IT connectivity systems. This is what David Brailer is working on for the NHIN national network.

HCT: *How do you think we can go about securing physician adoption?*

MJC: For adoption of EHRs in large groups and IPAs (independent practice associations), pay for performance is probably almost enough incentive. Although uptake will still be slow, pay for performance allows them to submit data on their performance and to collect incentive payments for this, covering part of the cost of the IT needed to do the reporting. Indirectly, it allows them to earn some extra money to pay for their investment. Looser IPAs, ones that are not bound as a single business entity, and small groups and solo practitioners will need economic incentives on a pretty significant scale. The best estimates are that it will cost approximately $25,000 a year for two to three years for the initial capital investment and for the operating losses during the transition period and for incentives to make the whole thing worthwhile for physicians.

We need data standards, and vendors that produce products certified for those standards so that physicians can know that products they purchase will operate using the data standards – and will actually exchange data with other systems. In terms of more general adoption of EHRs, you have to include nursing homes, healthcare agencies and other major provider groups beyond hospitals and physicians. In that larger world, safety net providers and those with very low margins will need some economic help in the financing, and all of them need help at least in the first two or three years. MedPAC voted in January as a recommendation to Congress that Medicare should pay for the use of IT for the first couple of years to get the capacity in place.

HCT: *Do you think security is a barrier?*

MJC: No, too many groups have fully adopted medical records in place and functioning well for that to be a serious barrier.

HCT: *What do you think is on the horizon in the next five years?*

MJC: For large medical groups, I suspect that at the end of five years they will be at the 80/20 rule, where 80 percent of them will have EHRs. A subset of IPAs that are close-knit economic entities will also have installed EHRs. We need to change the national leadership agenda to include more financing assistance for small group physicians – I think that you will only be at around 40 percent at the end of five years. ■

5

Increasing Efficiency & Performance

Once an organization establishes measurable clinical objectives, systems can help determine performance against defined benchmarks and track progress. The increased standardization and documentation improves the efficiency of clinical and administrative teams by increasing the accuracy of patient information, reducing turnaround time for care delivery, enabling real-time access to information, and increasing patient throughput and volume.

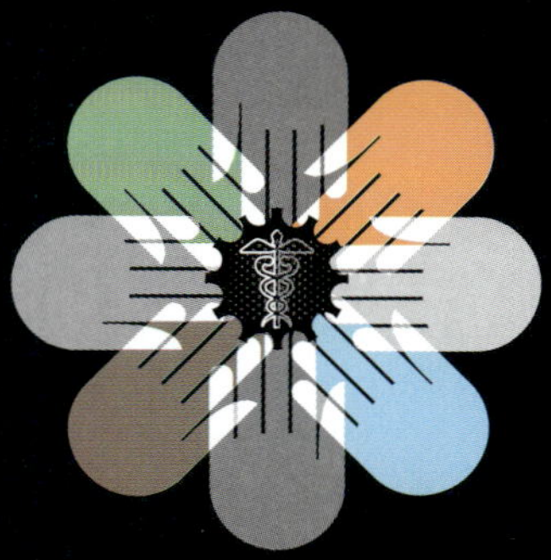

Claims Management and Legacy Integration

To strengthen the connections between patient systems and payer claim systems, healthcare organizations need to integrate their technologies by modernizing their legacy systems.

[Rick McNabb, Accenture]

In most provider offices today, the patient accounting system is the beginning of the electronic healthcare transaction. When patients arrive, their information is automatically entered or updated in the provider's patient accounting system. Physician notes on the patient's examination are reviewed by an assistant who turns key aspects of the patient's visit into a claim (e.g., clinical and financial information), which is then transmitted via the accounting system to the payer for reimbursement.

Currently information flows between the provider and the payer as claimable events. When a claim is created, only then is clinical and financial information sent to the payer.

Because insurance companies now require more detailed information for claims processing, transposition and interpretative errors are more likely to occur between the provider's chart reviews and data entry, and the payer's claim coding standards. The provider's administrative staff can cut corners to save time and avoid hassles, or code claims that favor the patient's benefits.

Due to the lack of integration between payers' and providers' systems, the quality and transmission of information is less than desirable. Payers spend too much time assessing claim submissions, providers aren't compensated as rapidly as they'd like and patients often can't make prompt or informed decisions about their care.

Bringing Technology to the Point of Care

Electronic integration can minimize these flaws. By improving the links among the EHR, patient accounting and the payer systems, information events can be created based on patient health events instead of merely financial events. A claim can be automatically populated with the correct data, resulting in a higher-quality, more timely flow of information. Payers and providers both can reduce administrative costs and errors and optimize patient care.

Payers and providers can strengthen the connections to each other's systems by upgrading the technology used within their own organizations. The reality, however, is that most companies have made considerable investments in their legacy systems, and the costs incurred from those installations will prevent many of them from purchasing entirely new systems. Very few establishments, if any, have the internal resources to create their own systems. In order to achieve legacy integration, this leaves most organizations with the only option of modernizing their legacy systems.

Healthcare providers are becoming more aware that system upgrades will soon be a necessity instead of a consideration. The Bush administration has set an ambitious goal of ensuring every American has an accessible EHR on a nationwide network within the next 10 years. It wants the healthcare industry to adopt technologies that deliver information to the point of care, especially by investing in EHR systems. The desired result, an interoperable health information infrastructure, will enable records to follow patients, clinicians to have access to information when decisions are being made and patients to become more involved in their own health decisions. This mandate, driven by the federal government's size and position as a healthcare provider and purchaser, will accelerate industry's adoption of information technology.

Opportunities for Improvement

By strengthening the connections between the EHR, patient accounting and payer systems, payers and providers can meet the government's mandate. As the quality and timeliness of data improve, new options for customer service and care delivery will also emerge, including:

- Explanation of benefits and an adjudicated claim at the point of care;

Rick McNabb is a partner in Accenture's Health & Life Science practice. He specializes in large transformation initiatives for healthcare operations, specifically large payer organizations. His focus has been creating and successfully implementing high-value/high-risk innovation ideas to the industry via technology enablement, process re-engineering and organizational change initiatives.

- Predetermination intelligence to assist the provider and patient when they make financial and clinical choices; the physician can view the patient's EHR and benefits to advise on available benefit options, drug formulary, preauthorization requirements and care delivery options; and
- Better self-service options for all stakeholders.

An ideal model to follow is similar to "e-prescription" solutions. Today the pharmaceutical business vies to obtain constant feedback on data generated from patient prescriptions. In a typical e-prescription situation, the provider enters a suggested prescription for arthritis into a handheld computer. In seconds, the computer screen displays the leading brand-name prescription's cost at $40, and the generic version's cost as half the price. The real-time information gives both the provider and patient real-time access to information that allows them to make intelligent choices involving both cost and care based on the patient's benefit plan.

Implications of Legacy Modernization

Historically at odds with each other, payers and providers will become more intertwined on the operations level and will benefit from the closer relationship. Payers will be more agreeable to compensate providers for higher-quality data. They will order end-to-end transactions, giving providers more incentives to contract with them and share the same automated systems. With updated legacy systems, the provider office will need less manual intervention and, therefore, less administrative support to maintain its reimbursement processes.

Because payers hold the most financial capital, they will be most responsible for legacy modernization. But they will reap the most benefits from an automated loop of information, which support improved medical outcomes and allows provider and payers to simplify their coding and reimbursement processes. The Bush administration's mandate means that quality of health information will become more critical during the next five to 10 years. As a primary stakeholder with the extensive repositories of data that can provide statistical outcomes on medical results, the payer will enjoy higher value-added propositions. If procedures have better statistical and financial outcomes, providers will become more dependent on payers to gain access to the data.

Successful Legacy Implementation

In recent years, legacy modernization has provided the most cost-effective approach for payers. Legacy modernization accords lower costs and higher comfort zones for payers with definitive levels of risk. By modernizing existing systems, companies have been able to reduce their information technology costs by 20 to 40 percent.

Healthcare leaders must resist the temptation to view healthcare records as an unconnected entity. Instead, they must take a more organic view and consider how their records will integrate with existing business processes.

A payer selecting an outside vendor should first evaluate its own technical strengths and weaknesses, and then select a vendor based on how the collaboration can improve its overall system. Then it must be willing to commit adequate funds. But simply throwing money at the vendor – paying generous fees without assessing the vendor's technological competencies and deficiencies beforehand – will likely be throwing money away.

Every successful innovation requires both leaders and followers. Leaders will take the risk and reap the early benefits, while the risk-averse will move forward at a later date when standards are determined and end results are a fixed outcome. Payers and providers have historically lagged behind in legacy integration because they have lacked a financial incentive. But now, with Europe taking the lead on the EHR initiative and the federal government becoming more intent on redefining the healthcare delivery problem, linking health records will soon be critical to the financial success both of payers and providers, instead of a selective option.

The Real-Time Conclusion

How can the payer world move forward? They must upgrade to real-time systems that record and utilize EHRs within the provider's accounting structures and the payer's own information databases. The ideal scenario of the future has a patient receiving an explanation of health benefits from the insurer while still in the provider's office. Each stakeholder will make intelligent use of real-time data – payers can interpret it, providers can use it to advise patients, and patients can use it to make reasoned care and financial choices.

The process of technological modernization involves considerable costs, not the least of which is the risk of early entry while standards are evolving – and the potential cost of retooling the system. No one wants to be the guinea pig when enforcement of electronic standards is still being debated. In other countries, nationalized care is modernizing healthcare systems to make electronic automation the status quo, albeit with government funding. But as the Bush administration moves forward on its plan for EHR nationwide, the for-profit healthcare industry must eventually upgrade its technology to account for real-time management of patient information. In the long term however, modernizing technology – most likely legacy integration – will reward the parties involved, with lower costs, higher-quality data, decreased errors, improved clinical and business work-flow processes and superior patient care and outcomes. ■

weblink

In the future, physicians will translate medical knowledge into consistent action in "Using EHRs to Reduce Practice Variation."

Utilizing Credit Scoring to Predict Patient Outcomes

One of the greatest challenges in predicting Medicaid eligibility is estimating the core components that are required to qualify patients.

[Tony Martin, Equifax]

In "Top Issues Confronting Hospitals, 2004," a research survey by the American College of Healthcare Executives, 480 CEOs responded to rank their three most pressing issues affecting their hospitals. Financial challenges was the most pressing, with 71 percent listing it in their top three, and within these challenges, Medicaid (78 percent) and bad debt (72 percent) were identified as the most specific concerns.

Medicaid is a concern because funding at the state level is being cut and Medicaid usage by patients has been on the rise since 1984. This trend creates a difficult situation for healthcare providers and chaos for the agencies that are charged with processing claims and verifying eligibility. For the providers, assigning resources to verify eligibility can be a taxing proposition since contact with the patient is needed to obtain the appropriate documentation required by the servicing agencies.

For a healthcare CFO, managing the hospital's bad debt is a constant challenge. Since a CFO's main responsibility is the financial health of its hospital, limiting the levels of bad debt is critical. These CFOs are challenged by multiple receivable factors such as managed care contracts, Medicare and Medicaid, but what keeps many up at night is caring for the uninsured and underinsured patient populations. By law, providers can't control who enters their facility and therefore can't contain their level of exposure.

Challenges in Predicting Medicaid Eligibility

One of the greatest challenges in predicting Medicaid eligibility is estimating the core components that are required to qualify the patient. The Medicaid eligibility guidelines are a sliding scale of household income by number of household members. The problem stems from finding reliable and proven sources of income and the number of household members. Currently there are two ways to obtain income information without contacting the patient. The first is through a demographic data provider that has household income as part of their deliverables. The second is through some form of an income prediction tool that includes either credit attributes, demographic attributes or both.

The problems with obtaining household income from a demographic source are hit rates (many demographic variables are sparsely populated), and the information contained is reported by consumers but not verified. While this is OK for marketing and other efforts where generalities are accepted, it cannot be utilized as a benchmark for decisioning.

Income prediction scores utilize regression techniques to find correlations between attributes from the data source and the income to create an algorithm or output that equates to a predicted income. These tools can be flawed if the income being modeled is reported versus verified income since we are attempting to predict the actual income. An example of the difference between reported and verified income is where a clerk verbally takes the word of the patient about income (reported) versus actually receiving a pay stub or tax record (verified) as proof of income. The other challenge in utilizing an income prediction score is in validating the score against verified income to ensure its accuracy.

As with utilizing demographic information for household income, the same holds true for utilizing demographic data for household size. In a recent test, we found in most of the patients being analyzed (greater than 60 percent), the number-of-household attribute was missing. Again if a provider is going to utilize an outside data source to assist in assigning resources, the predictive variables driving its decision strategy must be populated in the majority of cases.

Tony Martin is a consultant within Equifax Predictive Sciences, the modeling and analytical division, and has been with Equifax for over 10 years. He has consulted on many projects in the financial, insurance and healthcare industries, including custom analytics, risk and marketing custom models and generic scoring solutions.

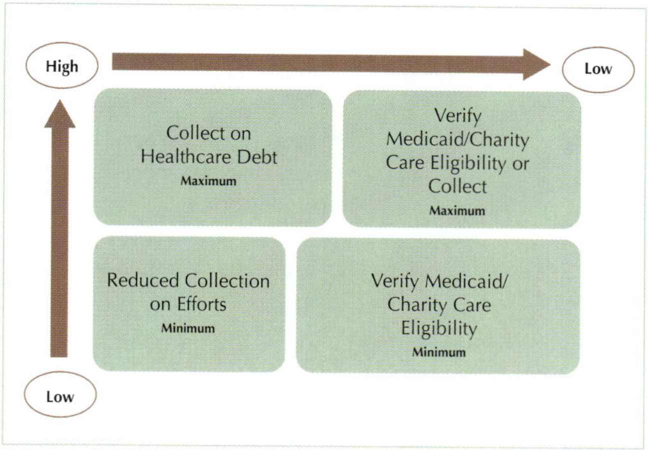

Figure 1 A Work Flow of Providers

The Hypothesis

Taking into consideration the providers' concerns and the challenges of predicting actual income, Equifax Predictive Sciences began to create a hypothesis. If proven correct, this hypothesis could assist providers in not only identifying which population has the highest probability of Medicaid eligibility but could also identify the population most likely to pay their healthcare obligations. This hypothesis was developed after multiple tests and strategies proved that credit scoring, specifically Equifax's Payment Predictor Healthcare score, does work in segmenting the self-pay population most likely to pay versus the population less likely to pay their balances.

The hypothesis: Combining the Equifax Payment Predictor Healthcare score with the Equifax Income Predictor® score to create a workflow for providers will enable them to effectively assign resources to a predicted outcome. The work flow is illustrated in Figure 1.

Figure 1 visually represents that if our hypothesis is correct, a provider would use the two scores in the following manner:

- Higher credit score combined with higher income prediction = maximum collection efforts.
- Low credit score combined with low income prediction = minimum collection efforts and attempt to verify household income and number in household to qualify for Medicaid or Charity Care.
- Higher credit score combined with lower income prediction = first attempt to collect on the debt, but take an approach that allows the patient the opportunity to submit verified data to qualify for Medicaid or Charity Care.
- Low credit score combined with higher income prediction = minimum collection efforts.

There is a significant advantage to proving this hypothesis versus utilizing a straight Medicaid/Charity Care prediction tool. We are attempting to remove the inadequacies with the data elements and are creating a solution that provides workflow strategies that tackle both bad debt and Medicaid issues for the provider.

The Analysis

To test our hypothesis, we needed to obtain data from providers where the Medicaid eligibility had been verified. Additionally, recreating the decisioning period was critical and could be accomplished by utilizing Equifax's archived database. Equifax archives its credit database on a monthly basis and for analysis purposes, our Predictive Sciences group can obtain credit scores and attributes at the point of service to analyze how predictive metrics would have worked had they been used at the historical point in time.

The first test performed was on a data set provided by a third-party collector of bad debt and provided the first supporting evidence that our hypothesis was correct. The collector provided a data set containing self-pay accounts, patient payment and balance information and verified Medicaid accounts. We appended our Payment Predictor Healthcare score and Income Predictor Score at the date of service points for the patients and matched that to the collector's outcome data to arrive at the calculations in Figure 2.

	Strategy A Collect	Strategy B Collect/Medicaid	Strategy C Medicaid	Strategy D Mail/WO	Strategy B&C
% Total Population	29.91%	18.67%	47.76%	3.67%	66.43%
% Number Payment	71.51%	10.92%	15.42%	2.15%	26.34%
% Medicaid Eligible	5.83%	20.87%	69.42%	3.88%	90.29%

- Strategy A = High credit score & higher income prediction (29.91% of the scored population, 71.51% of the patients that paid their obligations and less than 6% of the Medicaid-eligible accounts were captured in this population)
- Strategy B = High credit score & lower income prediction (18.67% of the scored population, 10.92% of the patients that paid their obligations and 20.87% of the Medicaid-eligible accounts were captured in this population)
- Strategy C = Lower credit score & lower income prediction (47.76% of the scored population, 15.42% of the patients that paid their obligations and 69.42% of the Medicaid-eligible accounts were captured in this population)
- Strategy D = Lower credit score & higher income prediction (3.67% of the scored population, 2.15% of the patients that paid their obligations and 3.88% of the Medicaid-eligible accounts were captured in this population

Figure 2 The Dual Score Strategy

Utilizing Credit Scoring to Predict Patient Outcomes

	Strategy A	Strategy B	Strategy C	Strategy D
Total Population	18%	28%	50%	4%
Number Payment	45%	37%	17%	1%
Number Amount Collected	50%	34%	15%	1%
Number Medicaid Eligible	5%	21%	71%	3%

- Strategy A = High credit score & higher income prediction (18% of the scored population, 45% of the patients that paid their obligations, 50% of collected dollars and 5% of the Medicaid-eligible accounts were captured in this population)
- Strategy B = High credit score & lower income prediction (28% of the scored population, 37% of the patients that paid their obligations, 34% of collected dollars and 21% of the Medicaid-eligible accounts were captured in this population)
- Strategy C = Lower credit score & lower income prediction (50% of the scored population, 17% of the patients that paid their obligations, 15% of collected dollars and 71% of the Medicaid-eligible accounts were captured in this population)
- Strategy D = Lower credit score & higher income prediction (4% of the scored population, 1% of the patients that paid their obligations, 1% of collected dollars and 3% of the Medicaid-eligible accounts were captured in this population)

Figure 3 Proving the Dual Score Strategy

To summarize the results, we found that the dual score strategy clearly identified the population on which to collect (Strategies A & B), the population on which to work Medicaid eligibility (Strategies B & C) and the population on which to perform minimal collection efforts (Strategies C & D).

While these results supported our original hypothesis, we felt the originating source, the third-party collector on bad debt accounts, restricted our story. We wanted to demonstrate the full benefit by testing it in the early-out environment. Therefore, we partnered with a large mid-Atlantic regional provider and obtained our second data set. Again we obtained a data set containing self-pay accounts, patient payment, balance information and verified Medicaid accounts with a date of service that covered a period of six months (July – December, 2004). We again utilized our historical archived credit database and appended our Payment Predictor healthcare score and Income Predictor score at the date of service points for the patients and matched that to the provider's outcome data to arrive at the data in Figure 3.

The results show that had this provider utilized the strategies described above, they would have maximized collection efforts on 46 percent of their population, which would have netted 84 percent of their patient collected dollars. Likewise, had they applied more discovery collection calls on the Strategy B population and verification calls on their Strategy C population, they would have identified 92 percent of their Medicaid-eligible population.

The provider in this example is currently testing these findings, and their results will be used as a case study later this year. Based on the fact that the hypothesis has held up in two different testing environments, we believe we have proven our original hypothesis and support this initiative on a going-forward basis.

Summary

Today's C-level executives are concerned with the level of exposure that caring for the uninsured and underinsured populations brings to their facilities. These executives need ways to service this population without finding themselves on the front page of newspapers for their collection tactics.

After two separate tests at different points in the revenue cycle, Equifax Predictive Sciences proved that combining our industry-specific Payment Predictor Healthcare score with our Income Predictor score could identify which populations a provider should collect on and which populations they should work as Medicaid/ Charity Care eligible. Providers should feel confident in moving forward with a scoring strategy to prioritize their efforts.

There are many healthcare vendors attempting to meet the Medicaid/ Charity Care-identification needs of providers but who may find growing pains without sound analytics behind their product offering. Our hypothesis was developed in the fourth quarter of 2004 but was not released publicly until sound analytical data supported our beliefs. This is the foundation on which our Equifax Predictive Sciences group has been built and on what it will continue to operate.

Background

In December 2003, Equifax Predictive Sciences released a research paper titled "The Unique Credit Characteristics of Healthcare Patients," in which a correlation was drawn between healthcare payment performance and overall credit payment performance. As a follow-up to that paper, Equifax Predictive Sciences utilized its research and development around multiple projects to summarize its hypothesis and findings with regard to utilizing credit scoring to predict patient outcomes. ■

Improving Your Revenue Cycle Performance Through Financial Management Solutions

EQUIFAX

Equifax Information Services LLC has been in the business of helping multiple industries improve their financial performance for more than 100 years. Working diligently over the past several years, we have successfully addressed the challenges of the healthcare industry's financial performance as well. We assist thousands of hospitals and healthcare providers nationwide in reducing bad debt and accounts receivable days, as well as increasing overall revenue efficiencies.

Our solutions identify potential fraud, assess risk and offer insight into managing differences in demographic information and financial interactions with patients. With our extensive credit and noncredit consumer databases, we have the information and expertise that addresses one of the major problems of the healthcare industry: cash flow. Through our solutions, you can objectively handle the financial portion of your patient relationship wherever it fits best in your revenue cycle, helping you avoid major process changes and meet your financial improvement objectives.

Equifax and the healthcare industry share the same vision: continuous improvement in patient care and protecting the patient mission. As a trusted steward of consumer information, Equifax has been awarded Cap Gemini's ISO 9000 certification of our procedures for monitoring the quality, integrity and stability of our consumer database. Additionally, to the extent applicable to a particular product or service we provide, we operate subject to the guidelines of the Fair Credit Reporting Act, the Fair and Accurate Credit Transactions Act, the Gramm-Leach-Bliley Act and the Health Insurance Portability and Accountability Act. Inquiries to the credit database from healthcare providers are kept private to be viewed only by the consumer, and we have a long-standing policy to protect sensitive healthcare information. Patient privacy is a cornerstone of our services.

We have also focused heavily on accessibility of our solutions. We have formed strategic alliances with industry-leading, forward-thinking healthcare service providers such as McKesson Corporation, HDX® Healthcare Data Exchange LLC (a subsidiary of Siemens Medical Solutions), Search America and ImageVision.Net. McKesson Provider Technologies addresses the industry's needs with a full range of transaction-based services from point of service to statements and claims. HDX provides integrated and Internet solutions for address verification, fraud/risk identification and scoring within the revenue cycle point-of-service and back-office work flows. Search America offers online/integrated, point-of-service payment and charity advisement using credit scoring as a base for their solution. ImageVision.Net incorporates scoring and detailed credit information into their HealthPay24® Financial Counseling workflow module to help healthcare providers collect more effectively on current and prior charges at the point of service, set accurate payment plans, identify Medicaid and Charity Care-applicants and recognize when sending a statement will suffice in collecting a patient debt.

Whether your organization has an aggressive point-of-service collection strategy or handles the entire A/R in a patient accounting function, knowing patients' propensity to pay can improve your cash flow, reduce days in A/R and expedite assistance filings such as Medicaid and Charity Care. From a cost perspective, you can prioritize patient accounting resources, minimize costly collection methods and even maximize the economics of outside collection agency contracts. Take advantage of our expertise, world-class analytics and consulting services to identify your greatest return on investment opportunities. ■

Equifax Inc. is a global leader in turning information into intelligence. For businesses, Equifax provides faster and easier ways to find, approve and market to the appropriate customers. For consumers, Equifax offers easier instantaneous ways to buy products or services and better insight into and management of their personal credit.

Richard F. Smith
Chief Executive Officer

J. Dann Adams
Group Executive, North America Information Services

Steven P. Ely
Group Executive, Equifax Personal Solutions

Owen V. Flynn
Group Executive, Equifax Marketing Services

Equifax Inc.
1550 Peachtree St., N.W.
Atlanta, GA 30309
Phone 404.885.8000
www.equifax.com

Business Contact
Jennifer Coxwell
Phone 770.995.0340
Fax 770.339.4253
jennifer.coxwell@equifax.com

Revenue Cycle Enhancements Associated With EHR Systems

Streamlining the revenue cycle and combining financial processes with an EHR can significantly improve a hospital's financial performance.

[Sue McBride, Accenture] [Elizabeth Guyton, Accenture]

Health industry leaders agree that an EHR and the integrated information system by which records will be accessed, modified and used to better inform treatment decisions are powerful and essential tools. These tools will improve patient safety, enhance the quality of services delivered to patients and make the most efficient use of beds, medical staff and other hospital resources. This can yield qualitative and quantitative benefits of reduced length of stay, staffing efficiencies, improved compliance with established medical practices, easier regulation reporting and simplified physician referrals and prescriptions. Revenue cycle enhancements can help build a persuasive business case to justify the expense of implementing an EHR.

Background and Current State

The federal government, recognizing the need for a nationwide EHR, and aware of the expense and complexity of such a project, has outlined The President's Health Information Technology Plan, an ambitious agenda to assure that the EHR will include most Americans within the next 10 years. The plan calls for the design and adoption of standards by which medical information will be stored and shared electronically while assuring privacy and security. The Department of Health and Human Services has been collaborating with the private sector to develop voluntary standards and a comprehensive medical vocabulary that are prerequisites for a nationwide EHR. The government's proposed fiscal year 2005 budget assigns $100 million toward funding demonstration projects that will enhance healthcare technology. What's more, the federal government – one of the largest buyers of healthcare – plans to create incentives and opportunities for healthcare providers to use electronic records. The plan's developers envision a future when each patient's comprehensive health information is available at any point of service where the patient authorizes access.

Hospitals are beginning to realize that an EHR implementation can directly enhance the revenue cycle by streamlining key processes such as admission and scheduling, eliminating many repetitive tasks and dramatically improving charge capture, billing and collections. These revenue cycle improvements can have substantial dollar value, increasing the ROI of an EHR implementation. For example:

- Both clinical and financial benefits from an EHR implementation in a small practice were demonstrated by Bergen Medical Alliance. Using EHR software that automatically reminds providers when they omit entries for visit documentation, such as associated diagnoses that payers require for claims processing, Bergen Medical Alliance improved its overall financial performance by saving costs for manpower and transcription while enhancing revenues by timely billing and thorough charge capture.[1]
- Small-practice benefits of EHR implementation include reducing drug costs and preventing adverse drug events.[2] Additional gains are reaped from the accuracy and completeness of notes, which give physicians more confidence that charges are justified by documentation, sparing huge fines from Medicare for coding or charging irregularities.[3]

Overall Implications of EHR To Revenue Cycle Functions

EHR offers the potential for health organizations to simplify registration, scheduling, eligibility, charge capture and claims manage-

Sue McBride is a senior manager in Accenture's Revenue Transformation practice. She has over 15 years of experience in healthcare operational management and consulting. She is the national lead for the Patient Access solution and has led large-scale multihospital system revenue cycle transformation projects. **Elizabeth Guyton** is a partner with Accenture and national leader of the Revenue Transformation practice for the health industry. She has over 18 years of healthcare management experience concentrating in the areas of accounts receivable and financial management at the facility and multifacility levels.

ment processes. By redesigning processes to take advantage of new technology, a hospital can streamline and accelerate the entire revenue cycle. Many tedious and labor-intensive processes such as transcribing, requesting and entering patient information, coding and billing can be eliminated or dramatically simplified. Reducing staff time needed for these tasks can mean retraining the hospital staff for more sophisticated, fulfilling and potentially revenue-generating jobs.

EHR can contribute bottom-line results in terms of reduced days in accounts receivable, lower denial rates and reduced write-offs. An electronic financial history will become part of each patient's health record and will foster similar gains in efficiency and enhanced financial return. With comprehensive financial and eligibility information available at the point of service, patient interactions will change from information gathering to opportunities for information analysis and conferring about treatment options. More highly trained patient-facing employees can help patients review and evaluate their own records. Patients have the capability for self-registration in many cases, and in general are able to take a more active role in their own healthcare.

Specific Functional Enhancements To the Revenue Cycle

Let's look more specifically at the revenue cycle processes that could be streamlined or improved by implementing an electronic health record.

- Scheduling;
- Medical necessity check;
- Registration;
- Coding and charge capture; and
- Billing and collections.

Scheduling

One of the ways EHR would enhance the revenue cycle is by streamlining and shortening the time it takes to schedule a new patient or a repeat patient. Since the information is electronic and linked among related functions and processes, the scheduling staff is able to schedule an event, compiling a core standard set of patient-level and visit-specific data. The reason for the visit or the diagnosis as well as the insurance information would be collected and entered into the system. This comprehensive information, available at the time of scheduling, would be available for others to utilize in their plan for patient care (e.g., forecast utilization, create diagnosis-specific plans of care, etc.). Physicians' office staff, too, can use the system to schedule a patient for a hospital visit. Either way, the core set of data, including the reason for care/diagnosis is known to all at the very beginning.

Medical Necessity Check

Knowing the diagnosis up front also means knowing in advance if the treatment will be paid and if so, by whom. There needs to be a medical reason for every patient's treatment, based on a list of diagnoses that are deemed payable (or not) as an outpatient or an inpatient. Integrating the medical necessity check into the process clarifies in advance whether the treatment will be covered and what tests and documentation are needed to support the diagnosis. Defining financial responsibility in advance greatly increases the efficiency of the claims process, minimizes denials and results in a more satisfactory patient experience.

Registration

An EHR implementation can link disparate revenue cycle information and functions so that accurate and current patient information is available for use by physicians, clinicians and administrative personnel. As each has a different use for this information, the EHR can consolidate and compare information from different sources, centralizing it in a comprehensive database. Many revenue problems occur in the registration process; current information about the patient's demographics, insurance information and coverage rules can remedy most of them. Each patient's correct primary and secondary medical insurance can be quickly verified. If the patient's physician is within the health system, the registration process can quickly determine the reason for the patient's visit, what authorizations or referrals are necessary based on the diagnosis code and insurance plan and whether the patient has insurance coverage for the prescribed treatment.

In an electronic environment, the patient can have real-time access to his or her own demographic information and can view and update the record. This helps transform patients from passive consumers of health services, not involved in helping to determine what's best for them, into active planners who take more ownership of their health information and care. Today few patients even see their health records. That is rapidly changing.

Coding and Charge Capture

Charge capture likely offers the single most significant opportunity for leveraging an EHR to enhance the revenue cycle. In an outpatient clinical setting, providing appropriate documentation for the desired level of care poses a major challenge. In general, the more expensive medical interventions – identified by their codes – require the most stringent documentation. Physicians often lack the confidence in their documentation to support reimbursement for the actual service provided and, as a result, sometimes "down-code," choosing a reimbursement code with less stringent docu-

> **weblink**
> Read how business intelligence software helps organizations integrate data in "Getting Action From Your EHR Data."

mentation requirements. Since what is coded becomes the charge that is billed to the insurance carrier, under-coding results in lower compensation to the provider. With an electronic record and accompanying templates, physicians are better able to document with certainty the services they provide. In some instances, the computer system automatically creates the correct codes based on the available documentation and templates. When the fear of compliance is gone because the right documentation exists to support the correct coding, the provider's revenue increases as the coding reflects the intensity of services provided. Other care providers can use the templates as well. Specifically, documenting surgical supplies, implantables and procedures is facilitated by electronic documentation. As many high-dollar surgical supplies are "carved out" and paid for separately, comprehensive documentation is essential.

Central Utah Multi-Specialty Clinic, a 59-physician group with practices in nine locations treating 200,000 patients annually, earned significant additional revenue by using its EHR templates to recommend the appropriate evaluation and management (E/M) codes based on the level of care that was documented.[4]

Increased Revenue as a Result of Accurate Coding

	Year 1	Year 2	Year 3	Year 4	Year 5	Total
Increased revenue	$103,059	$283,413	$415,673	$457,240	$502,964	$1,762.349

In an electronic environment, there's no waiting to find information necessary for coding and capturing charges. In some cases, once the physician enters an order into the system, it gets linked to a charge description, then to a master charge list and the charge is added automatically to the patient's bill. No additional personnel are required to manually enter charges or to remove them if the procedure is changed or cancelled. The hospital can eliminate many steps and handoffs required to distribute and process paper charts. By linking EHR with their billing systems, hospitals can quickly and expeditiously submit claims to payers electronically. The claim goes out clean with appropriate coding and documentation to the payers, who pay more promptly, improving cash flow. Hospitals are also better able to match ancillary service claims to hospital-based outpatient visits.

An EHR implementation also improves coding for inpatient diagnoses and treatments. An important measure of accounts receivable performance is the amount of funds in DNFB (discharged not final billed). In this situation, the patient has been discharged, but the hospital is unable to bill for services rendered because of missing information. Usually, what's missing is verification of the patient's insurance coverage or coding of the patient's chart. The chart hasn't been coded for one of two reasons; either there wasn't enough information to add codes, or the transcription of the discharge summary or the operative note has not occurred. With an electronic record, transcription costs go down and the timeliness increases. In addition, the time needed to add appropriate codes is reduced, since both coding templates and the patient record are close at hand. Little time is lost in finding, transporting and filing paper charts. Claims get submitted more quickly and contain fewer errors and better supporting documentation, so they get paid more promptly.

In a paper environment, hospitals expend a great deal of effort transcribing information, double-checking it, calling up information from patient charts, filling in information gaps and then resolving denied claims when they get rejected by the payer for incomplete information. EHR makes the process of submitting a clean claim almost automatic. A case in point is the Virginia Mason Medical Center, which before the implementation of EHR sent out bills to patients on an average of 4.3 days after they were discharged. After implementation, patients and their bills left the hospital simultaneously. This brought revenue into the hospital faster and earned the hospital a significant bonus equal to the time value of the expedited revenue.

Finally, a physician benefit of better inpatient coding is more accurate physician profiles. Payers profile physicians based on their Medicare diagnosis related group (DRG) assignments of the patients they treat. Payers use this information to track trends and evaluate physicians on compliance and performance issues. The electronic record allows physicians to feel more comfortable that what the payer is seeing is accurate and realistically depicts their clinical judgments.

Billing and Collections

Electronic billing results in accurate bills submitted to patients quickly – in many cases, the same day the patient is discharged. The number of steps between a physician ordering a medical intervention, the hospital calculating the patient's financial responsibility and billing for it and the patient paying for it are much fewer than in a paper environment and cost much less to complete. Since the patient's financial responsibility was determined upon scheduling or registration, the patient receives no unpleasant surprises that can lead to collection problems. Bills get paid sooner with fewer complications. Both collection expenses and write-offs to bad debt decrease substantially.

Impacts of Streamlined Processes

The technology-enabled revenue cycle is able to streamline revenue processes; reduce the number of people involved in coding, preparing and submitting reimbursement claims to payers and bills to patients; and allow the hospital to bill faster and more cleanly.

One important cost-reducing impact to the hospital's bottom line is reduced denials. Medical claims may be denied for technical reasons, such as for containing information that is incomplete or inaccurate, or simply missing from the documentation. Having the patient's clinical and financial data available and templates to ensure that correct documentation is submitted with each claim reduces technical denials.

Likewise, an EHR implementation can reduce medical necessity denials by ensuring that claims are submitted with the right supporting documentation for the corresponding diagnoses. Medical necessity checks are performed at the time of scheduling. A denial is the payer's way of saying, "You haven't given us enough information to justify doing this test or procedure on our member." With an electronic record at hand, it's relatively easy for the scheduler or physician to determine right away whether or not the documentation and diagnosis justifies the treatment. When coverage rules preclude paying for the service on the basis of the provider's diagnosis and documentation, the patient will need to know that he or she will be responsible for paying the full charges for the test or treatment.

An integrated, electronic revenue cycle, with its capability to submit cleaner claims to payers quickly, can also reduce denials caused by failing to submit claims in a timely manner. Without EHR, hospitals routinely get up to 15 percent of their claims initially rejected by payers. Upon resubmission with information added and corrected, hospitals hope to achieve a 1 to 3 percent denial rate. The EHR can help achieve this minimum denial rate on the first go-around.

Denials of any kind are labor-intensive and expensive to remedy. Processing denied claims requires considerable time from highly trained and highly compensated staff to research each denied claim, confer with the payer, correct the claim and/or append appropriate documentation to the claim, and then resubmit it, often more than once. Substantial costs in manpower and time are spent in accounts receivable, often focusing on rework due to errors at the beginning of the cycle.

Example: The Ohio State University EHR has built-in compliance features and automatically supports Medicare compliance by prompting charge entry clerks when a modifier needs to be added to a particular charge and an advanced beneficiary notice needs to be implemented to inform a patient that Medicare will not pay for a specific test.[5]

A streamlined, integrated revenue cycle also reduces repayments to payers and, in the case of Medicare, fines levied against providers for submitting claims with noncompliant documentation or for ineligible services.

Example: Healthcare provider Heritage Behavioral Health's EHR implementation helped reduce repayments to payers for noncompliant documentation or ineligible services from $49,477 in 1994 to $774 in 2001.[6]

More accurate coding in outpatient clinics can help providers obtain higher reimbursements and receive fewer fines due to noncompliance.

Example: Primary Care Associates, a 120 patient-per-day practice in Cape Coral, Fla., saved $152,000 in fines from the Centers for Medicare & Medicard Services due to incorrect coding of claims.

Example: Central Utah Multi-Specialty Clinic, the largest independent multispecialty group in the state with 59 physicians and nine locations, was able to increase reimbursements by an average of $26 per patient, increasing revenue by $1.7 million over five years.[7]

Example: Three Rivers Dermatology in Fort Wayne, Ind., achieved a 30 percent increase in total billings as a result of more accurate coding for outpatient procedures.

Fast and accurate billing means that patient bills spend less time in accounts receivable.

Example: Reid Hospital and Health Care Services, a not-for-profit 240-bed hospital in Richmond, Ind., reduced average days a bill spent in accounts receivable from the upper 60s to the lower 50s after implementing an EHR.

Summary

The value of an EHR implementation to improve patient safety, enhance the quality of care and create efficiencies in the use and deployment of clinical resources is now well-documented and well-understood. Less well-understood but more quantifiable in terms of dollars saved or additional dollars earned are the financial benefits of an integrated, electronic revenue cycle to the provider's bottom line. Recent studies are demonstrating that streamlining the revenue cycle and combining financial processes with an electronic health record can significantly improve a hospital's financial performance. ■

Endnotes

1. *Masiello J; Optimizing Practice Efficiencies, presented at Bergen Medical Alliance, 2003.*
2. *Bates DW, Ebell M, Gotlieb E, Zapp J, Mullins HC; "A proposal for electronic medical records in US primary care,"* JAMIA, *Vol 10(1), Jan/Feb 2003.*
3. *Rogoski RR: "Having it Your Way,"* Health Management Technology, *May 2003.*
4. *Barlow S, Johnson J, Steck J; "The Economic Effect of Implementing an EMR in an Outpatient Clinical Setting," Journal of Healthcare Information Management, Vol 18(1).*
5. *Nicholas E. Davies Symposium Proceedings 2001. Ohio State: "The design and implementation of a computerized patient record at the Ohio State University Health System – A success story." HIMSS Chicago, IL.*
6. *Nicholas E. Davies Symposium Proceedings 2001. Award for behavioral health, Heritage Health Center Inc. HIMSS Chicago, IL.*
7. *Barlow S, et al. Ibid.*

5

Patient-Controlled Personal Health Records for Patients and Physicians

Providing information that is accurate, secure, private, comprehensive and up to date at the point of clinical decision making and care will assure the best possible outcome at the lowest cost.

[Marie Savard, M.D., American Healthways] [Jim Pope, M.D., American Healthways] [James K. Geraughty, M.D., NewQuest]

Bridging the Cultural Chasm

Despite the lack of decision- or health-support systems in healthcare today, patients and physicians alike are being held increasingly accountable for the healthcare decisions they make. Both lack access to the broad array of information in healthcare – including such things as specific clinical and patient information, practice guidelines and drug interactions – that is critical at every point of decision making and care to provide the best possible outcomes. And according to a report by the Markle Foundation, no single entity in our increasingly complex, fragmented and pluralistic healthcare system is capable of, or responsible for, collecting and maintaining all of the important health information about any one individual (*Achieving Electronic Connectivity in Healthcare: A Preliminary Roadmap*, Connecting for Health, July 2004).

It is now generally accepted that the healthcare system needs electronic connectivity in every aspect, and that this can best be achieved via a central, readily accessed electronic health record (EHR) and a patient-controlled personal health record (PHR). Given the formidable task of instituting complete EHRs with full connectivity among providers, it is unlikely to happen in the near future.

Compared to the technological complexity of creating standardized EMRs, the development of PHRs seems simple. Both however, are entwined in a cultural chasm that will prove challenging and that can only be addressed through health support systems that enhance the patient-physician relationship, exchange valuable information in ways that both patient and physician find convenient and useful, and that put the patient at the center of care.

Physicians have for so long been the ones in control of the medical record that delegating or sharing any of that responsibility will require as much of a shift in thinking and training as it will in systems. Likewise, patients are used to, and in many cases reluctant to shift away from, the notion that "doctor knows best," despite the fact that best practices are provided only about 50 percent of the time.

Personal health information is usually dispersed among multiple providers and participants. Health plans, generalist and specialist physician offices, hospitals, laboratories, pharmacies, pharmacy benefit managers and disease management organizations all collect some (and sometimes duplicative) information.

Patients with chronic illness and their caregivers need access to their medical information to actively manage their conditions in collaboration with their practitioners. But the reality is, they typically don't have easy access to such information – nor do they always know they need it. Patients need to be provided tools to integrate and manage all of their information across all providers and across time. Practitioners are poorly prepared for the necessary and imminent shift in information collection and management, collaborative patient participation and, ultimately, patient control.

Some providers, however, can play a significant role in setting the stage for what will be a huge paradigm shift in healthcare where patients move from peripheral positions of decision making to central positions of decision making and information control.

Disease management companies are uniquely positioned to facilitate both greater electronic connectivity between multiple providers and patients/caregivers, as well as support, prepare and facilitate the patient and practitioner for the paradigm shift in decision making and information control. As experienced health coaches with access to a broad array of clinical information, disease managers can teach patients how to be the model patients for the 21st century – fully informed, involved patients managing their health conditions in collaboration with their practitioners.

Marie Savard, M.D., is an internist, noted author and creator of a patient-centered PHR system. **Jim Pope, M.D., F.A.C.C.,** is CMO for American Healthways, where he is responsible for outcomes initiatives, medical informatics, quality improvement, accreditation and program medical integrity. **James K. Geraughty, M.D.,** is the CMO for NewQuest, parent company of HealthSpring of Tennessee.

Disease management collects a vast amount of clinical information and puts it in the hands of patients and physicians in ways that patients can understand and physicians and patients can use. Disease management organizations can serve as the conduits of electronically collected, organized and stored clinical information to practitioners and patients, thus helping them build and populate their EHR/PHR.

Disease management supports and enhances the patient-physician relationship and educates people with chronic conditions about the best ways to partner with their physicians and optimally manage their diseases. Think of disease management as everything that happens between the time patients leave the doctor's office and the time they return. Disease management reaches out to people in whatever way they deem most convenient and supports them in the same way they live with their disease, which is 24 hours a day, seven days a week, 365 days a year; not just the five, 10 or 15 minutes they get with their physicians during a typical office visit. Support can be as simple as advising someone with diabetes what they should or shouldn't eat when they go to their favorite restaurant. Or it can be as potentially life saving as advising a cardiac patient who is experiencing shortness of breath to consult the doctor.

Using claims and other data, disease management is capable of identifying thousands of patients with any disease and engaging them in structured and repeated interactions. Those interactions build personal relationships and trust.

Disease management works from within the system, but it doesn't wait for patients to show up in the doctor's office or the emergency room. Using claims and other data, disease management is capable of identifying thousands of patients with any disease and engaging them in structured and repeated interactions. Those interactions build personal relationships and trust, resulting in the kinds of changes that get and keep people healthier. Such interactions lead to a vast array of clinical information stored electronically that can be readily transmitted to the patient and their practitioners (EMR and PHR respectively).

The healthcare system necessarily must move to more evidence-based practices to eliminate the quality gap in healthcare. So far evidence-based information has been disseminated almost exclusively through the physician. But with the advent of the Internet and the more empowered healthcare consumer, patients can have access to evidence-based information to guide them in their shared decision making.

Some physicians have been initially skeptical of disease management services, but as our system moves to a more "pay-for-performance" model of reimbursement and recognition, doctors will ultimately see the value of informed, involved and responsible patients partnering with them to achieve the best and most cost-effective outcomes.

Given that our healthcare system continues to make more demands on doctors without giving anything in return, it's easy to understand their frustration and their reluctance to latch on to what they may feel is just another "cure *du jour*." Even in our technological age, many physicians still don't have the technological infrastructure to support these demands, much less take on additional information from other sources. HealthLeaders magazine reported that fewer than 15 percent of all physicians use the advanced technologies available, mostly because they're cost-prohibitive, but also because of the uncertain return on investment and the inherent difficulties associated with implementation. Much of that will change as the federal government pursues various solutions, incentives and changes in reimbursement policies.

And while disease management companies are already heavily invested in state-of-the-art technologies, they must do a much better job of leveraging that technology to meet the needs of physicians and patients and work even more closely with them during this paradigm shift in healthcare.

Disease management is not just opening the door of possibility, but is leading the way to innovation in all aspects of information technology – including the commitment to help bring greater connectivity to patients and practitioners by supporting and contributing to the development of an EHR/PHR.

Case in Point

As part of a pilot program, HealthSpring of Tennessee and its disease management partner American Healthways, are working collaboratively with the Sumner Medical Group (SMG) to develop an EHR that provides the most pertinent and up-to-date information possible to physicians and patients when they need it: at the point of care and healthcare decision making.

weblink

Read how EHRs enhance collaboration in "EHRs Drive Dramatic Change in Clinical Practice" in this book.

HealthSpring already was experiencing good clinical and financial results with its disease management program, HealthSpring Cares, but it saw the potential for even better outcomes through further and closer integration with physicians. The resulting pay-for-performance pilot with SMG includes a dozen primary care physicians and approximately 1,400 patients – most of them Medicare Advantage members – in the HealthSpring Cares disease management program. The pilot provides for an active exchange of information between physicians and chronic care nurses to track patient interactions and adherence to standards of care. The goal is to more closely align the health plan, the patient and the provider with the goals of the disease management program and drive further improvements in health outcomes, in patient and physician satisfaction and in healthcare cost reductions. Participating physicians are eligible for a 20 percent performance bonus based on improved quality and outcomes measures, and patients are more accepting of the program because they are introduced to it by their physician.

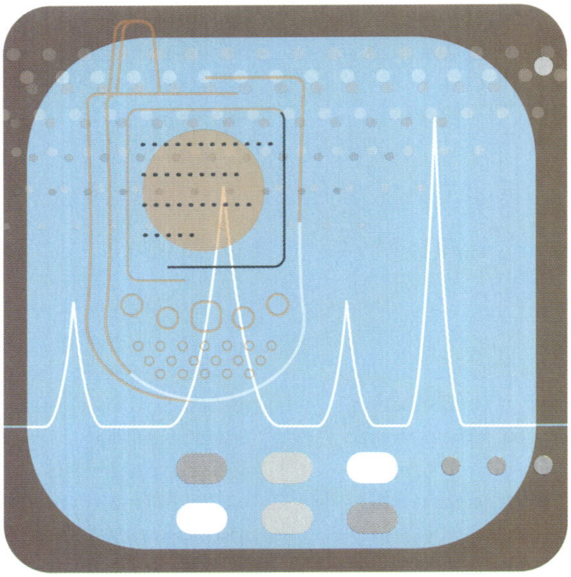

HealthSpring and American Healthways provide a nurse at SMG who is responsible for communicating with the entire healthcare team. They have established a process to provide a one-page abstract at the end of each office visit, which is shared with the HealthSpring Cares nurse manager, who is now contacting patients by phone on behalf of the physician's office rather than HealthSpring. A synopsis of the nurse care call is then relayed back to the physician – another data point for the EMR. Work is under way to transmit this information electronically and in real time, providing the physician and the disease management nurses both with up-to-date and vital information.

Most of the patients in the program recognize their nurse manager's voice when she calls. Janet DePriest is the disease management nurse assigned to the program. She says patients often share certain things with her that they may feel uncomfortable sharing with their physicians, and it's her job to take the time necessary to help them work through it, help them know the right questions to ask their doctor and to help interpret what the doctor has said. Physicians at SMG note that DePriest is often able to discover social factors or problems that patients are sometimes reluctant to share with their doctor. Patients are also much more likely to tell DePriest than they are their doctor when they don't fill or don't take their prescribed medication.

"I have people tell me all the time that they can't talk to their doctor about certain things, and so we talk, and I try to help them devise a plan of what they're going to say once they get to the doctor's office, and I tell them these things aren't going to embarrass the doctor, and we sort of develop a plan," DePriest says. "Sometimes people are uncomfortable questioning the doctor so they say their nurse told them to ask. They don't want to question the doctor, but it's OK for me to."

DePriest also stresses with patients the importance of keeping track of their health to share with their doctor at the next visit – in essence she is helping patients take the first steps to building a PHR. She has steadily helped increase the number of patients in the program who are keeping logs of their blood sugars, letting them know that it helps their doctors better regulate their medication. If something unusual is happening with a patient, DePriest explains to them the importance of logging the details of that as well. She lets them know that the more detailed they can be with their doctor, the better decisions the doctor can make.

"I let them know that it's going to help the doctor if they can tell him not just that their sugars are low, but that they're always low around 11 o'clock at night, and it always happens the day they skip their lunch. Or if they're feeling dizzy, it's going to be a lot more helpful to the doctor if he knows they were dizzy three times this week when standing at the kitchen sink. These kinds of details really help put all the pieces together," DePriest says.

Plus, now that the physicians at SMG have the potential to share in the financial reward for helping improve clinical outcomes, they see the disease management provider as part of the team instead of part of the problem.

The physicians at SMG are no different from their peers across the country, who, a recent study by Duke University Medical Center found, are being overwhelmed by the needs of patients with chronic diseases such as high blood pressure, heart disease and diabetes. According to the study, published in the May/June 2005 issue of the *Annals of Family Medicine*, new team-based approaches to care, changes in healthcare reimbursement and informed and proactive patients are essential to meet the healthcare needs of the burgeoning chronic disease population.

According to HealthSpring, early indications are that its attempt to realign the system is driving improved clinical quality measures and, as a result, cost savings that appear to be far in excess of the pilot program's costs. The next step is adopting new technologies that will drive further integration and more online collaboration between the physician practice and the disease management provider.

Similar to provider networks across the country, some form of EHRs exist in only about half of all physicians' offices in the HealthSpring network. HealthSpring's vision is to generate enough savings as it rolls out more pay-for-performance pilots to pay for more investment in technology and to encourage physicians to reinvest performance bonuses into technology within their practices.

The ultimate goal is to create an open data exchange, giving physicians in-office access to American Healthways' EMR, Population Works, and making sure physician offices' EMRs can talk to PopulationWorks. As simpler, more automated and better integrated systems are being developed, the focus must remain on what's important to the physician and the patient at the point of care.

Disease management organizations also are ideally suited to educate patients about how to become informed and proactive consumers interacting with their information and making informed decisions about their care. American Healthways is developing a program that will actively teach patients how to become better consumers of healthcare – showing them how to collect, manage and store their medical records and information, how to set and monitor target goals for health conditions and how to better collaborate with their physicians – assuming much more responsibility for their health information, health decisions and healthcare outcomes.

Summary: Keep It Simple and Focused

Modern society produces and disseminates information at a faster clip than even the most educated employees at our country's largest and most sophisticated corporations can keep pace (McKinsey Quarterly 2005). Almost daily there are new, and often conflicting, reports about drug therapies, diseases, medical treatments and scientific breakthroughs. Every month approximately 30,000 new medical journal articles are published around the globe. The "information superhighway" that was supposed to help simplify our lives has in many ways added to the overload. What physicians, patients and their caregivers need most are tools and systems to help them cut through the clutter and stay focused on what's important at the moment decisions are being made and care is being delivered.

Just making medical records available electronically isn't going to do it. Patients have to become engaged and involved in their own care. PHRs encourage that, but healthcare consumers must be taught how to start and keep track of their PHR. Physicians need support to track and follow up with patients between office visits. The good news is that work has already begun and it doesn't have to wait on the development of widespread, widely adopted EMRs.

Disease management companies are uniquely positioned to facilitate greater electronic connectivity between multiple providers and the patient/caregiver as well as support, prepare and facilitate the patient and practitioner for the paradigm shift in decision making and information control. ■

What physicians, patients and their caregivers need most are tools and systems to help them cut through the clutter and stay focused on what's important at the moment decisions are being made and care is being delivered.

Success Through Human Connections

Technology is often seen as **the solution** for what ails healthcare in the United States. At American Healthways, we believe technology is not the solution, but a critical solution enabler. Because while technology will enable a National Health Information Network that will connect stakeholders more readily and reduce the costs of traditional paper-based connections, each stakeholder also must be properly motivated and their interests aligned if improved health, improved quality and reduced costs – the desired outcomes – are to be achieved.

Unique Perspective

American Healthways' perspective in this arena is unique. As a coordinator and integrator both of care and data, American Healthways provides medical management services to nearly 2 million people while seamlessly interfacing data from more than 50 health plans, more than 400 employers and governmental entities both at the state and federal levels.

Our business – our *only* business – is helping people lead healthier lives by bridging the well-recognized gaps in healthcare, supporting the patient-physician relationship and motivating sustainable behavior change. The outcome is improved health and patient safety, first and foremost, directly resulting in cost benefits and productivity gains. Our nurses – supported by proprietary advanced technologies, proven standards of care and evidence-based medicine – fill the healthcare system gaps between patient, provider, employer and payer. American Healthways is paid to produce both clinical and financial outcomes, existing as one of the few true pay-for-performance health services providers today.

Population Solutions

Our experience tells us that additional improvements in the healthcare system depend on the successful alignment of stakeholders to ensure positive outcomes delivered at scale through the intelligent and appropriate use of technology. American Healthways is working strategically with Microsoft to create new data and service integration solutions based on Microsoft technologies and American Healthways' disease and care management expertise. Together American Healthways and Microsoft have the opportunity to create meaningful human connections in healthcare through software connections that enable an efficient, effective and affordable point of integration for all stakeholders. American Healthways is in a natural position to serve as that point of integration, providing relevant information to health plans, providers, patients and employers precisely when they need it to make the most appropriate healthcare decisions possible.

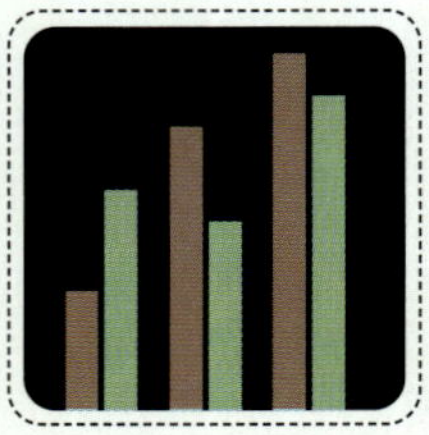

American Healthways is in a natural position to serve as that point of integration, providing relevant information to health plans, providers, patients and employers precisely when they need it to make the most appropriate healthcare decisions possible.

To that end, American Healthways is developing and deploying solutions – such as **health risk assessments, physician pay-for-performance** programs, advanced **provider EMR integration, consumer PHR integration and remote patient monitoring services** – that address the health risks and conditions of 100 percent of the population, not just those with chronic disease.

Our proprietary **health risk assessment** model provides employees and their dependents with a personal health risk score as well as the information and support they need to maintain or improve their health status. Participants receive detailed and actionable information about their health, including biometrics, body mass index, cholesterol, triglyceride, glucose and nicotine levels in addition to overall physical and emotional health indicators.

This clinical health information supports and motivates behavior change and more effective self-health management by enabling employees and their families to make informed decisions about their health and their healthcare. The health risk score also allows American Healthways to measure and report objective and verifiable annual changes in participant health status. By enabling participants to identify, understand and address their health risks, our **Health IQ** programs have helped lower participants' annual healthcare claims.

When combined with American Healthways' **chronic disease management programs**, the health risk assessments allow for the incorporation of objective biometric data with existing claims, lab and self-reported data, helping to more fully engage our members, improve our interventions and further improve health outcomes.

Our StatusOne **high-risk care management program** identifies individuals at highest risk of incurring significant medical costs within the next 12 months and creates a customized care-support system focused on high-intensity, one-on-one nurse interventions.

For senior populations, American Healthways is working strategically with the **Massachusetts Institute of Technology AgeLab** to focus on ways technology can improve the quality of life and health outcomes for the aging. At the same time, American Healthways is bringing its proven solutions to **Medicare Advantage** and to the **Medicare** fee-for-service population under the new **Medicare Health Support** chronic care improvement program authorized by the Medicare Prescription Drug, Improvement and Modernization Act of 2003.

Future Perfect

American Healthways' mission is to be a meaningful contributor to the necessary, and possible, transformation of healthcare delivery from a system that is siloed and disconnected, to a system that is aligned around evidence-based standards, healthy behavior and positive clinical and financial outcomes. Because of our unique position as care managers, we have access to data and information that no other single stakeholder has, and we have synthesized it in ways that allow us to deliver our services efficiently and at scale, assuring the delivery of the right message by the right resource to the right person at the right time.

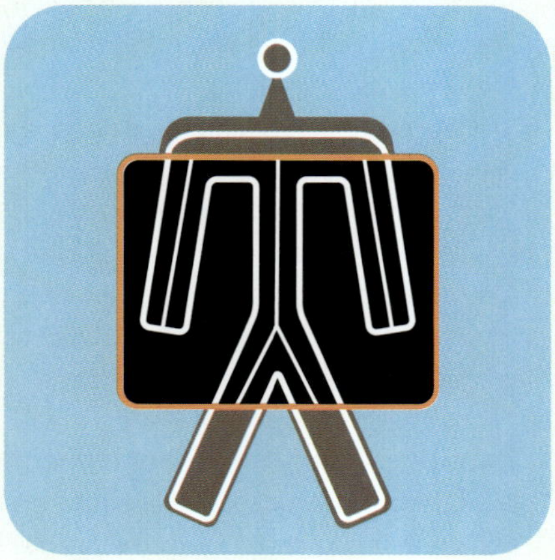

Leveraging the appropriate technologies, American Healthways will continue to evolve a solution that enables stakeholders to support quality, affordable healthcare that is driven by an outcomes focus, rather than by counting units of service. This approach will enable:

Employers to manage their investment in employee healthcare appropriately and to understand the return on their investment by connecting premium spend with health and productivity outcomes.

Providers to access information and services that allow them to best serve their patients according to their unique situations and recognized standards of care, and to have a meaningful care-support process in between office visits to ensure patients are following through with their evidence-based care plans. This integrated approach provides for less variability in outcomes and critical information support for successful pay-for-performance models.

Payers to manage populations and risk effectively by using mass customization services to tailor the appropriate benefits for the member's unique situation and by guiding provider services toward a consistent standard of quality.

Consumers to access a comprehensive base of information – including their own health information – tools and services to help them practice healthy behaviors, and to engage in positive, empowered and successful interaction with the healthcare system.

Opportunity

With healthcare benefits and their costs pressuring **employers'** competitive position – and in some cases, their profitability – employers need innovative systems that inform and empower their health and productivity decisions. **Government** needs similar systems to be able to address and afford quality healthcare for current and future generations. At the same time, **consumers** must be informed and empowered to make the kinds of healthcare decisions they're now being asked to make.

American Healthways believes that for such systems to be effective and sustainable, they must be aligned around improving health. American Healthways seeks partners that understand this important distinction and who want to actively work together to build and test such systems. Working together to design, build and implement these enhanced, integrated care models will, we believe, restore confidence that the health of our nation, and its workers, will be a firm, competitive social and economic advantage through the 21st century. ■

AMERICAN HEALTHWAYS

American Healthways, Inc. is the nation's leading and largest provider of disease management, care enhancement and high-risk care management services proven to improve the quality of healthcare and lower costs.

Ben R. Leedle Jr.
President and CEO

Mary Chaput
Executive Vice President
and CFO

James E. Pope, M.D.
Executive Vice President and
Chief Medical Officer

Donald B. Taylor
Executive Vice President
and COO

American Healthways
3841 Green Hills Village Dr.
Nashville, TN 37215
Phone 615.665.1122
Fax 615.665.7697
info@amhealthways.com
www.americanhealthways.com

Business Contact
Mike King
SVP Business Development
Phone 615.263.7911
mike.king@amhealthways.com

EHRs, Automating Coding And Advanced Analytics

Adopting the EHR and integrating it into other elements of the data universe of our healthcare system will generate positive outcomes at every link in the transaction chain.

[Andrea Allmon, Ph.D., Fair Isaac Corporation] [Jean de Traversay, Fair Isaac Corporation]

The move to create a nationwide system of EHRs (electronic health records) comes at a particularly critical time in the history of our healthcare system.

Annual per capita costs continue to soar but without a demonstrated increase in improved benefits to patients. The population is aging, leading to a concomitant increase in those suffering from chronic diseases. And fraud is a growth industry.

For these and many other reasons, our healthcare system needs to embrace integrated systems built around an EHR, or face a future of continued cost escalation, unconscionable waste, burgeoning inefficiencies and a growing epidemic of sicknesses and deaths from inappropriate treatment of patients. The trend can be reversed. The healthcare industry needs to think of every medical-related encounter as a transaction. How to optimize the transaction throughout the whole continuum of processing? It's not just the doctor; it's the clinic, the pharmacy and the payer, as well as transactions arising from ancillary services.

The Rosetta Stone for Integrating Disparate Systems

How can this work? Previously disparate systems need to be integrated to improve patient care, reduce errors, gain insights into trends in clinical care and identify fraud, abuse and errors in claims before they are paid. The Rosetta Stone: intelligent analytics, which can turn terabytes of data into useful, actionable knowledge in nanoseconds.

The American Health Information Management Association issued a white paper in June 2005 to recommend automated coding software to enhance productivity, effectiveness and anti-fraud activities. The paper reports that when combined with the EHR, automated coding could streamline the way that healthcare organizations gather data and bill for services. When integrated and enhanced with intelligent analytics, the system could become a powerful tool for pre-payment and post-payment audits and predicting potential fraud; it could solve multiple problems simultaneously.

Evidence abounds for advancing the EHR and integration. It starts with studies showing that medical personnel don't have the time to fill in all the boxes on claims. Some claims lack detail because they are simply linked to a percentage of payment. As with financial transactions, validity of the information on the bill or claim will be important to payment integrity and the most important long-term goal of our healthcare system: improving patient care.

Examples From the Financial Sector

Establishing integrated, highly efficient systems has been a proven benefit to the financial sector, which has standards for electronic transactions around the world. You can be in Kuala Lumpur and get cash from a bank in California, plus be alerted to potential fraud if the transaction doesn't fit your profile and history. The same approach can work in healthcare with EHRs managing every claim as a detailed, data-rich transaction that fits into a bigger universe of many other transactions just like it, all being constantly analyzed for appropriateness, new trends and aberrations.

Pharmacies are already at the forefront of this evolution because they operate in the closest thing to a credit card-like system. In this environment, analytics can intercede during the rapid authorization process to prevent fraud. Also information captured on the pharmacy side will be a core element in representing the patient's condition to any provider, anywhere, when accessing the EHR.

Dire Need for Consistent Information

Connecting for Health, a public-private collaboration that was launched in June 2002, notes that the current system is economically ineffi-

Andrea Allmon is director of healthcare operations and product management for Fair Isaac's predictive software products for the healthcare industry. She led the development of the industry's first prepayment fraud detection system that has resulted in millions of dollars of savings for leading healthcare payers. **Jean de Traversay** is director of analytic science for Fair Isaac's predictive software products for the healthcare industry. He has an extensive background in commercial health insurance and in clinical research.

cient and clinically dangerous. It says that emerging technologies offer an unprecedented ability to provide accurate and actionable medical information in a secure and private format when and where it is needed – whether by patients themselves, or by the clinicians who care for them.

Access to consistent, quality information can also have a positive impact on improved adherence to prescription regimens, another potential area for proactively controlling costs while reducing human suffering. Studies by the Case Management Society of America note that more than half of all Americans fail to follow their prescriptions, which can decrease the quality of their lives and life spans while increasing healthcare costs throughout the system (e.g., the annual cost of a prescription versus the cost of bypass surgery). In fact, non-adherence to prescriptions costs the U.S. healthcare system some $100 billion a year. Studies by the American Heart Association estimate that non-adherence causes more than 125,000 deaths in the U.S. each year among those taking cardiovascular medications.

Avoiding Deaths From Medical Errors

The Institute of Medicine notes that up to 98,000 people die in hospitals each year as the result of medical errors. Elderly U.S. patients are prescribed improper medications in about one out of every 12 physician visits. More than 57,000 Americans die needlessly each year because they do not receive appropriate healthcare (different from medical errors or lack of access) according to a study from the National Committee for Quality Assurance.

Moreover according to the Institute of Medicine, more than 500,000 people are injured annually in the United States due to avoidable adverse drug events. The institute stresses the importance of linking medical records electronically to ensure more prompt and accurate diagnoses, more appropriate treatment decisions and the avoidance of adverse consequences. This will become increasingly important as the population continues to age and patients begin to see multiple providers with more frequency.

Fraud on the Rise

Estimates of annual losses resulting from all types of healthcare fraud are staggering, and range from 3 to 10 percent of national healthcare expenditures. This translates to $54 billion to $179 billion based on 2004 expenditures of $1.79 trillion projected by the Centers for Medicare & Medicaid Services. In 2002, the Office of the Inspector General of the U.S. Department of Health and Human Services identified $12.1 billion in fraudulent claims paid by Medicare. The system will see additional costs after Jan. 1, 2006, when Medicare Part D of the Medicare Modernization Act becomes effective, making voluntary prescription drug benefits available for the first time to more than 40 million Medicare beneficiaries.

The Benefits of Integration and the EHR

If we integrate the clinical side, pharmacy, payment histories, financial models and other forms of relevant data, the richness of the information will provide benefits and positive results on every front: patient treatment and satisfaction, medical reimbursement, transaction accuracy, best practices and reduced fraud.

The Center for Information Technology Leadership estimates that the use of electronic systems for ordering medicines could deliver national savings of $86.8 billion annually after full implementation and would result in significant direct financial benefits for providers and other stakeholders.

The Journal of the American Medical Informatics Association estimated that the use of electronic systems for ordering medicines has already reduced the incidence of serious medication errors by 86 percent. Intelligent analytics, with pharmacy data, can help monitor the regimen to ensure it's appropriate. It can also detect suspicious activity and billing and policy errors in pharmacy claims at the point of sale, prior to payment or immediately after payment.

The benefits will even translate to favorably impacting one of the more frustrating aspects of visiting a provider: having to fill out a detailed patient history on a fifth-generation photocopy of a typed form with each new visit while having to retell your story to multiple people as you work your way through the doctor's office or hospital.

The Bigger Fraud, Abuse and Errors Issue

The EHR and integrated systems will enable the analysis of millions of interactions in a fraction of a second, using both incoming and historical data. Neural networks can then create a multidimensional picture of the healthcare and pharmacy delivery system. Users can quickly identify fraudulent activity, including fraud types that previously could not be detected, new and unknown fraud patterns as well as subtle and complex trends by looking at each claim in relation to deep contextual information, such as the patient's and provider's histories. For example:

- Wrong tests (e.g., pediatrician giving an allergy test; OB/GYN running a prostate-specific antigen test);
- Double dipping (two bills for the same patient on the same day or consecutive days);
- Upcoding (an expensive procedure not indicated by the patient history);
- Nonstandard procedures (hemorrhoidectomy by a dermatologist); and
- A prescription that doesn't tie into the diagnosis and patient history.

The History of Advanced Decisioning Systems

Advanced analytics has been used in a number of industries for decades. One of the more successful applications today is the detection of fraud in the financial services industry.

Credit card fraud is perceived as a huge problem, yet the use of advanced analytics has reduced annual losses to $788 million, which is dwarfed by healthcare fraud, totaling an estimated $54 billion to $179 billion a year. The technology leaders in healthcare, including payers, understand the potential return on investment and have started using an adaptation of the software that proved so valuable in spotting and stopping credit card fraud. Since this decisioning technology is highly evolved, success is coming quickly; case studies are emerging that demonstrate positive results in detecting fraud in the more complicated and intricate world of healthcare reimbursement.

Saving Money Throughout the Claims Process

Fraud, abuse and errors occur in every aspect of the healthcare system: hospitals, doctors' offices, laboratories, dental facilities and pharmacies. A doctor may get away with billing twice for the same surgery on the same patient in the same day, for example, or a dentist may abuse the system by filling cavities on perfectly healthy teeth or dentures. But with adoption of an EHR standard, organizations armed with the latest intelligent software can combat such deviance with dramatic, cost-saving results.

Healthcare payers using advanced decisioning applications find themselves a step ahead of the game. Once data analysis is performed by the system, claim outcomes appear in the form of scores, each coming with explanations to justify the score. Claims adjusters, fraud investigators, case managers and other personnel are able to focus their review on claims with the highest likelihood of fraud, abuse or error. Scoring criteria and thresholds can be used to automatically determine the priority given to individual claims. This allows healthcare payers to operate more efficiently from a personnel standpoint in addition to reducing costs lost to fraud, abuse and errors.

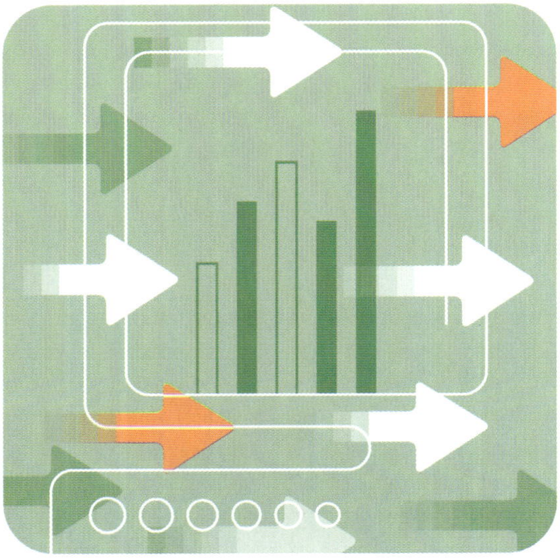

Advanced decisioning systems really flex their muscles through profiling technology. The profiling technology compresses terabytes of claims and claims-related data into essential informational packets, allowing predictive models to perform detailed analyses of such information in a matter of seconds. And since the profiling technology is dynamic, the system is able to detect fraud with increasingly greater accuracy over time and with additional aggregate data, giving organizations a greater opportunity to catch fraud, abuse and erroneous claims before the checks are cut. As a result, the most advanced payers employ both prepayment and postpayment analytics and watch the benefits flow to the bottom line.

Prospective and Retrospective Detection

Systems should be both prospective and retrospective to ensure the reduction of healthcare fraud, abuse and erroneous payments in all stages of the claims process. Used in a number of cutting-edge business applications, such as airline security and infectious disease control, predictive models are able to discover patterns and discern otherwise cryptic relationships among complex data.

Once claims are already paid, the time, the effort and expense needed to attempt to recoup losses from fraud rise exponentially. So it's in the best interest of healthcare payers to detect such claims before they're paid, whenever possible. And with advanced decisioning systems, claims that are most at risk for fraud, abuse or error can be quickly detected with very high accuracy.

Advanced analyses enable healthcare payers to reap extraordinary benefits after payment as well. The intelligent processes of these analyses enable organizations to successfully review suspicious providers without expending laborious hours chasing red herrings. And when payers utilize post-payment analysis, they are able to detect fraud that's only apparent over time, and not necessarily detected in smaller data sets.

Industry-Specific Detection

Advanced decisioning systems can expertly analyze claims for fraud or error from every part of the healthcare sector, including medical, pharmacy and dental. Predictive models then allow organizations to detect unusual medical practices and charges that are inconsistent within a given peer group, so orthopedic surgeons are compared to and against one another, oncologists to other oncologists, chiropractors with other chiropractors. A sophisticated blend of predictive models and expert decision logic are used to understand a provider's practice patterns to determine the appropriate peer group for comparison. In one case, advanced analytics discovered a psychiatrist seeing 112 patients in a single day – for 75-minute procedures and a total of 140 billable hours in one day.

Benefiting the System

As validated by an increasing body of evidence, every positive step taken to adopt the EHR and integrate it into other elements of the data universe of our healthcare system will generate positive outcomes at every link in the transaction chain. Payers will succeed in cracking down on fraud. The system will run more smoothly and efficiently. The cost savings to payers will enable more affordable coverage plans and reduce costs to employers while improving quality of care. While advanced information technology programs and analytic tools have been used successfully for years in other industries, now is the perfect time for organizations throughout the healthcare continuum to agree on their own IT standards, starting with the EHR, automated coding and advanced analytics. ■

Making the Right Decisions Easy

Fair Isaac's leading healthcare solutions for healthcare payers and providers include advanced analytics, business rules, analytic applications and business consulting to propel the healthcare industry to higher levels of business efficiency, profitability and innovation.

Payer organizations use Fair Isaac's healthcare analytics and patented dynamic profiling technologies to identify not only fraud and abuse, but also processing errors, billing issues, internal policy and system flaws – before payment is issued – leading to reduced risk and improved operating costs. Fair Isaac's enterprise decision management platform provides the flexibility to deliver solutions using business rules or analytics and business rules in combination. Many healthcare organizations are using this technology to develop customized applications for automated decision making in areas such as member management, underwriting, marketing, care plan management and eligibility and enrollment.

Healthcare providers are using Fair Isaac's business rules-based solutions to identify drug interactions, improve clinical care and manage complex schedules. Systems that ensure compliance with evidence-based medical guidelines and eliminate redundant and unnecessary tests are used to ensure quality care and cost-effectiveness. Rules and analytics are used in combination at admission to ensure that billing and coverage information is assessed to minimize later paperwork problems, confirm that identity is correctly established and that the correct billing processes are initiated.

Solutions for Providers and Payers

Fair Isaac Blaze Advisor

Consistently ranked as a leader in the top right of Gartner's "Magic Quadrant for Business Rules Engines," Blaze Advisor provides a complete set of tools for developing, deploying and maintaining business rule applications and services. Powerful analytic models can be integrated into Blaze Advisor to maximize decision-making power. It is used by providers to check for drug interactions, enforce clinical care guidelines, reduce unnecessary tests and increase administrative efficiency. Leading solutions' companies such as IDX, Misys, and MEDecision embed Blaze Advisor as part of their various offerings to healthcare providers.

Blaze Advisor is also used by payers to manage eligibility, enrollment, HIPAA compliance, coverage and claims.

Patient Decision Manager

Patient Decision Manager generates patient-specific payment strategies at the point of admission using analytical processes, business rules and credit scores. Providers can increase payments and reduce bad debt while verifying patients' identities to reduce fraudulent use of insurance coverage.

Payment Optimizer Solution

Payment Optimizer® solution is the first fraud, abuse and error detection system for healthcare payers that provides both prepayment scoring and postpayment analysis to reduce fraud losses and ensure payment integrity in pharmacy and medical claims.

Model Builder and Predictive Science

A complete development environment for building predictive analytics, Model Builder is the same tool used by Fair Isaac's own analytic experts. Our Predictive Science custom modeling services use Model Builder to deliver sophisticated models for predicting risk, fraud and more.

Find Out More

Fair Isaac offers products and services can help you make profitable decisions across your entire organization. Contact us to find out more. ■

weblink

Learn more about how the Payment Optimizer® solution can catch fraud before payout in the GEHA case study at www.fairisaac.com/hct.

Fair Isaac Corporation (NYSE: FIC) is the leading provider of decision management solutions powered by advanced analytics. Fair Isaac solutions reduce fraud, manage risk and reduce costs for healthcare companies worldwide.

Tom Grudnowski
Chief Executive Officer

James Taylor
Vice President Product Marketing Enterprise Decision Management

Jim Kalustian
Client Partner and Vice President, Healthcare Services

Anu Pathria, Ph.D.
Vice President, Healthcare and Insurance Analytics

Fair Isaac Headquarters
901 Marquette Avenue
Suite 3200
Minneapolis, MN 55402
Phone 612.758.5200
www.fairisaac.com/hct

Business Contact Group
Enterprise Decision Management Sales
edm@fairisaac.com
Toll-Free 888 FICO EDM
Phone 408.535.1500

5

The Business Case for EHR

Making an understandable and convincing business case for EHR means careful consideration both of the quantitative and qualitative benefits associated with implementation.

[R. Wesley Champion, Accenture] [Judith M. Wilczewski, R.N., Accenture]

An EHR infrastructure provides substantial opportunities to favorably impact clinical care and improve the bottom line. The most obvious improvements include improving patient safety by reducing incidences of adverse drug events, reducing unnecessary clinical practice variation to enhance clinical outcomes and enabling timely and effective information sharing that leads to quicker and better decisions for care delivery and increases the accuracy of data and revenue capture.

Successful EHR development requires a structured work plan and timeline that includes a comprehensive benefits analysis (identifying both organizational and broader market "wins"), a project measurement process and plan to address the organizational changes that are necessary to realize anticipated results and benefits.

EHR implementation begins with defined organizational goals and objectives that are tied to discrete elements of the implementation work plan. Discrete elements that must be considered include: a clear understanding of the role that technology plays in achieving organizational goals and objectives, a precise definition of anticipated quantitative and qualitative benefits, sufficient planned technical functionality to support electronic enablement, a collaborative process to assure EHR integration across complex organizations and a road map and timeline for system design and operations re-engineering – all to achieve the desired level of integration with realistic expectations about when value will be realized.

Quantitative or Financial Benefits

The first step is to uncover the benefits that provide a financial upside for the organization and also provide additional revenue to help underwrite the EHR effort. These quantitative benefits can be directly measured in the financial statements of the organization, unlike a cost deferment or quality enhancement. They include:

- Revenue enhancements (revenue capture, pay-for-performance, volume, market share);
- Cost reductions (productivity, utilization, transcription, forms, inventory);
- Cash acceleration; and
- Cost avoidance (cost associated with adverse drug events – morbidity, mortality, liability).

Realizing benefits assumes a high level of operational commitment in tandem with full implementation of targeted applications. This commitment may require a re-engineering and standardization of key operational processes before or in parallel with system design and build. Specific system requirements (functionality, integration, interfaces, etc.) as well as transformation enablers (defined accountabilities, roles, infrastructure, processes and mechanisms for ongoing management and maintenance) need to be defined for each benefit (see Figure 1).

Benefits That Reduce Future Costs

There are also quantitative benefits that result from EHR implementation that are not immediately measurable in financial statements. These are usually cost deferments on changes and processes that need to be managed in the present to help avoid cost increases in the future.

An example of such non-measurable financial benefits is the cost of pharmaceutical supplies, which are subject to price increases and represent a substantial and growing cost burden for all medical organizations.

R. Wesley Champion is a partner with Accenture and the national leader of Strategy and Transformation Services, Health & Life Sciences practice. He has over 17 years of healthcare consulting and management experience, concentrating his efforts in large-scale organizationwide improvement, strategy and change management activities in hospitals and multihospital systems. **Judith M. Wilczewski, R.N.,** is a senior manager of Accenture's Provider, Health & Life Sciences practice and one of the practice leaders for operational and benefit aspects of Clinical Transformation.

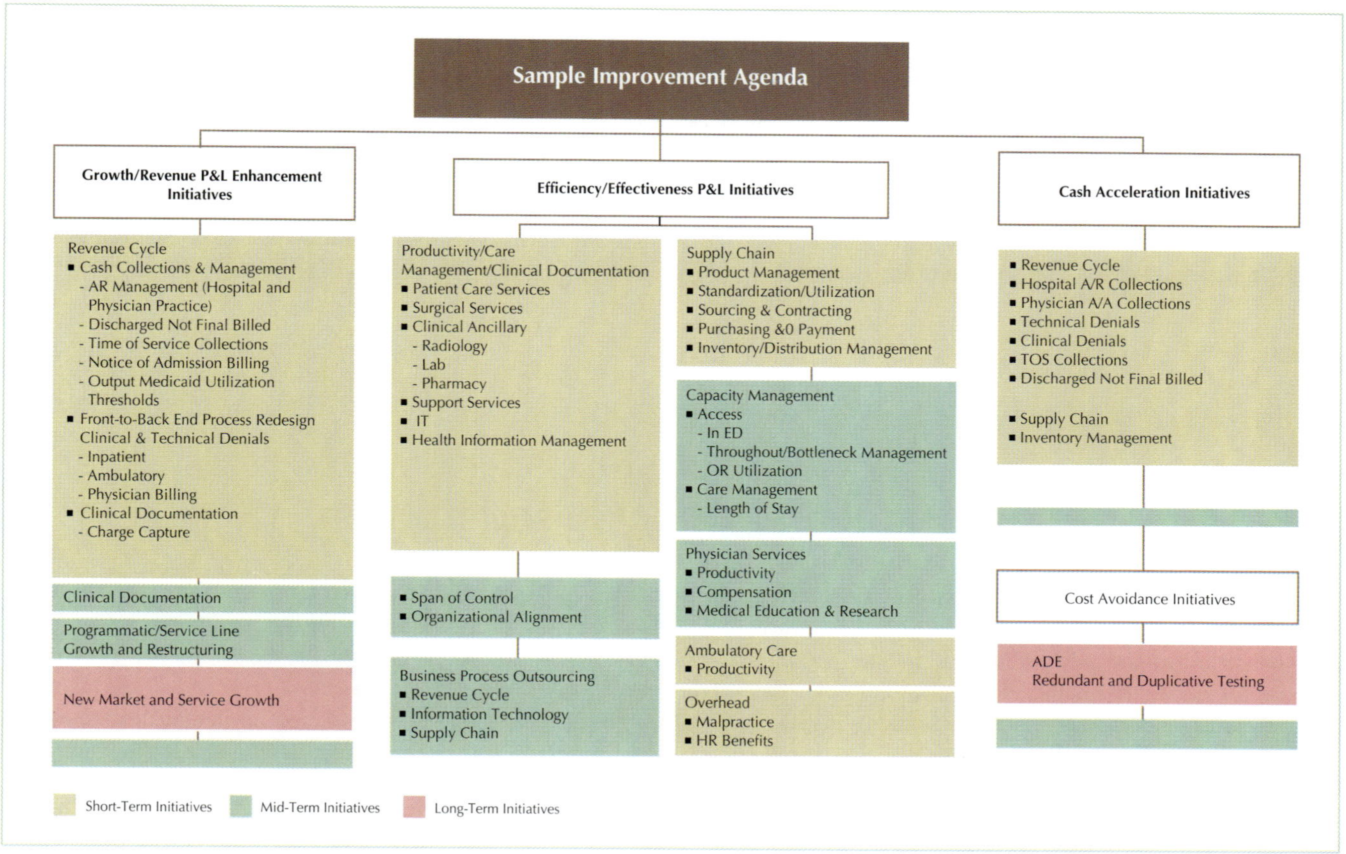

Figure 1 Sample Improvement Agenda

Qualitative or Nonfinancial Benefits

Market pressures to deliver and demonstrate high levels of quality, customer service and financial performance are increasing. Organizations such as the Institute of Medicine (IOM), The Leapfrog Group, Centers for Medicare & Medicaid Services (CMS), Joint Commission on Accreditation of Healthcare Organizations (JCAHO) and others are explicitly defining, demanding and publicly reporting measures of quality. Though qualitative benefits look beyond the numbers at all factors that influence the quality of the services offered by the organization (clinical practices and patient safety) and general personnel and operational issues, many, if not all, of these benefits will generate a significant financial benefit; for example, quality-based pay-for-performance incentives via CMS and some commercial payers.

There are three main aspects of qualitative benefits: clinical quality and patient safety; operational efficiency and effectiveness; and physician and staff satisfaction.

Clinical Quality and Patient Safety

Mechanisms critical to realizing optimal outcomes include reduction of unnecessary clinical practice variation, timely access to information and the ability to communicate and synthesize information to improve decision making (for medical diagnosis and treatment). Technology plays a critical role in enabling this work.

For example, a reduction in medication errors can be supported by implementation of a closed-loop medication use process. This process links together technical mechanisms to reduce prescribing errors (computerized physician order entry, or CPOE), dispensing errors (pharmacy applications) and administration errors (electronic medication administration record and bar coding).

Adding standardization (standardized order sets) creates the vehicle for reducing unnecessary variations in clinical practice – such as consistently prescribing the drugs (type and dosage) that correspond to the patient health profile via rules, alerts and reminders (i.e., critical lab values and allergy information) that result both in qualitative and quantitative benefits.

The business value of these qualitative benefits includes reduction of costs associated with adverse drug events (morbidity, mortality, liability), reduction of costs associated with avoidable clinical practice variation (medication use management, reduction of redundant or duplicative testing), enhanced revenue related to improved charge capture and elimination of costs associated with paper documents (forms, transcription, storage).

Operational Efficiency and Effectiveness

The increased standardization of clinical practice, work flow and documentation improves the performance and efficiency of clinical teams and operational departments by increasing accuracy and legibility of patient information and orders, reducing turnaround time for care delivery (orders and results), enabling real-time access to information and interventions, automating checks and balances to monitor adherence to performance criteria and increasing patient throughput and volume (backfill), etc. In addition, reducing the number of manual processes increases productivity and may reduce the number of people in the organization needed to provide requisite levels of quality, particularly the number of agency or contracted employees who tend to have the most negative impact on the bottom line.

Operational management will welcome the improved financial impact resulting from increased efficiencies.

Physician and Staff Satisfaction

Operational efficiency and effectiveness are integrally linked with physician and staff satisfaction.

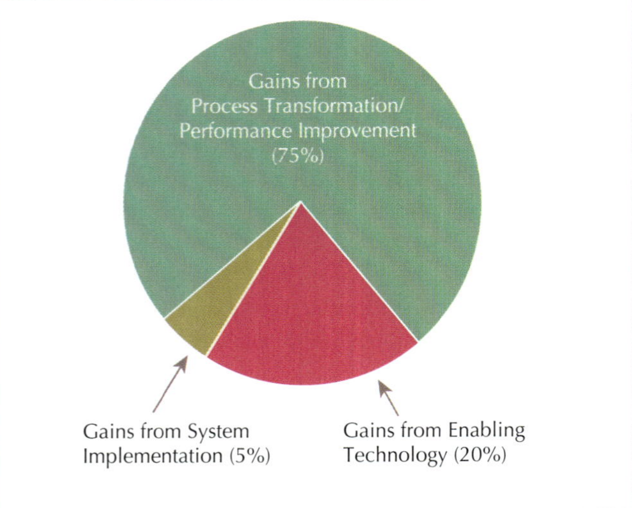

Figure 2 Representative Contribution to Goal Achievement

Standardizing what pops up on the screen when a patient is admitted not only improves the quality of documentation and an organization's services, it also improves the quality of the clinical work experience for physicians, nursing teams and clinical staff. By eliminating redundancies, streamlining work flow and increasing productivity through real-time access to information, less time is spent on manual and often redundant processes, information retrieval, documentation and confirmation calls and the quality of decision making is markedly improved.

Less time spent with paperwork through better clinical processes increases the time that clinical staff spend with patients, contributing both to patient and clinician satisfaction.

Less time spent with paperwork through better clinical processes increases the time that clinical staff spend with patients, contributing both to patient and clinician satisfaction. This is an important factor in any EHR program because many of the benefits originate with and are linked directly to physician practice and work flow. Any successful implementation will depend in large part on physician support of the goals and resulting process changes.

The business value of these qualitative benefits includes elimination of costs associated with paper documents (forms, transcription, storage), reduced incidental overtime and turnover and increased patient throughput, among others.

Magnitude of Benefit

Organizations must consider two key factors when calculating anticipated EHR-related return on investment. The first consideration is that the magnitude of anticipated benefit depends on the scope of planned technology enablement (i.e., emergency department versus acute care versus both ED and acute pharmacy applications versus POE versus both pharmacy and CPOE, etc.) The second consideration is that the magnitude of anticipated benefit depends on an organization's willingness to move beyond the narrow realm of benefits tied directly to implementation of the technology.

Understanding the Relationship Of Benefits to Technology

Whether quantitative or qualitative, benefits associated with information technology implementation are classified into three distinct categories:

- Technology-dependent: Benefits not possible without implementation of technology such as the closed-loop medication use process.

- Technology-enabled: Benefits that can be realized without technology but are accelerated, enhanced and/or sustained by technology (such as standardized order sets or standardized clinical documentation); technology enhances and accelerates the benefits of reducing variation by increasing availability and access and incorporating rules, alerts and reminders to speed and improve the results.
- Technology-independent: Benefits that have little or no direct relationship to technology, such as improving existing processes that help realize efficiencies and reduce costs.

It is our experience that the percentage of total benefit increases exponentially when moving from dependent to enabled to independent. Also clients who pay attention to all three of these categories achieve the greatest return on investment. Often benefits classified as "independent from technology" are excluded from the EHR business case. But the goal is to generate value (qualitative and quantitative) and create a funding source to finance the transition to an EHR system, so this benefit category can play a critical role (see Figure 2).

Technology-independent benefits may already be on the table or may need to be identified. Often EHR implementation provides the focal point necessary to marshal interest and resources more broadly to cover all three benefit categories.

Leveraging Technology to Create Value

Successful EHR implementation requires the integration of the project goals and process changes with the design, structure and deployment of the information system that stands behind the program. The clinical transformation – including the targeted benefits, the streamlined work flow processes, alignment of the physicians and other EHR enablers – can create the desired value only if all linked to the information system design (required workflow processes, IT system functionality and operational and physical design).

EHR implementation also requires integrating the ability to drive value and effectively execute the project. While project management focuses on kick off, design, build, test, conversion, train and go-live (often with the primary focus on technology), the ability to reap maximal benefit is contingent upon an organi-

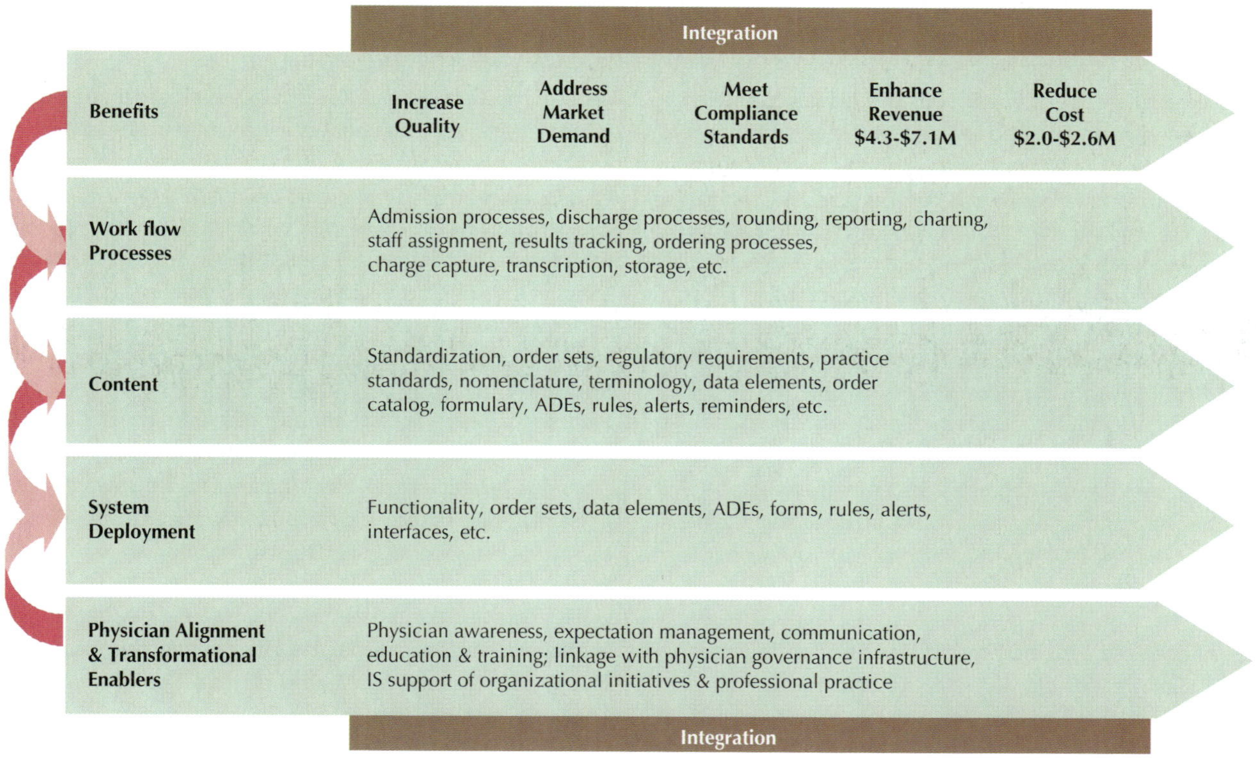

Figure 3 Global example – Linkage of benefit type to work flow process redesign, content development, system deployment, physician alignment and transformational enablers required.

zation's ability to drive value by integrating target benefits, work flow process redesign, content development and system deployment, with physician alignment and transformational enablers, (see Figure 3).

Measure and Manage Project Goals

Depending on an organization's view, while all of the aforementioned benefits are important, any one of the benefits may be key to driving EHR implementation. Many people in an organization may be motivated by the qualitative or nonfinancial benefits, but all organizations base an initial decision to pursue EHR on a clear and sober analysis of the costs and benefits.

For the client considering EHR implementation, the process usually begins with the question, "What is the ultimate goal?" Regardless of the motivating factors driving the decision to pursue EHR, it is important to balance needs with desires and to manage expectations. Doing so will help the organization develop a clear understanding of what can be achieved with EHR, what is required over and above technology to achieve project goals and when realization of benefit can be expected. Once all of this is articulated, defined and communicated, a detailed implementation plan must be developed, along with a rigorous mechanism for measurement, reporting and accountability for results to ensure that the project remains on track.

To fully realize the desired benefits, EHR implementation requires a high level of commitment and ownership by the clinical staff. Hurdles in the transformation process include:

- Committing to increased standardization (evidence-based order sets, documentation templates);
- Adjusting work flows to optimize EHR benefits; and
- Coping with the initial negative impact on productivity; and
- Need for extensive training and support before, during and after implementation.

On the technical side, EHR implementation also places rigorous demands on information system performance (network and system stability, response time, effective downtime procedures and point-of-care hardware).

Establishing a Collaborative Approach

At the beginning of an EHR program, organizations are often all over the board with departmental overlaps, process redundancies, incompatible legacy systems and inefficient infrastructure management – to name just a few issues. A collaborative approach is key to a successful EHR implementation process. Representatives from all involved departments should be involved to articulate their needs and to generate and maintain wide acceptance for EHR implementation.

A complete EHR program may have over a dozen initiatives that both include financial and service quality issues: reducing overtime, drug prescriptions, compliance with patient care standards and managing hospital backfill. To pinpoint areas where EHR can deliver maximum benefits, cost and revenue structures should be analyzed, potential efficiencies identified and current and future costs determined. Differing requirements need to be integrated, and both the potential quantitative and qualitative benefits laid out. Once the clinical teams working on the front lines with patients see what EHR can achieve, the EHR benefits become a driving factor in the positive transformation of the organization.

To pinpoint areas where EHR can deliver maximum benefits, cost and revenue structures should be analyzed, potential efficiencies identified, and current and future costs determined.

Summary

Assuring the success of EHR implementation starts with careful analysis of the potential costs and benefits. The quantitative (financial) benefits (dependent, enabled or independent of the implementation of technology) can be directly measured and can provide an exponential increase in benefits when realized together. Qualitative (nonfinancial) benefits focus on service quality, patient safety, personnel and physician satisfaction and operational efficiency and effectiveness, but may also have a significant positive financial effect. ■

Transforming Healthcare With Connected EHRs

Today new medical advances in the healthcare industry are dramatically changing the way care is provided to patients. At the same time, healthcare organizations are under pressure to cut costs, increase productivity and improve patient care. Connected healthcare applications, including electronic health records, that address these issues and streamline information and communications at the point of care are critical. These applications require a network infrastructure that is "medical grade" to satisfy the requirements of patients and the highly specialized professionals who rely on them.

The Cisco® Medical-Grade Network provides a foundation for healthcare organizations to enable a wide variety of applications. Built on industry best practices and standards, the Cisco Medical-Grade Network provides the underlying architecture designed to meet the specific needs of health care.

- Utilizes intelligence to triage information, delivering the right information to the right people at the right time;
- Integrates vital equipment and devices into a converged infrastructure, streamlining communications and care;
- Protects with self-defending network security; and
- Connects people and information in real time regardless of location or device, creating efficiencies and responsiveness.

Solutions

Managing a clinical environment today involves paper – lots of it. Clinical information stored in paper charts is difficult to access, takes up costly space dedicated to chart storage and can impact quality of care. **Connected Electronic Health Records** provides effective distribution of information to caregivers at the point of care to support higher-quality care with increased efficiency. Physician productivity and clinical efficiency can be improved by automating common activities including prescribing, capturing charges, dictating, ordering labs, viewing results, providing patient education and taking clinical notes over the network. Clinicians have access to patient charts and medical histories without having to search files or wait for chart pulls. Connected electronic health records over secure wireless or the Internet provide remote access to medical records from satellite sites, or even from home.

In many cases, the electronic health record includes images as well. **E-Radiology** applications implemented over the Medical-Grade Network extend the reach of diagnostic imaging capabilities for radiologists and clinicians in the hospital or at remote locations. The networked availability of images and patient records at remote locations provides for more effective consultation and faster diagnosis and treatment.

Effective communication is also critical for quality care. **The Cisco Clinical Connection Suite** (nurse call, patient monitoring, location-based services, collaborative care) simplifies the process of communications and helps clinicians find what they need when they need it. The solution combines Cisco Medical-Grade Network technologies – IP Communications, Wireless Mobility, Security – with industry-leading partner applications to drive faster, smarter healthcare by directing, locating and prioritizing information for clinicians and their patients, optimizing work flow increasing productivity and enhancing the patient's experience and care.

Cisco Systems, Inc.

Founded in 1984, Cisco Systems, Inc. is the worldwide leader in networking for the Internet. Since the company's inception, Cisco engineers have been leaders in the development of IP-based networking technologies. This tradition of IP innovation continues with industry-leading products and solutions. ■

CISCO SYSTEMS

Cisco Systems, Inc. is the worldwide leader in networking for the Internet and the development of IP-based networking technologies.

John Chambers
President and
Chief Executive Officer

Cisco Systems, Inc.
170 West Tasman Dr.
San Jose, CA 95134-1941
Phone 408.526.4000
www.cisco.com

Business Contact
Kacey Carpenter
Healthcare Marketing Manager
Phone 408.527.0371
kacey@cisco.com

The Impact on Healthcare Costs For American Companies

Because U.S. healthcare challenges have created a competitive gap for American companies, many are calling for the transformation of the healthcare industry.

[Jeffrey Rideout, M.D., M.A., F.A.C.P., Cisco Systems]

Nearly 100,000 Americans lose their lives each year to preventable medical errors.[1] More than 45 million Americans – about 15 percent of the total population – are uninsured.[2] Getting evidence-based care in many situations is not much better than a coin flip[3], and medical costs are now the country's second leading cause of personal bankruptcy.[4]

None of these trends is improving. In fact, most are getting worse. At current rates, it is estimated that 28 percent of the American workforce will be uninsured by 2013.[5] Unfortunately the shock value of these numbers seems to be wearing off without any change in sight.

Healthcare's impact on national productivity is equally alarming. In June 2005, General Motors announced it was laying off 25,000 employees to reduce costs, specifically citing surging healthcare expenses.[6] Ford spent $3.2 billion on healthcare in 2003 for 560,000 employees, retirees and their dependents. This cost added $1,000 to the price of every Ford car and truck built in the United States – up from $700 in 2000.[7]

The rising healthcare tab means Ford has less money to invest in new products. "Our foreign competitors don't share these problems," Ford Motor Co. Vice Chairman Allan Gilmour said in a speech in July 2004. "These healthcare challenges have created a competitive gap that, if unchecked, will drive investment decisions away from the United States."[8]

High U.S. Healthcare Costs, But a Care Shortfall

The United States spends more on healthcare than any other industrialized country – as much as 44 percent more than Switzerland, the country with the next highest per capita expenditure. In 2000, U.S. per capita healthcare spending was 83 percent higher than that of neighboring Canada and 134 percent more than the median of $1,983 for the 30 industrialized countries in the Organization for Economic Cooperation and Development.[9]

Despite this spending, Americans are not necessarily getting better care. In a national study on quality of care published in 2005, RAND Corporation found that American adults were receiving about one-half of recommended medical services; that is, services shown in scientific literature to be effective in specific circumstances and agreed upon by medical experts.[10]

RAND's study found quality deficits across chronic, preventive and acute care. Recommended care for managing chronic conditions (such as diabetes and hypertension) was provided 56 percent of the time. Preventive care (such as flu shots, mammograms and smoking cessation counseling) met quality standards 55 percent of the time. Recommended care for acute health problems (such as pneumonia and urinary tract infections) was provided 54 percent of the time.[11]

These deficits in care pose serious threats to the health of the American public and translate into thousands of preventable complications and deaths each year. According to one estimate from the Agency for Healthcare Research and Quality, 1.12 million problems with patient safety occurred in 1.07 million hospitalizations, about one per hospitalization.[12]

Industry Comparison Shows Low U.S. Healthcare IT Investment

While there are many contributing factors to the healthcare dilemma Americans now face, it is undeniable that investment in healthcare information technology (HIT) has been lacking relative to nearly every other U.S. industry. In a 2000 McKinsey report on annual U.S. IT spending per employee, healthcare ranked in the bottom five of 59 industries surveyed, at just $1,156.[13] The average U.S. IT investment per capita in all U.S. industries is seven

Jeffrey Rideout, M.D., M.A., F.A.C.P., is vice president of Internet business solutions group, healthcare practice, for Cisco Systems. He is also the company's corporate medical director. Dr. Rideout, a board certified internist, previously was chief medical officer and SVP for Blue Shield of California. A former Rhodes Scholar, Dr. Rideout graduated from Harvard Medical School.

	Cumulative Implementation years 1–10 (in billions)	Annual steady state, starting year 11 (in billions)
Stage 2		
Benefit	$141	$21
Cost	0	0
Net value	$141	$21
Stage 3		
Benefit	$286	$44
Cost	$320	$20
Net value	-$34	$24
Stage 4		
Benefit	$613	$94
Cost	$276	$16
Net value	$337	$78

Figure 1 Net Value of Healthcare Information Exchange and Interoperability

times higher than that invested in healthcare. Banking, for example, invests nearly 10 times as much as healthcare per employee. While getting cash from an ATM in Moscow might be important, getting the right medication can be a matter of life or death at home in the United States.

Moreover much of the money being spent, unfortunately, is not supporting clinical care. Harvard Medical School researchers reported in early 2005 that the United States spends $399 billion per year on healthcare bureaucracy – essentially the waste in a fragmented, paper-bound, uncoordinated system of care.[14] Of the nearly 30 billion healthcare communications that occur each year, more than 90 percent are handled by paper, surface mail, fax or telephone.[15]

Technology Can Drive Healthcare Savings

Technology-enabled clinical processes have been shown to dramatically reduce medical errors, complications, readmissions and mortality rates when properly implemented, while improving efficiencies. The stakes are huge. E-prescribing applications help automate prescription orders and refills. Assuming a 70 to 75 percent adoption rate, e-prescribing could save the United States $29 billion a year.[16] If computerized physician order entry (CPOE) and electronic health records (EHR) were added in a stand-alone environment, the savings would be $44 billion.[17] The savings climb another $78 billion if these applications – the full EHR suite – are implemented by your local doctor's office and are interoperable with other doctors' offices.[18] Each technology has also been associated with improvements in patient quality and safety.

In a *Health Affairs* paper, the Center for Information Technology Leadership (CITL) divided EHR into four deployment stages and forecasted savings over the next 10 years (see Figure 1). The first stage relies on telephone and traditional mail communication, providing the foundation for future deployments. The second stage adds faxes and scanning. According to the CITL study, the implementation cost of stage-two capability is nothing. The cumulative net value benefit over 10 years would be $141 billion, with a steady state annual benefit of $21.6 billion starting in year 11.[19]

The third stage allows for the sharing of nonstandardized data. At this level, additional complications often arise due to incompatible vocabulary and proprietary file formats. As a result, analysis indicates that the net value of implementing stage three EHR would be negative $34 billion over 10 years. It would cost $320 billion to deploy, only partially offset by a benefit of $286 billion. Starting in year 11, however, the steady-state annual benefit would be nearly $24 billion.[20]

Stage four is where business and government need to be to take full advantage of potential savings. At this level, all messages are standardized and coded for complete sharing of information through the system. In effect, this would mean having a universal translator for healthcare information; different segments of the healthcare industry, ideally on a global scale, would need to agree on terms and how they related to each other. Analysis indicates that deployment over 10 years would cost $276 billion. The benefit to the United States, however, would be $613 billion, for a net value benefit of $337 billion. The steady-state annual benefit would be $94 billion starting from year 11.[21]

Technologies Being Deployed Now

A key function of EHR is CPOE. According to CITL, the typical physician using an advanced ambulatory computerized physician order entry (ACPOE) system would save close to $28,000 per year. Advanced systems cost nearly five times as much as basic ACPOE, but produce more than 12 times greater financial returns.[22] (See Figure 2.)

Another key feature of most EHRs, also available in more "stand-alone" applications, is e-prescribing. Solutions from companies such as Allscripts Healthcare Solutions allow physicians to order a drug and route the prescription to a pharmacy directly from the exam room with a personal computer or handheld device such as a personal digital assistant. Most e-prescribing includes drug reference information, drug alerts, automated prescription refills and electronic prescription transmission.

Medco Health Solutions, Inc., TPI Health Systems and Cardiovascular Associates conducted a study in 2003 to demonstrate the efficiency of e-prescribing. At the start of the study, 29 percent of prescriptions resulted in pharmacy callbacks, with 86 percent of those pertaining to refill or renewal questions. These calls were costing more than $175,000 in medical assistant time and lost revenue opportunities.[23]

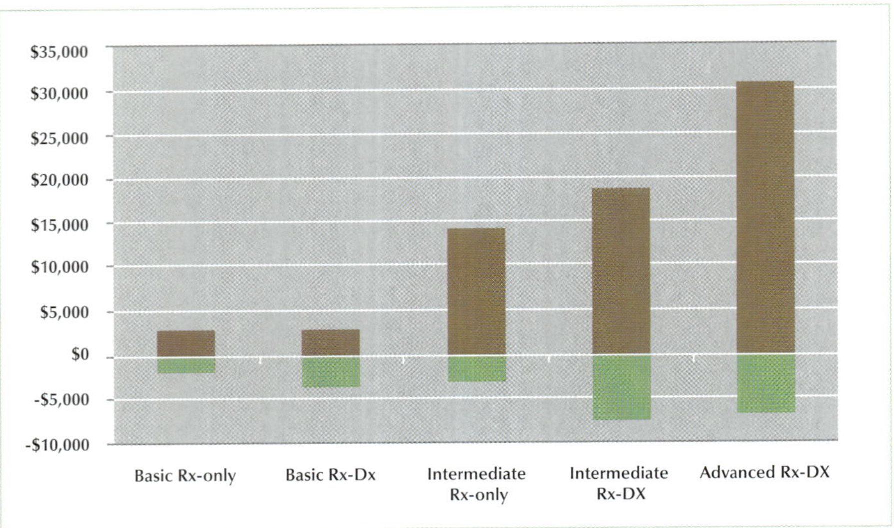

Figure 2 Annual Cost Benefit of ACPOE in the First Five Years

Within three months of implementing a new e-prescribing platform and improved training procedures, inbound pharmacy calls fell 36 percent and the number of outbound calls to manage renewals declined 50 percent. Financial savings equated to approximately $3,000 per physician per year, or about $66,000. The return on Cardiovascular Associates' investment in the technology and training was positive, with a payback period of less than six months.[24]

While EHRs are used largely in the background, patient-physician messaging could change how care is given. Since the days of Hippocrates, doctors have asked patients questions and prescribed care based on those answers and their own findings. While physician-patient messaging does not change the dynamics of this interaction, it does allow the two to be in different rooms or different states.

Using secure messaging, patients are able to get treatment for common ailments such as a sore throat or follow up on an acute condition. When interoperable EHR and e-prescribing are already in place, the doctor is able to view the patient's complete medical file and order prescriptions which complement rather than conflict with medication she is already taking. The patient does not need to leave her office to visit the doctor and can pick up her prescription on the way home from work.

Blue Cross and Blue Shield plans in California, New York, Florida, Massachusetts, New Hampshire, Colorado and Tennessee are now paying $24 to $30, including any co-payment, for online consultations. Blue Cross of California has made the program available to 160,000 of its 6 million health plan members. In February 2005, Empire Blue Cross and Blue Shield began testing the payment system with New York doctors at the Columbia University and Weill Cornell Medical Centers. Kaiser Permanente, the nation's largest nonprofit managed care company, has tested physician-patient messaging in the Pacific Northwest and is starting the program this year in Hawaii and Colorado as part of Kaiser's $3 billion information technology program.[25]

Pushing Pay-for-Performance

Large employers are also encouraging the adoption of healthcare IT. Cisco Systems provides healthcare benefits for more than 60,000 employees and dependents worldwide. An analysis of claims histories highlighted that 14 physician groups in the San Francisco Bay Area accounted for roughly 10 percent of the company's ambulatory care visits. One group, the Palo Alto Medical Foundation (PAMF), is a recognized leader in using technology to improve care delivery, having already implemented EHR with CPOE, e-prescribing and a physician-patient messaging service called PAMFOnline.

To encourage employee usage, Cisco committed to paying the $60-per-person subscription fee for the PAMFOnline service for one year, starting in February 2005. As a condition of this payment, employees and their dependents are providing feedback on their usage of the system, including satisfaction, use of services and "presenteeism" in the workplace.

Cisco is using feedback from this pilot to design and deploy more pay-for-performance programs at other medical groups and clinics that serve a high number of Cisco employees and dependents. Though hospital visits are less frequent, parallel pay-for-performance plans for hospitals are also being considered, as an analysis of 2003 data showed that five hospitals in the San Francisco Bay Area accounted for 64 percent of all Cisco regional hospital visits.

Government Should Play an Active Role

While Ford, Cisco and most other American corporations are calling for the transformation of the U.S. healthcare industry, no company or group of companies can do this on its own. Government leadership in the form of shaping standards and righting the economic equation is needed to implement the necessary changes.

Current studies show that the adoption of technology in healthcare primarily benefits private payers and government, not the physicians or hospitals that pay for implementation. This needs to change quickly. With 45 percent of all U.S. healthcare spending coming from government sources,[26] the federal government has the weight to promote the adoption of healthcare IT.

In the first nine months of a Medicare pay-for-performance demonstration pilot, quality at more than 270 hospitals rose about

6 percent, as measured by hospitals' rate of compliance with a series of medical best practices. On the heels of these findings, Senators Charles E. Grassley (R-Iowa) and Max S. Baucus (D-Mont.) introduced a bill in June 2005 that would authorize Medicare to expand the pay-for-performance concept nationwide.[27]

The U.S. government also needs to implement a national standards certification process that will reduce the adoption risk for physicians and hospitals. Currently there are more than 200 different EHRs from which to choose, with no guarantees regarding their functionality, longevity or interoperability.[28] Imagine making a purchase decision if you are a one-person physician's office with no reserves, no IT expertise or staff and an expected pay back window of two to three years. It is not surprising that adoption rates are low.

The federal government must be encouraged to do even more about certifying standards, relaxing Stark provisions, providing meaningful financial relief and incentives for clinicians adopting healthcare IT, and clarifying state versus federal issues in current HIPAA regulations. By creating a strategic partnership between the public and private sectors, the United States can begin to take full advantage of exciting technologies such as EHRs, e-prescribing and patient-physician messaging.

Other sectors of the economy have long seen that information technology, when viewed comprehensively and deployed effectively, can replace old problems with new possibilities.

Now it's time for healthcare to do the same. ■

Endnotes

1. *"To Err Is Human: Building a Safer Health System." Institute of Medicine, 1999. www4.nationalacademies.org/news.nsf/isbn/0309068371?OpenDocument*
2. *DeNavas-Walt, C., B. Proctor, and R. J. Mills.* Income, Poverty, and Health Insurance Coverage in the United States: *2003. U.S. Census Bureau. Aug. 2004.*
3. *"The First National Report Card on Quality of Health Care in America." RAND Corp., 2004*
4. *David U. Himmelstein, Elizabeth Warren, Deborah Thorne, and Steffie Woolhandler. "Illness And Injury As Contributors To Bankruptcy."* Health Affairs, *Feb. 2005; http://content.healthaffairs.org/cgi/content/full/hlthaff.w5.63/DC1*
5. *Todd Gilmer, Richard Kronick. "It's The Premiums, Stupid: Projections Of The Uninsured Through 2013."* Health Affairs, *April 2005. http://content.healthaffairs.org/cgi/content/abstract/hlthaff.w5.143?ijkey=C.oW5ICDr801o&keytype=ref&siteid=healthaff*
6. *"Downsizing at General Motors Comes as No Surprise to Workers." Jeremy W. Peters;* New York Times, *June 8, 2005; www.newratings.com/analyst_news/article_863999.html*
7. Detroit News, *July 2004. www.detnews.com/2004/autosinsider/0407/23/c01-216906.htm*
8. *Ibid.*
9. Health Affairs, *May 2003. www.healthaffairs.org/press/mayjune0301.htm*
10. *Dana P. Goldman, Elizabeth A. McGlynn. U.S. Healthcare: Facts About Cost, Access and Quality. Rand Corp, 2005.*
11. *Ibid.*
12. *Ibid.*
13. *McKinsey Global Institute, U.S. Productivity Growth 1995-2000 (1999 data)*
14. *David U. Himmelstein, M.D., Steffie Woolhandler, M.D., M.P.H. and Sidney M. Wolfe, M.D. "Administrative Waste in the U.S. Health Care System in 2003: The Cost to the Nation, the States and the District of Columbia, With State-Specific Estimates of Potential Savings."* International Journal of Health Services, *Vol. 34-1, pp. 79-86, 2004. www.pnhp.org/news/IJHS_State_Paper.pdf*
15. *Michael Menduno, "apothecary.now."* Hospitals and Health Networks, *July 1999, 35-36. www.ehealthinitiative.org/initiatives/policy/HouseWaysandMeansTestimony06172004.mspx*
16. *National Center for Policy Analysis: www.ncpa.org/newdpd/index.php*
17. *www.citl.org/research/ACPOE_Executive_Preview.pdf*
18. *www.ehcca.com/presentations/hitsummit1/middleton.ppt*
19. *Jan Walker, Eric Pan, Douglas Johnston, Julia Adler-Milstein, David W. Bates, and Blackford Middleton. "The Value Of Health Care Information Exchange And Interoperability."* Health Affairs, *Jan. 2005.*
20. *Ibid.*
21. *Ibid.*
22. *"The Value of in Computerized Provider Order Entry Ambulatory Settings," CITL, 2004. www.citl.org/research/ACPOE_Executive_Preview.pdf; see also www.ehcca.com/presentations/hitsummit1/middleton.ppt and www.healthvision.com/knowledge/resources/CHCFonACPOEvalue.pdf*
23. *"Use of Six-Sigma Techniques in Evaluating Readiness for and Impact of e-Prescribing Technology," MGMA Connexion, 2003.*
24. *Ibid.*
25. New York Times, *March 2, 2005*
26. *Centers for Medicare & Medicaid Services, Office of the Actuary, National Health Statistics Group. www.cms.hhs.gov/statistics/nhe/historical/chart.asp*
27. *"Cisco: Paging Dr. Info Tech," Tim Mullaney;* Businessweek, *July 11, 2005. www.businessweek.com/magazine/content/05_28/b3942108_mz063.htm*
28. *EMR Consultant, 2005, http://emrconsultant.com/phys_start.php*

weblink

Learn how France is modernizing its healthcare systems to improve affordability in "The French Perspective."

Unparalleled Insight Drives Improvement in Hospital Operations, Planning & Marketing and Patient Care

Healthcare organizations run on information. Not only do they produce incredible amounts of information every day on everything from supply costs to patient outcomes, but they also require information to benchmark their performance against their peers and to identify opportunities for improvement.

Solucient is the leading expert at turning information and data into actionable insights and is the most trusted source in the healthcare industry for decision-making tools and services that drive business growth, manage costs and help deliver quality care.

Healthcare providers need better methods and tools to understand and quantify their business and clinical issues – whether it's determining which investment will yield the greatest result or identifying key best practices to control costs as they deliver high-quality patient care. By transforming data that spans the continuum of healthcare into information that can be acted upon immediately, Solucient ensures its customers are accurately measuring, managing and improving their overall performance.

The following are some examples of Solucient's proven track record as an innovator in supporting growth and quality in healthcare.

Data-Based Marketing

Solucient has led the way in combining vast quantities of demographic information with inpatient, outpatient and disease data, resulting in powerful marketing and planning tools like The Market Planner® Plus and The Market Impact Modeler. These products enable hospitals to accurately predict healthcare demand, target high-growth opportunities, forecast the impact of new and emerging technologies and justify capital expenditures.

The Market Impact Modeler forecasts trends in technology as far out as 15 years. Hospitals can use these tools to plan for consumer demand for treatments based on new technologies by forecasting patient resource and use rates in hospitals. The Market Impact Modeler is the most effective method of forecasting the impact of a specific technology, such as the drug-eluting stent, on a particular service line. It combines Solucient's expertise in modeling local healthcare utilization rates and long-term population growth data with the Health Technology Center's (HealthTech) comprehensive, clinically relevant and unbiased research on the expected impact of new medical technology.

For example, data from The Market Impact Modeler showed that despite steady population growth, the use of drug-eluting stents to treat clogged arteries will significantly reduce the number of cardiac inpatients over the next several years. When HealthTech predicted a decrease in discharge rates for heart attack patients due to the adoption of drug-eluting stents, Solucient combined this prediction with demographic and technology forecasting data to provide a more accurate projection of how these two factors would affect local markets. The resulting data indicated that the impact of drug-eluting stents would outweigh the effect of population growth during the initial adoption period. But as drug-eluting stents become the norm, the effect of demographics will again dominate – as will other technologies that affect the same patients. Solucient's ability to dovetail data and information provided valuable insights to trends and forecasting.

CentraState Health System of Freehold, N.J., used The Market Planner® Plus and Solucient's ACTION O-I™ operational benchmarking tool to identify and quantify its market and operational opportunities. Through detailed analysis with The Market Planner Plus and ACTION O-I, CentraState was able to project expected future demand for inpatient cardiovascular services and craft a well thought-out and quantitative plan to ensure a strong return on investment.

Solucient is the leading expert at turning information and data into actionable insights and is the most trusted source in the healthcare industry for decision-making tools and services that drive business growth, manage costs and help deliver quality care.

Meeting the Demands of Your Healthcare Consumers

Today's healthcare consumer, more than ever, is armed with a wealth of information on health-related topics, as well as the performance of healthcare organizations. Understanding the changing needs and demands of these consumers is essential to delivering quality care.

Solucient provides several tools that tap into rich marketing segmentation information – stratifying consumer groups by age, gender and socioeconomic status – all within Solucient's HealthView Plus™ tool to identify how healthcare consumers will respond to marketing, and when, where and how they will use specific services.

Solucient's crmView™ is a customer relationship management (CRM) tool that allows organizations to collect customer data and build their own CRM databases. crmView lets healthcare marketers build relationships with prospects and customers, generate mailing lists, track customer interactions and measure return on investment against campaign costs and revenue.

It combines the industry's leading consumer research with Internet reporting and HouseholdView™, Solucient's proprietary healthcare segmentation system. HouseholdView divides healthcare consumers into 56 separate segments, based on household demographics and composition, allowing marketers to develop specific messages for precisely targeted audiences.

BJC Healthcare of St. Louis, Mo., wanted to track revenue generated as a result of its marketing campaigns. They used Solucient's crmView to create a database of all their marketing activities matched to clinical and non-clinical information on specific customers going back several years. Each customer's experience with the hospital was recorded in the database and linked back to the relevant campaign. By using crmView to launch more than 300 direct marketing campaigns, BJC Healthcare has been able to convert campaign respondents into customers at a rate 25 percent higher than the rate at which control members have been converted.

Assessing Performance, Charting an Improvement Pathway

In response to growing public pressure to reduce medical errors and increase access to care while operating more cost-effectively, Solucient offers an ambitious and complete performance assessment tool: The Solucient Polaris™ Suite. This powerful tool can help organizations understand their operational and strategic initiatives, manage resources and identify trends in growth opportunities.

As the flagship of Solucient's powerful clinical decision support tools, which include HBSI EXPLORE® and Solucient's Core Measures Solution, the Solucient Polaris Suite also gives users access to a network of hundreds of other healthcare professionals to share and compare information on best practices, process and techniques for overcoming challenges. These clients can analyze and compare complication, mortality and readmission rates and compare patient outcomes for clinical services against national, regional and peer groups.

Benchmarking Toward Excellence

Recognizing the need for hospitals to prosper despite the growing pressures of public reporting and pay-for-performance, Solucient has pioneered a comprehensive database for the industry.

Solucient's ACTION O-I is the largest comparative healthcare information database in the industry, with financial and operational data from more than 850 healthcare organizations across the country. With Solucient's ACTION O-I program, hospitals and health systems can compare operational and financial performance across the industry at the system, hospital and department level to help identify key opportunities for improvement and analyze and support budgets, staffing projections and other decisions.

ACTION O-I gives hospitals a clear window into their own financial and operational performance, and provides an opportunity for facilities to benchmark themselves against their peers of similar size, payer mix, geography, patient population and other measures across the nation.

St. Tammany Parish Hospital of Covington, La., used ACTION O-I to help increase productivity and reduce cost in the endoscopy lab, particularly in staffing levels, skill mix and use of overtime. Improvement initiatives based on data from ACTION O-I helped the hospital to reduce overtime from 5.78 percent to 3.69 percent, and R.N. skill mix was reduced from 85 percent to 50 percent. Overall staffing also decreased from 8.19 to 4.15 worked hours per patient. These factors combined for a direct cost reduction of $340,000 per year. Most importantly, ACTION O-I helped St. Tammany create a process that involved staff, management and physicians in maintaining the quality of care while improving productivity and cost performance.

Take the Next Step

Discover how Solucient can help your hospital drive business growth, manage costs and help deliver quality care. Contact your Solucient sales representative, or visit our website at www.solucient.com. ■

Solucient®
Insight to Better Healthcare

Solucient is the leading source of healthcare business intelligence, enabling providers, payers and pharmaceutical companies to drive business growth, manage costs and help deliver quality care.

Nancy Nelson
Chief Executive Officer

Tom Wilkas
Chief Financial Officer

Matthew Bates
Senior Vice President,
Products & Technology

Kaveh Safavi, M.D., J.D.
Chief Medical Officer

Solucient, LLC
1007 Church St., Ste. 700
Evanston, IL 60201
Toll-Free 800.366.PLAN
(800.366.7526)
Fax 847.332.1768

Business Contact
Christopher N. Clemmensen
Vice President of Marketing
Phone 847.424.4219
cclemmensen@solucient.com

Moving Pay-for-Performance to Pay-for-Value

It is unlikely that current pay-for-performance models will have a lasting impact – given patients have consistently shown equal interest in knowledge, outcomes and compassion.

[Kaveh Safavi, M.D., J.D., Solucient]

Pay-for-performance seems to be part of every healthcare pundit's prediction of emerging trends. Yet there is cynicism about the persistence of current models.[1] In large part, this stems from the fact that the words "pay for performance" mean everything, and yet nothing, at the same time.[2]

More importantly, the term performance is often used synonymously with clinically correct care, and the associated best possible outcomes. There is an implicit belief that payment will be tied to clinical competency. The inference is that you will get paid more if your clinical performance is ideal, or less if it is not ideal. Hence a number of schemes have been deployed that tie a doctor's or hospital's payment to some aspect of care outcomes (did the patient survive?), process (was the right test or drug ordered?) or structure (did the hospital have a computerized order entry system?). These experiments are noteworthy, but not likely to become widespread or permanent until the current dialogue shifts to a pay-for-value concept.

From Performance to Value

Pay-for-performance in its current iteration is inherently provider-centric. It assumes that providers or other experts are in the best position to know if a care experience was valuable to a patient. The current model suggests that the provider, such as doctors or hospitals, will get more money if they perform better. In reality, payment is determined primarily by the patient or those that pay bills on their behalf, such as health insurers, not the provider. Payment is based primarily on the purchaser's concept of value for services. In an imperfect market such as healthcare, the price of services is influenced by a variety of external factors. These factors include introduction of a third party that pays the majority of the bills, the politics of federal entitlement programs and the role of the employer as a health insurance sponsor. It is quite plausible that a hospital delivering patient care in a technically flawless manner, following the most up-to-date guidelines, best practices and evidence-based medicine will not receive any higher level of payment than it would if its quality of care was less exceptional.

One of the challenges of the current indirect system of payment is that value to the ultimate consumer of healthcare – the patient may not be the same thing or have the same value to the intermediary who pays the bills. However, the recent demise of mandatory primary care "gatekeepers" as a cost containment strategy architected by third-party payers, shows how the third-party payer ultimately acquiesces to the thing most important to their real client – the patient.

Think about what you will pay today for housing or education. How much more would you pay for the promise of perfect performance? It depends on how much you make and what else you spend your money on. Alternatively consider airline tickets. How much more (or less) would you be willing to pay for the airline that promises "fewer plane crashes than before?"

This issue is particularly relevant in light of the analysis of Anderson and Reinhardt in 2003. They demonstrated that the primary reason U.S. per capita healthcare costs are substantially higher than the rest of the developed world is due to the price of services in the U.S., not the number of services.[3] That analysis is reflected in a thoughtful commentary by Bruce Vladeck that suggests that the national concern with cost will not really be addressed by focusing on eliminating unexplained variations in utilization of services.[4] Perfect quality is not likely to change the dynamics that ultimately set prices. Therefore providers should not expect that better clinical performance will result in improved ("higher") prices.

Kaveh Safavi, M.D., J.D., is chief medical officer at Solucient. He has 20 years of healthcare experience, most recently as senior vice president of Solucient's clinical business unit. Prior to this, he served at Alexian Brothers. Dr. Safavi received his M.D. from Loyola University and his J.D. from DePaul University.

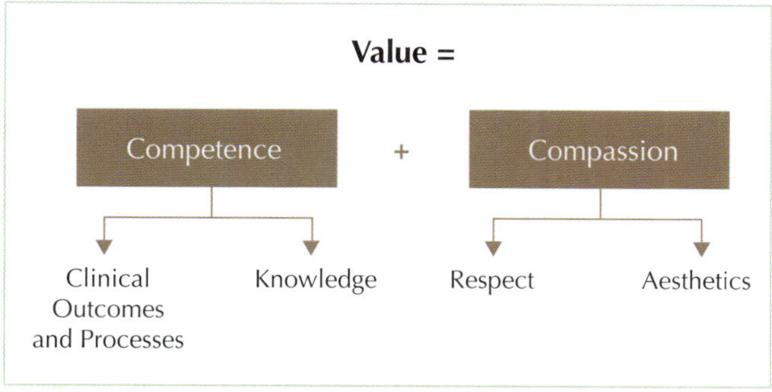

Figure 1 Components of Value

What Is Value?

What do patients pay for? They pay for what they value. A patient's perception of a good care experience includes, but is more comprehensive than, clinical performance or quality.

Significant research has been conducted on what patients want from their healthcare providers. It appears they want both competence and compassion.[5,6]

Competence alone is not enough. This is corroborated by the fact that hospitals that excel at empiric measures of performance, such as outcomes, may not be considered the best by referring doctors or patients and vice versa. One only needs to compare the Solucient 100 Top Hospitals multiyear winners, with *U.S. News and World Report's* Best Hospital Honor Roll winners and J.D. Powers' Distinguished Hospital Program winners.

Further research on patient attitudes on healthcare supports this information. Patients are interested in how well doctors explain alternatives, how well healthcare providers listen to them and the quality of the environment in which they receive their healthcare. Patients equate cleanliness and order in the environment with quality, suspecting that if a provider doesn't care about keeping their office or hospital hallways clean, then they may be just as lax in their care of the patient.

Assuming all these variables enter the equation, the next question is, which variable is most important? Contrary to expectation, clinical outcome may not be the most important variable in determining quality of care. Particularly for office-based care, the perception of quality is correlated to how well the physician answers a patient's questions and explains the patient's illness.[7,8] For hospital care, the dominant factors seem to be responsiveness of staff and cleanliness of the environment.[9,10]

What Does This Mean for Providers?

If value ultimately influences how much money people will pay relative to everything else they can do with their money, then providers must seek to maximize a patient's perception of value. In addition to improving clinical performance, providers must strive to optimize all aspects and channels of delivery of value. In many cases, value may not be significantly affected by maximizing clinical care alone. Even large change may not confer much incremental value. This is a sign that the other elements of the equation must not be overlooked.

Healthcare providers should begin to think equally about strategies that improve all aspects of the healthcare experience. The popularity of entrepreneurial "concierge" medicine and ultra-fast CT cardiac screening tests support the hypothesis that non-clinical factors can have dramatic influence on a patient's willingness to pay for services not measured by traditional approaches to quality. Said another way, being a good doctor may not be good enough to win and keep your patient's business.

What if There Is No Money to Pay Anyway?

The American healthcare system may have a price structure so out of line with the rest of the world that it is unlikely that prices received by providers will go up substantially even if care or performance improved. That does not mean there will not be pressure on providers to maximize value. There is likely to be some price difference within geographic markets – at least at the margin for privately insured patients – so that providers may be able to gain by being a high-value provider. Market share

If value ultimately influences how much money people will pay relative to everything else they can do with their money, then providers must seek to maximize a patient's perception of value.

weblink

Read how patients can learn how to respond to early indicators of chronic diseases in "Driving Care Management Home: EHR and Patient Self Monitoring."

is likely to continue as a significant competitive issue in most urban areas.

In addition, as technology allows providers to be physically separated from patients, provider competition may become more regional and national in nature, raising the bar for rural providers as well. Finally, as patients pay more out of pocket – particularly for discretionary services – competition may emerge for their "retail" healthcare expenditure that will be driven by value as defined by the patient.[11]

What About Efficiency?

Payers often speak in terms of rewarding efficiency. This is an artifact of our disconnected third-party payment system. Ordinarily purchasers don't pay for efficiency; they pay for value realized.

In the meantime, expect third-party payers to define performance in terms of efficiency if for no other reason than to stimulate efficient business practices. Either way, providers will need to focus on doing better with less.

For healthcare providers, this means if you are efficient, you can do more with what patients (or their insurers) are willing to pay. In this way, you provide your services with more value relative to their dollar spent on care. This notion fits well with the broader concept of value. The investment needed to increase the quality and compassion of an organization – whether it is new diagnostic technology or better-trained staff – will be funded out of efficiency. In the meantime, expect third-party payers to define performance in terms of efficiency if for no other reason than to stimulate efficient business practices. Either way, providers will need to focus on doing better with less.

Where Do We Go From Here?

To date, pay-for-performance has been limited to a very provider-centric notion of technical quality and competence. In the short term, this narrow view is helpful in that it will help transform a qualitative and highly opaque care system into a more quantitative and therefore more transparent one. This will begin to give patients some tools with which to measure the clinical competence aspect of their healthcare experiences. Patients and payers that respond are much more likely to be persuaded to pay based on value received. This much broader notion will require providers that want to succeed to go beyond the facts they learned in medical school and pay equal attention to other aspects of the healthcare experience. ■

Endnotes

1. *Wessel D. "Rx for Healthcare May Include Carrots."* Wall Street Journal. *Feb. 3, 2005, A2.*
2. *Safavi, K. "Pay for Performance: Fad or Forever?" Available at: www.HCTProject.com. 2004.*
3. *Anderson G.F., Reinhardt U.E., Hussey P.S., Petrosyan V. "It's the Prices Stupid: Why the United States is so different from other countries."* Health Affairs. *May/June 2003; 22(3):89-105.*
4. *Vladeck B.C. "Everything New is Old Again."* Health Affairs *Web exclusive, Oct. 7, 2004.*
5. *Schneider C.E.* The Practice of Autonomy: Patients, Doctors, and Medical Decisions. *Oxford University Press. 1998;195-206.*
6. *Smith T. "Can Patient Choice Shape Organizational Behaviors to Provide Patients with What They Want. Qual Saf Healthcare." 2003;12:473-476.*
7. *Laine C., Davidoff F., Lewis C.E., Nelson E.C., Nelson E., Kessla R.C., Delbanco T.L. "Important Elements of Outpatient Care: A Comparison of Patients' and Physicians, Opinions."* Ann Intern Med. *1996;125:640-645.*
8. *Mangione-Smith R., McGlynn E.A., Elliot M.N., Krugstad P., Brook R.H. "The Relationship Between Perceived Parental Expectations and Pediatrician Antimicrobial Prescribing Behavior."* Pediatrics. *1999; 103:711-718.*
9. *CAHPS II Investigators and AHRQ. HCAP + PS Three-State Pilot Study Analysis Results. Dec. 22, 2003. www.cms.hhs.gov/quality/hospital/3State_Pilot_Analysis_Final.pdf.*
10. *American Hospital Association and Picker Institute. "Eye on Patients Report" Jan. 27, 1997. www.amhpi.com/eyeonpatients*
11. *Herzlinger R.* Market-Driven Health Care: Who Wins, Who Loses in the Transformation of Americas' Largest Service Industry. *Addison-Wesley, 1997.*

Healthcare Performance Management Solutions From Cognos

Performance Management is a business imperative, particularly for healthcare providers. Healthcare executives are dealing with an increasing volume of business questions, the answers to which are usually found across disparate information systems. Cognos performance management solutions help healthcare organizations pull together those diverse pieces of data into a more complete picture of their business performance to support better business decision making – just as electronic medical record solutions pull together patient information from multiple sources to support better clinical decision making. With this information in hand, healthcare organizations are in a better position to answer fundamental questions:

- How are we doing?
- Why?
- What should we be doing?

Scorecarding, business intelligence, financial consolidation and planning technologies answer these questions. Knowing what happened without finding out why is of little use to a healthcare provider. Knowing why something happened, but being unable to plan and make the necessary changes, is likewise of limited value.

A Performance Management system automates and preserves senior management intent, making the organization's strategy and priorities everyone's priorities. It provides these three core values:

- Information delivery – understand the business;
- Performance oversight – manage the business; and
- Performance effectiveness – improve the business.

Healthcare providers are using Cognos Performance Management to manage operational performance, improve patient safety and increase clinical effectiveness.

By managing, measuring and analyzing day-to-day operations, they have been successful in reducing patient wait times, increasing staff during expected service uptakes and maximizing medical equipment and facilities usage. With up-to-date, cross-departmental information at their fingertips, healthcare staff is more accountable to make informed decisions and implement necessary operational adjustments in "right time." Cognos' industry-leading solutions have also helped numerous healthcare organizations worldwide cut costs and comply with government regulations.

> With up-to-date, cross-departmental information at their fingertips, healthcare staff is more accountable to make informed decisions and implement necessary operational adjustments in "right time."

Success results from transforming the vast amounts of disparate health and patient data into information assets, allowing healthcare providers, suppliers and other important stakeholders to effectively collaborate and make critical, informed decisions designed to:

- Increase patient satisfaction;
- Reduce patient wait times;
- Improve nursing care;
- Optimize staff deployment;
- Reduce labor costs;
- Maximize reimbursement;
- Reduce supply costs; and
- Enhance accountability and teamwork. ■

COGNOS®
THE NEXT LEVEL OF PERFORMANCE™

Cognos, the world leader in business intelligence and corporate performance management, delivers software and services that help institutions drive, monitor and understand corporate performance. Founded in 1969, Cognos employs over 3,400 people and serves more than 23,000 customers in over 135 countries.

Rob Ashe
President and
Chief Executive Officer

Cognos Inc.
3755 Riverside Dr.
P.O. Box 9707
Station T
Ottawa, Ontario
Canada
K1G 4K9
Phone 613.738.1440

Cognos Corp
15 Wayside Rd.
Burlington, MA 01803
Toll-Free 800.426.4667
Phone 781.229.6600
www.cognos.com/healthcare

Business Contact
Bill Stevens
Senior Director Life Sciences
Phone 214.259.6270
healthcare@cognos.com

University of Pittsburgh Medical Center Adopts Performance Management

Enterprisewide deployment helps a complex organization get a new view of its entire operation – achieving new efficiencies, maximizing resources and cutting costs

[James Fitch]

Like all healthcare organizations, the University of Pittsburgh Medical Center (UPMC) faces the challenges of optimizing performance in many areas, from revenue cycle management to improving patient care. By applying the concepts of corporate performance management (CPM) it has made tremendous improvements in each.

Benefits of Corporate Performance Management

CPM is a management approach that organizations can use to measure and manage performance by combining their processes, methodologies, metrics and systems. CPM gives healthcare organizations access to new data, key insights and ways to manage their organizations. It lets decision makers at all levels take quick action to use resources more efficiently, address organizational issues and ensure the highest-quality patient care. Many of the world's largest companies and major public sector organizations have embraced CPM.

CPM can help organizations answer their fundamental business questions: How are we doing? Why? What should we be doing?

Some vendors have been expanding their standards-based technologies built for ease of integration and a partner ecosystem to offer a complete CPM system. This whole-product approach comprises:

- Technology – through an integrated platform;
- Best practices – planning, reporting and metrics templates;
- Solutions – covering departmental, industry and enterprisewide performance management needs; and
- Partner ecosystem – building performance management solutions on the same platform.

Through CPM, organizations can bring clarity to what are often complex processes and establish a common understanding of their performance. This enables decision makers to act with more confidence.

A Complex Organization Searches For a Simpler Reporting Solution

For UPMC, the size and diversity of its business further complicated the challenge of implementing performance management. With $6 billion in annual revenues, UPMC is the largest integrated healthcare delivery system in the region and includes a network of 18 hospitals, 400 outpatient sites and physician practice offices, and several nursing, personal care and long term-care facilities.

Growth through acquisition left UPMC with multiple data repositories, billing systems and other core processes. Reporting meant time-consuming manual compilation of data in spreadsheets. As a result, senior management often had to wait for key data, such as census reports, and had low confidence in its accuracy.

Implementing Performance Management Across the Enterprise

To raise performance to new levels, UPMC recently standardized on Cognos performance management solutions for enterprisewide reporting and analysis. More than 1,100 users at UPMC rely on the software to speed daily census reporting, track receivables, and improve overall delivery of patient services. The software lets them make dynamic adjustments to performance and respond to their ever-changing needs. UPMC leaders report benefiting from faster access to vital information, better use of resources and new efficiencies across a wide range of critical processes.

An Effort Driven From the Top

Key executives at UPMC – including the CFO and COO – made performance management a priority for the organization, and their sponsorship of the effort helped it keep moving ahead. The organization moved from an initial three-week proof of concept to a more broad-based development that addressed "top pain points" from four major business units. The solid results from these initial

James Fitch is a journalist and business writer based in Boston who writes about emerging technologies, healthcare trends and education in the U.S. and U.K. In each case, he provides a critical, objective perspective on the bottom-line business results achieved by technology.

efforts, as well as the very positive reaction from users, led to enterprisewide adoption of the software, and subsequent rollout to UPMC's hospitals and other facilities over nine months in 2004–2005.

"Right from the start, we had an extremely committed team, from the executive level on down," recalls Chuck Watson, director of enterprise business applications at UPMC. "The committee included representatives from key businesses as well as IT."

An Enterprise-Level Effort Yields Real Results

From the back office to the front lines of patient care, UPMC is improving performance and gaining new control over its complex, diversified operations. "With Cognos, now we have transparent, cross-functional access to information that lets us effectively monitor and manage our performance – and take the steps necessary to optimize healthcare delivery," says Mr. Watson. "We're making tangible performance gains, particularly in terms of time savings and better staff utilization. The software helped us continue to reduce the number of accounts receivable days (A/R) from 42 to 35 in fiscal 2005."

A New Vision of the Entire Enterprise

UPMC can now do consolidated, automated reporting – without needing to move data from multiple locations. "We wanted a solution that would give us a unified picture of our key data without having to move it to a central repository," says Terri Mikol, manager of client services and decision support at UPMC. "We knew that the challenge of relocating key data was much more than we wanted to take on at this point. Down the line, we'll be working toward that level of centralization. But for now, we need to be able to leverage our data no matter where it happens to reside."

Sophisticated Tools That Are Easy to Use

Like all healthcare organizations, UPMC wanted to make life easier for its staff – putting new capabilities at their fingertips without complicating their work. "We wanted a sophisticated toolset that non-IT personnel could work with quickly and easily – replacing static reports with interactive, visual data that they can slice and dice," recalls Ms. Mikol. "If the software was hard to deploy, learn or use, it wouldn't work for us."

Deploying Across the Enterprise

During deployment, UPMC tapped the expertise of a consultant, who provided quick answers to technical questions at key junctures. "The whole process went very smoothly," says Mikol, who reports that the whole process took approximately two weeks.

Training Provides Critical Guidance

Ms. Mikol is clear that UPMC's business units are driving implementation of performance management, not the IT group. "We let the operations move at their own pace, taking on the tools when they're ready," she says. To ensure acceptance, at the end-user level, UPMC provides in-house training to its users, leveraging its existing training approach and solutions. "We have a very set way of training staff," says Ms. Mikol. "When you introduce sophisticated software, you want to make sure that everyone is taking complete advantage of all the capabilities that they have available to them. So training is important to help get the most out of any software."

Making Performance Management Part of Every Day

The response from end users at UPMC? "They're very impressed with what they can do with the performance management software," says Ms. Mikol. "They like how they can get data into new formats that make more sense to them and let them interpret and analyze it better. And they like the accuracy of the data, which is much more accurate than when they used to download data from various sources and manually merge it in a spreadsheet."

As the number of users expands during UPMC's incremental roll-out, the IT group continues to manage requests for functionality, establish a priority queue and train new users throughout the organization. Acceptance of the new software capabilities has been a non-issue, according to Mr. Watson. "When you have a performance management effort driven by senior management, acceptance really isn't an issue. Besides, our users know that performance management helps them do a better job, makes their lives easier, and in the end, helps us deliver better patient care. Isn't that what any healthcare organization wants to be doing?"

Achieving Results in Critical Areas

UPMC users rely on performance management solutions to streamline monitoring, reporting and analysis:

- Executives now have accurate census reports at their fingertips, enabling them to spot trends and take action;
- Financial analysts can monitor revenues and receivables, reducing A/R days;
- UPMC's Institute for Performance Improvement can monitor, measure and improve critical quality metrics, like infection control; and
- Management can see an overview of hundreds of physician practices and drill down into the details when necessary.

UPMC reports that the biggest performance increases come from easier access to critical information. For example, in the past, several UPMC analysts took until mid-afternoon every day to prepare the census report. "Now the CFOs and presidents of our hospitals can see the previous day's numbers at 9 a.m. – automatically, every day – via a detailed but easy-to-use hospital dashboard," says Ms. Mikol. "So they can make adjustments and change the way they're allocating resources. Plus those analysts can now turn to more strategic work than simply compiling data. Performance management helps us achieve new efficiencies in many ways." ■

5

EHR and Pay-for-Performance

Pay-for-performance programs use incentives to encourage evidence-based practices that promote better outcomes and ultimately transform the healthcare system.

[Maureen O'Neal, Accenture] [Roxanne Walther, Accenture] [Cindy Urbancic, Accenture] [Kathleen T. Lennon, Accenture]

Health plans, large employers and government agencies are driving the move to a pay-for-performance (P4P) healthcare environment in the United States. P4P focuses on outcomes of healthcare treatment, essentially linking reimbursement to quality. Most organizations, however, are not prepared for the significant P4P reporting requirements. A key enabler of P4P goals is the implementation of an EHR to collect, track and deliver evidence of patient outcomes.

P4P Drivers

The use of P4P in healthcare is being driven principally by the purchasers of healthcare services, including health plans, large employers and government agencies. Provider participation in national and local P4P programs is on the upswing. Additionally the public is determined to address medical errors and patient safety.

Multiple industry studies focusing on medication errors and patient safety have uncovered a high incidence of problems. Moreover the current reimbursement system does not offer the best incentives to deliver quality, and in some cases has resulted in misaligned incentives among providers and payers. Providers do not have direct financial incentives to follow clinical practice guidelines. Many different payment structures have been tried, but none rewards preventive services or chronic care management. Fee-for-service approaches reward time and activity but penalize quality initiatives that reduce the length, intensity or frequency of service utilization. Capitation rewards efficiency, but fails to encourage innovative quality programs that require additional resources. Salary systems reward stability but do not distinguish between under- and over-utilization, and do not foster innovation.

As both public and private program purchasers emphasize a link between reimbursement and quality, P4P is being positioned as a provider payment methodology of the future.

Model Programs

There are several indications that the time is right for P4P in healthcare. As of November 2004, there were 84 P4P programs covering 39 million beneficiaries. By March 2005, there were 104 programs. Based on continuing governmental, health plan and employer interest, as well as growing consumer demand and emerging new sponsors, some predict that the number of P4P program sponsors could reach 160 by 2006.

A number of initiatives are under way to encourage and reinforce the delivery of evidence-based practices that promote better outcomes and ultimately transform the healthcare system.

The federal government is supporting P4P on several fronts. The Medicare Modernization Act financially encourages hospitals to report a standardized set of quality measures. The Centers for Medicare and Medicaid Services has initiated several pilot P4P programs. And Medicare recently launched a public website, Hospital Compare, that shows how most of the nation's general hospitals perform compared with state and national averages, as well as against their peers on 17 widely accepted quality measures.

Other private organizations driving P4P initiatives include the Leapfrog Group, Bridges to Excellence, the Integrated Healthcare Association, and the Sharp Community Medical Group IPA.

Maureen O'Neal, R.N., is a senior manager with Accenture's Health & Life Sciences Practice and has clinical and administrative experience focused on designing and implementing operational improvements in community-based and multisite health systems. **Roxanne Walther, R.N.,** is a partner in Accenture's Health & Life Sciences Practice with over 25 years' experience, specializing in all aspects of hospital operations and patients care services. She is a leader in the benefits identification aspects related to technology implementation. **Cindy Urbancic, R.N.,** is a senior manager in Accenture's Health & Life Sciences Practice and has over 20 years' experience in clinical care delivery and operations management and serves as Project Director for large-scale business transformation and clinical transformation engagements. **Kathleen T. Lennon, R.N.,** is a senior manager in Accenture's Health & Life Sciences Practice and one of the firm's leaders in clinical solution development and delivery. As an industry expert, she has spoken at national conferences and published articles on patient flow integration and transformation.

Common Features

Many of the pay-for-performance programs in the market today are designed to align payment and quality, facilitate adoption of information technology (IT), and reduce clinical practice variation by creating an infrastructure for evidence-based medicine. Accordingly, they have several common features:

- Measures based on accepted evidence-based standards, developed with active involvement of clinicians and encompassing several dimensions: clinical outcomes, compliance with clinical process standards and cost management;
- Mechanisms for continuous improvement (versus meeting static thresholds);
- Specific incentives promoting the development of providers' information systems and reporting capabilities. This is, in part, a recognition of the level of importance that the market is placing on the use of EHRs;
- Incorporation of a consumer component such as patient satisfaction measures; and
- Mechanisms to shift market share based on quality performance, such as decreased co-payments for patients who use high-quality providers and public reporting of quality performance data.

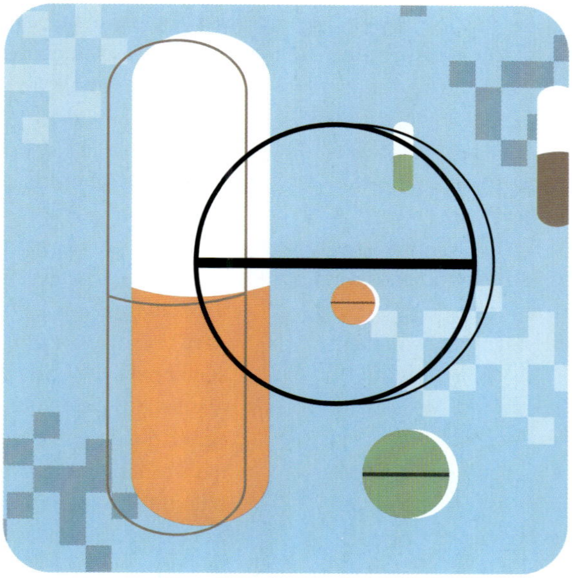

In general, pay-for-performance programs are placing increasing reliance on national norms and evidence-based medicine. There is a trend toward standardized, nonproprietary measures. While many of the measures in place are designed for use with chronic conditions, there is an emerging effort to develop a core set of measures that will be useful in primary care.

Technology Requirements

For the most part, health organizations today use a manual, paper-based approach to retrospectively report their performance on quality measures as specified by P4P programs. This approach is cumbersome, costly, labor-intensive and subject to errors. In addition, it does not facilitate changes to clinical decision making at the point of care. Particularly as P4P programs move beyond process-based to outcomes measures, reporting cannot be accomplished through manual means over the long term, and must eventually be supported through information technology.

To support the quality and patient safety requirements of pay-for-performance programs, secure information in data systems will need to be available in standardized electronic formats. Advanced business and clinical intelligence applications that compile discrete arrays of outcome and performance data must be developed. Healthcare providers will need to move from manual, paper-based processes to the adoption of longitudinal EHRs that enable them to collect, access and analyze patients' information at the point of care. EHRs also provide tools and decision support to manage care. The availability of patient-level clinical data and information to care providers in multiple settings like skilled nursing, home care and the doctor's office can decrease duplication of services and errors, and improve coordination of care.

The growing availability of clinical information technology is starting to make it possible for health organizations to gather the clinical data necessary to administer sophisticated P4P programs. But in developing EHR to make P4P work, providers run into a number of barriers and questions.

The technology infrastructure to support interconnection among hospitals, physicians, inpatient and outpatient services, independent labs and test centers, home health agencies and other parts of the healthcare provider community is sorely lacking. For P4P to work, all those providers need some level of timely access to consistent and current patient information. This access will improve the ability to manage care across the continuum, reduce redundancies in testing, identify patient clinical trends and evaluate outcomes of hospital care in a post-acute environment.

At present there are no good systems, applications or processes in place that allow the required information to be captured readily and consolidated or warehoused in a manner that meets reporting requirements. Under most current records systems, almost all patient information must be pulled manually from disparate applications, compiled and put into a form accepted by the government or payers. It is a labor-intensive, costly and time-consuming process.

EHR links specific data elements together. If a patient comes in with an acute myocardial infarction (AMI), for example, P4P reporting would require information on the type of intervention administered; the time when the medication, procedures or tests were given; and the clinical impact of the treatment. The initial results – vital signs, electrocardiogram (EKG), lab tests – might be available in the ER, but P4P requires more complete results that might not be ready for several hours or even days. And those results might reside in separate computer systems, on a lab report or even in the chart at the patient's bedside. A P4P system needs to capture information about what's happening across the whole spectrum of care, not just in the ER or the doctor's office.

EHR and Pay-for-Performance

The ultimate goal is to create a system that effects changes in care delivery – that gives providers timely and accurate information that allows them to modify or improve patient care based on having access to what happened to that patient yesterday or last week or last month. Ultimately P4P looks to EHR to deliver the data that allow clinicians to make decisions at the point of care. The clinical information systems used to support the EHR should have the capabilities to enable the care process with continually updated evidenced-based practice mechanisms, patient safety guidelines (i.e., medication interactions), documentation fields that are aligned with performance measures being tracked and the ability to pull concurrent information and data.

Clinical information system vendors are trying to respond, but as yet there is no off-the-shelf solution. Vendors are in the early stages of creating the enabling technology and functionality to support P4P requirements.

Even if an off-the-shelf solution were available, there are other barriers to overcome. Some hospitals are delaying participation because they don't have the necessary results to be eligible for the bonuses being offered in many programs. When hospitals look at core measures from those programs and how to raise performance, they usually need to face the reality that success means making changes in how people practice.

As these pilot programs evolve and expand, P4P requirements are continually changing, making it difficult for hospitals to keep up. It's difficult for everyone to get on same page, even with tasks as basic as how to code a specific event.

Requirements also vary by payer. The Centers for Medicare & Medicaid Services requires information on five clinical conditions. California collects clinical measurements but also incorporates a consumer component; patient satisfaction measures. In addition, the state looks at how many actual dollars organizations are investing in information technology. There is a trend toward standardized, nonproprietary measures, but we are not there yet. Requirements are inconsistent for each of the clinical systems currently involved in P4P models.

The key in developing EHR is to devise technology that doesn't vary if measures change from A to B.

Action Guidelines

Health organizations need to determine their organizational readiness for P4P programs and improve their ability to comply with program requirements. They need to assess their capabilities and build the necessary organizational commitment to the concept. They then need infrastructure, processes and tools to support and drive quality outcomes, compliance, measurement and reporting in a P4P environment. Some of the key success factors are as follows:

- **Collaboration.** Payers and providers must be able to overcome any historical mistrust. Together they must define measures upon which quality ratings and bonus payments will be based, determine the financial formulas and timelines for reimbursement and potentially change the contracting processes. Only through collaboration will providers overcome their resistance and payers achieve the necessary buy-in and support.
- **Continuous and proactive planning.** Health organizations need to develop the organizational infrastructure, culture and professional resources to support P4P approaches and compliance with measures. Organizations need mechanisms for continuous improvement (versus meeting static thresholds). They need to plan carefully to ensure that the savings derived from P4P outweigh the administrative and program costs.
- **Clinicians involved in program design and implementation.** Hospitals and payers need to get the necessary support from physicians and other clinicians whose performance may be impacted by the program. They need an adoption strategy to get buy-in around evidence-based practice.
- **Evidence-based guidelines.** Health organizations need to establish a culture and process to decrease the variance in care and standardize clinical practices through adoption of evidence-based practices.
- **A rigorous follow-up process.** Health organizations need to evaluate program performance and track direct and indirect consequences to ensure that changes in quality – not just cost – are being effected. Payers and providers will need to respond to results and guide improvements in performance. They will need to evolve the programs over time to incorporate consumer behavior changes.
- **A substantial commitment to clinical information technology.** Health organizations must determine how to fund and implement clinical information technology to enable the process of collecting and reporting data on performance. Focusing care delivery on the production of outcomes rather than on just producing services will require developing new care management capabilities. This could include disease registries, electronic information systems capable of producing quality and outcome metrics and longitudinal trending analyses.

Summary

The use of performance measures is definitely growing and, increasingly, performance measures will be publicly reported and will influence consumer behavior. Consumerism, payers' frustrations with escalating costs and the imperative to improve patient safety will mandate greater monitoring of quality performance, with or without the payment component. So providers need to be prepared, regardless of whether they're currently involved in a P4P contract. Preparation means the timely creation and deployment of an electronic health infrastructure that facilitates the collection, transmittal and analyses of the performance data that will drive these programs. The ultimate destination is certain: Providers will need to be prepared for an era of greater accountability and performance tracking. ■

Healthcare in Germany Today

Germany is driving a unified view of patient information across the country, which will ultimately reduce costs and improve overall patient service.

[Dr. Harald Deutsch, Accenture]

Germany follows the Bismarck model of healthcare based on contributions both by employees and employers to a partially duplicated health insurance system. There are two parallel health insurance systems. Statutory health insurance funds (once called sickness funds) have a market share of 85 percent. They are nonprofit and are organized by geographical region, trade and company. They have different contribution levels, but all are required to cover a broad range of benefits. In 1994, Germany created a program that forced statutory health insurance funds with wealthier members to contribute a portion of their payroll revenues to a national pool, which then distributes it to the poorer ones.

The majority of Germans have incomes under $40,000 per year and are obliged to take statutory health insurance. For the wealthy, private health insurance can be purchased and offers more extensive coverage, but this is not automatically an advantage. Only 15 percent of Germans are fully insured by private insurance companies. Private insurers also offer additional coverage services (e.g., single bed in hospitals, dental care, etc.) for members of statutory health insurance funds.

The German government does not "own" payers or providers; however, it has legislative authority to regulate healthcare. The German provider sector consists mainly of hospitals, hospital chains and physicians in competition to deliver care to citizens. Over 75 percent of hospitals are owned by public institutions and are nonprofit – with about two-thirds owned by cities or states but not the federal government (the federal government only owns army hospitals). The last third are nonprofit hospitals owned by churches or other social organizations. Twenty-five percent are private hospital chains; this share has increased steeply, having comprised only 10 percent five years ago.

Doctors employed by these hospital organizations are public service employees. General practitioners, however, are required to join regional associations, which pay them from regional funds. These associations have administrative responsibilities and negotiate with payer organizations on behalf of physicians.

Services rendered by general practitioners are paid by patients' insurance companies. Prices are regulated, so that competition is determined by the services offered and the quality of those services, rather than price. There are also associations of regional insurance carriers that work collectively to negotiate with provider organizations for general terms of pricing and volumes of service.

The result is a country where almost all citizens have health insurance and there are virtually no shortfalls of service, such as waiting lists for difficult operations or people lacking needed care. Furthermore quality of medical services is good and meets qualified standards of Organization for Economic Cooperation and Development countries.

Challenges: Setting the Stage for E-Health in Germany

The German healthcare system is not without problems. As more and more Germans demand high levels of health services, there is a growing need to increase efficiency of distribution. In addition, citizens have little control over the medical services they receive and what they pay for these services. The result is continued pressure on insurers and a growing consensus that Germany needs to limit and manage the services paid by administrative bodies, and shift the burden to citizens.

The German government wants people to pay a larger portion of discretionary care costs and is also pressuring providers to become more efficient in managing healthcare. However, because the German healthcare system is decentralized, there is no one origin of patient data, so redundancy is a huge problem.

The lack of centralization is hurting e-health initiatives. In the United Kingdom, the centralized National Health Service

Dr. Harald Deutsch is a partner within the German Health & Life Sciences practice of Accenture. For more than eight years, he has been working in the consulting area with a focus on public health. Prior to consulting, Dr. Deutsch worked in several positions within the diagnostics industry.

has the authority to define exactly what will happen during a given timeframe. This helps create a blueprint for infrastructure and a business case for the whole system. In Germany, however, this blueprint is missing because no group has taken ownership in absence of final responsibility.

The result is that e-health in Germany will be built incrementally. To date the only application focus has been around e-prescriptions. This application involves routing a prescription electronically from the doctor's office via the patient to the pharmacy and then through the pharmacy's back office, making the process fully automated. There is no actual plan for additional applications and the financial consequences for the entire EHR operating model have not been adequately addressed.

is driving e-health through the introduction of a new health card, which is supposed to allow easy access to patient records and other data for anyone involved in a patient's care. At the beginning of 2003, German Chancellor Gerhard Schroeder stated that electronic healthcare cards (eHCCs), also referred to as e-patient cards, for patients and EHRs would be a priority of his administration and would be achieved by 2006.

The Federal Ministry of Health and Social Security responded to Schroeder's call for action by assembling a group of technology companies with the "bIT4health" project to implement eHCCs. Responsibility for the rollout falls to the individual health insurances for their members; they are supposed to roll out in 2006 and 2007. The new system will be designed to provide an elec-

Since these processing costs have historically been paid by insurers through reimbursement, insurance companies stand to benefit most from streamlined e-prescribing if they are able to adjust their reimbursement accordingly.

tronic key to the cross-institutional, cooperative efforts of Germany's 80 million patients, doctors, dentists, hospitals and pharmacies, as well as the related infrastructure. The card alone, however, is not enough to pave the way for a true, national EHR.

Overcapacity challenges German hospitals. The average hospital stay in Germany is 10 days – significantly higher than other Western European countries or the United States. Capacity will continue to be a problem, as it is widely expected that only 2,000 of the 2,800 German hospitals in operation last year will survive this decade. This is likely to lead to pressure to reduce hospital stays and stays will further be reduced by primary care services shifting to ambulatory forms.

Another problem is the lack of cooperation between the primary sector and hospitals. Physicians tend to work independently, without knowledge of each other or patients in common. This creates layers of redundancy, duplicate diagnoses and multiple therapies. German physicians are trying in vain to introduce evidence-based medicine; however, this type of cooperation will not be possible until a collaboration platform is established.

The statutory health insurance system has also come under pressure during the last decade. As the government tries to cut the cost of healthcare, co-payments for medical treatments have been increasing and are likely to increase further in the future. According to "OECD Health Data 2003," Germany's health spending was at 10.7 percent of the GDP, which is considerably lower than that found in the U.S., but still a high percentage of the GDP.

The Introduction of e-Health in Germany

The German e-health initiative was founded to meet some of the challenges to the current system and is similar to what is already occurring in other European countries. The German government

Financing Mechanisms

The financial dimensions of the German e-health initiative are substantial. IT infrastructure and rollout costs for the e-health and professional cards alone are estimated at €1 billion to €1.7 billion. Although no figures are yet available to estimate the cost of funding the necessary applications to tie electronic systems together or the cost of operations, training or compatibility investments into IT systems, estimates are in excess of €10 billion.

So who will pay for this massive undertaking? Germans believe the costs of e-health will be borne mostly by insurers, who supposedly will save money by eliminating manual processing and redundancy. An example of how this might work can be seen in current specifications for Germany's e-prescription system, which eliminates the paper trail for prescriptions. The multiple steps involved in getting prescriptions from doctors to patients to pharmacies will be dramatically reduced. Since these processing costs have historically been paid by insurers through reimbursement, insurance companies stand to benefit most from streamlined e-prescribing if they are able to adjust their reimbursement accordingly.

Providers may also pay for the evolving EHR, but in an indirect way. A new law recently introduced in Germany reduces providers' bills by 1 percent if the providers do not participate in an integrated care model. This has motivated hospitals and entrepreneurial physicians to explore different contract models to reduce redundancy costs and increase cooperation between general practitioners and specialists such as oncologists, orthopedists and cardiologists. The money withheld from nonparticipating physicians is then used to fund organized forms of cooperation. It is expected that these funds will someday fund EHR initiatives to encourage electronic collaboration.

Current State

The only part of a German EHR that has been defined so far is infrastructure to support the e-health card initiative. The basic application definitions for eHCCs, which drive centralized patient data, have been created and infrastructure requirements such as new terminals, hardware and card readers have been defined but not yet implemented.

E-prescription, the first "killer app" of the e-health system, has been defined to some extent; specifications have already been written with RFPs currently out to create a cost benefit analysis for the entire project. It is widely expected that within a year, the first infrastructure project will begin and application packages will be awarded to winning vendors shortly thereafter.

In Germany, some precursors to electronic data exchange are already in place. For example, the government currently requires all hospitals to send bills and commercial transactions electronically to insurers. For hospitals to be reimbursed, they must transmit data electronically. Most hospitals in Germany also have modern ERP systems and many are currently introducing electronic messaging system to transmit information electronically between providers. This will provide an easier way to share patient information and will serve as a prototype for an electronic health record.

A similar application project is currently in the works in Scandinavia in which standardized email systems are being used to securely communicate medical information. This system, however, does not use the type of central data repository required for an EHR. It simply allows information to be easily read and understood by medical record applications through a standardized interface. eMDLetter, like other applications, requires full implementation of the e-health card before it can be introduced.

Barriers to Implementation

There are several barriers to overcome before Germany can introduce a national EHR. One of the biggest is the lack of a complete blueprint, specifically in the areas of applications and functionality for the whole platform. Without a clear vision, the project will be extremely difficult to manage.

In addition, buy-in must be obtained from physicians, which may be difficult due to the current reimbursement structure. Because physicians are currently reimbursed by regional associations instead of directly by insurance companies, insurers do not necessarily know which physicians provide the most profitable or efficient health services. Implementing e-health will add transparency to the process, allowing insurers to examine physicians' bills and prescriptions. German physicians are not accustomed to this level of scrutiny and are therefore resisting the introduction of electronic processing. They are also reluctant to help pay

Because physicians are currently reimbursed by regional associations instead of directly by insurance companies, insurers do not necessarily know which physicians provide the most profitable or efficient health services.

medical records, at least internally. Of all the players involved in Germany's e-health initiatives, hospitals are probably the furthest ahead with some sort of clinical information system in place.

Although hospitals are ahead of the game, minor players within the healthcare system will require the necessary infrastructure upgrades to drive EHR initiatives forward. For example, on the primary care side, there is less existing infrastructure; physician associations claim only 75 percent of all Germany's general practitioners have Internet access.

eMDLetter will probably be the second application to be created once e-prescribing is implemented. eMDLetter will be Germany's first stab at an electronic medical record, creating a standardized for a system that is seen as initially offering the biggest benefits to insurance companies. Physicians will need to be sold on efficiency gains to overcome their current resistance to change.

The work being accomplished around e-prescribing illustrates many of the barriers to EHR implementation in Germany. The infrastructure for e-prescribing will come first because it is fairly easy to implement; however, because the application landscape has not been defined, the business case for infrastructure is missing. Critics of the proposed e-prescribing system question how infrastructure can be built if there is no plan yet for specific functionality. There is also ambiguity about the process for implementing e-prescription and when it will occur. The exact delivery timeline is shaky because it will follow infrastructure, which can only occur after e-health cards are in place.

One way of addressing the issue of infrastructure is to actually build infrastructure that can accommodate multiple applications; however, this is time-consuming and expensive. Because no one organization has ownership on a strategic or operational level, there is no project management platform in a professional sense, so problems such as missed deadlines and spiraling budgets are bound to occur.

Germany's e-health initiatives may also be delayed because current integration is growing from the bottom up. A new law was enacted last year to deregulate the healthcare system and make it easier for corporations, hospitals, insurers and practitioners to conduct business in a regional, contractual way. This caused many healthcare groups to investigate ways to organize medical processes regionally, supported by IT and powered by investment funds offered by the government. The result has been a myriad of applications that are beneficial to regional groups but lack the required standardization or scalability to comply with the future architectural needs of an integrated EHR.

Next Steps

Healthcare reform is expected to once again become a hot topic, most likely by late 2006. Optimistic experts believe that by rising in importance, many of the barriers discussed here will be addressed, if not resolved. Also by that time, many European countries, such as Austria, will have introduced e-health. Germany will want to keep pace with the other countries and will spend considerable effort to resolve any outstanding issues in making e-health a priority. However, it must be noted that large governmental technology projects of the last years have suffered difficulties; for example, TollCollect (traffic control), Hercules (armed forces IT) and digital police radio. These projects have damaged German political credibility and have cost billions of tax funds, reducing the appetite for repetition by the political elite.

The next steps for a German national EHR are clear. The rollout of Germany's health professional card (eHPC) is expected in 2005 or 2006, so every physician, nurse and healthcare professional will have the necessary keys and standardized identification tools to access patient health records. Then, in 2006 or 2007, the e-patient card will follow. The first applications will probably occur regionally, and will be developed and tested in integrated care models in pilot projects around Germany. Those that are successful might well develop to building blocks of a national EHR that enables cooperation between hospitals, general practitioners, insurers and pharmacies.

Since the German health system has built-in competition, Darwinistic evolution of successful applications may lead to stronger final results than the central governmental authorities could have planned.

The problem is getting started. Because most of the European Union features standardized infrastructure and German infrastructure targets are ambitious in terms of functionality, Germany will lag behind most of Western Europe, including France, the U.K., Netherlands and other countries with centralized healthcare governance.

The application landscape is bound to be rich as competitors race to build solutions that are compatible with Germany's EHR, with many worldwide, global players already waiting to see how it will evolve, including Microsoft, IBM, SAP, Siemens, Deutsche Telekom and large global players in the smart card business.

Once implemented, the German system may be the best in the world. Functionalities like electronic health cards, double access rights for patients and health professionals and other features make Germany's infrastructure more ambitious than most other national solutions. Since the German health system has built-in competition, Darwinistic evolution of successful applications may lead to stronger final results than the central governmental authorities could have planned. So over the long term, trade-offs of decentralistic governance may well be judged differently than they are today.

Summary

The German healthcare system faces a host of challenges. Tying together disparate patient data and streamlining processing are problems that can be solved through technology. The real challenge lies in uniting German healthcare players to create an action plan for a national EHR. The current drive to introduce eHCCs will create a partial framework and e-prescribing will present an opportunity to learn lessons for future application development. The greater issue, however, is how to champion a project of this scale and diversity without centralized management. The world will be watching with keen interest. ■

Overview of EHRs in the United Kingdom

At this point, the U.K. is ahead of many other countries in articulating and taking action on the most challenging elements of public health provision and the role of information in the future of healthcare.

[Archie Galbraith, Accenture]

A distinguishing feature of healthcare in the United Kingdom is that it is essentially free to the patient at the point of service. The U.K. government is charged to design, manage and fund a centralized healthcare system that addresses every aspect of care delivery including office visits to a general practitioner, hospital services, outpatient treatment, prescription drugs, in-home care and social services. An EHR in this context is the fundamental information source and flow, crossing organization boundaries, reflecting the life of the patient and the life cycle of their healthcare. Such an EHR must collect and manage patient demographic and medical information in consistent ways so that it can be combined and analyzed with provider information to ensure that the right care is delivered in a connected manner, providing the optimal outcomes for the patient. Information on episodes, treatment and outcomes becomes part of the "real time" planning, management and funding that is emerging as an essential element of health system management.

The underpinning technology that supports the EHR must be seen to be secure and interoperable to permit accessibility of the information to a broad base of staff that supports patients across all sectors of health and social care. The goal of a population-wide, comprehensive, interoperable EHR is not yet a reality. Citizen EHRs have been accepted by the E.U. as a standard to be achieved in all European countries regardless of their funding model or infrastructure, which most countries are seeking to achieve in their own ways. Whether or not it will eventually be implemented in all its glory or sustained over time is not yet known, but it represents a direction of travel towards a patient-centric, connected healthcare approach reflecting the demands of modern healthcare.

Three critical factors or principles make a broad, comprehensive EHR possible:

- Making information available;
- Making people accountable for healthcare delivery and performance; and
- Linking results with rewards.

The United States faces a significant challenge to progress against these principles in a universal or national way due to the fragmented health market; this will make development of such a broadly defined EHR very difficult.

EHR Reflects Social Policy

An EHR is only part of the tool kit required by a modern, population-wide approach to healthcare. Far more fundamental has to be the definition of the healthcare direction and priorities established by the government or purchasing body on behalf of its citizens or members. We must determine what we as a community believe is right to offer our members in terms of healthcare. To what standards of access, quality and outcomes will we strive? For example, should we deliver care funded by taxes or other social funding that costs the patient nothing at the point of service, or should the costs be borne by insurance, employers and/or employees? The answer to these questions determine the model of care – a plan for how care will be delivered, where and by whom. After that must come a logical model or model of information. Who needs to know what so that healthcare can be delivered in the manner we have defined? Which items of information need to be combined in order to run the health system we've just described? Once those determinations are made, the technical architecture is designed and built to support the logical model.

Archie Galbraith leads Accenture's European Health practice and its Global Electronic Health Records team with operations in Australia, the U.K., the U.S., France, Spain, Singapore, South Africa and Ireland. Previously he was deputy director of NHS' Development Group, where he led work across all health sectors including changing ways of working within acute care hospitals and supporting the development of multi-agency protocols.

Overview of EHRs in the United Kingdom

It is this logical and hierarchical approach that drives the sources of funding and how the money will be spent.

Once we've determined that we are going to deliver care to everyone in our community, regardless of income, actions must deliver on that promise. If patients cannot afford cars to drive to a local hospital, means must be found to get them there or the care to them. We must set up a method of care delivery that is both affordable to the nation and accessible to the individual. In the years to come, care of chronic disease is going to become a larger proportion of healthcare. Patients will need access to a broader range of services from a much wider network of service providers. Information must be accessible and exchangeable among patients, physicians, nurses, clinicians, social workers, welfare workers, public housing workers and others, because all of them have a part to play in keeping clinically ill people as healthy as they can be and at home.

Though access is still imperfect and incomplete, patients can, for example, review the activities and current standing of their local hospitals and compare their performance against national standards.

Overview of the U.K. Healthcare System

Several years ago, the United Kingdom's National Health Service (NHS) set out a vision of "a health service fit for the 21st century." The plan recognized that although the NHS has delivered major improvements in the nation's health, it still "falls short of the standards patients expect and staff want to provide." In particular, survival rates in the U.K. for diseases like cancer and heart disease were below those in many other countries. There were long waiting lists for people needing medical service, and availability of certain treatments and medications had become a "post code lottery." This failure to meet patient and staff expectations was exacerbated by an increase in demand for healthcare, changes in medical knowledge that make possible more complex and expensive treatments, an acute shortage of doctors and underfunding of healthcare services.[1] Adding to the problem, the NHS remained – until recently – a system lacking national standards or clear incentives to improve performance. It perpetuated old-fashioned demarcations in staff and barriers between services. The NHS further suffered from a complex mix of centralized policy and priority setting with a semi-autonomous local management capability and disempowered patients.

An independent review of the NHS concluded that, in order to meet people's expectations and deliver the highest quality care over the next 20 years, the U.K. would need to devote more resources to healthcare, and implement corresponding reforms to ensure that all resources are used effectively. The review also called for doubling the previous spending on information and communications technology to support the new healthcare model. "The strategy will enable NHS professionals to have the information they need both to provide that care and to play their part in improving the public's health. The strategy also aims to ensure that patients, caregivers and the public have the information necessary to make decisions about their own treatment and care, and to influence the shape of health services generally."[2]

During the last 10 years, the health system in the U.K. has established the legitimacy of access to clinical information, performance comparisons and minimum standards. Though access is still imperfect and incomplete, patients can, for example, review the activities and current standing of their local hospitals and compare their performance against national standards. The scrutiny based on the reimbursement and clinical audit process requires physicians in family practices to report the treatments they have prescribed based on their diagnoses and to evaluate their effectiveness. They increasingly receive guidance on leading medical practices and which drugs or therapies are recommended by government-sponsored organizations. A national strategic framework spells out what kind of care is appropriate for key disease groups. Diabetics know in advance what type of care they should expect. Cancer diagnosis and treatment, where time can be a critical factor, must meet specified time constraints.

These care requirements and acceptable wait times are built into the performance measurements for medical practices and public hospitals. For example, it is now required that a family practitioner be able to offer a patient an office visit within

weblink

Read how healthcare can be provided in the home in "Telemedicine and Telehealth – Expanding the Continuum of Patient Care."

48 hours of receiving the call for an appointment. Emergency rooms must see walk-in patients within four hours. Providers are monitored and evaluated partly on their ability to meet these time requirements. Providers report their compliance with access guidelines and other performance metrics to their funding authorities on a regular basis. Since performance is linked to rewards and payment, hospitals that experience a slip in performance will experience a commensurate slip in payment. Hospitals are currently rated using a star system – zero to three stars. A three-star hospital gets access to more money and more self-determination than fewer-starred hospitals. A zero-star hospital faces the potential of government-mandated replacement of its chief executive and management team.

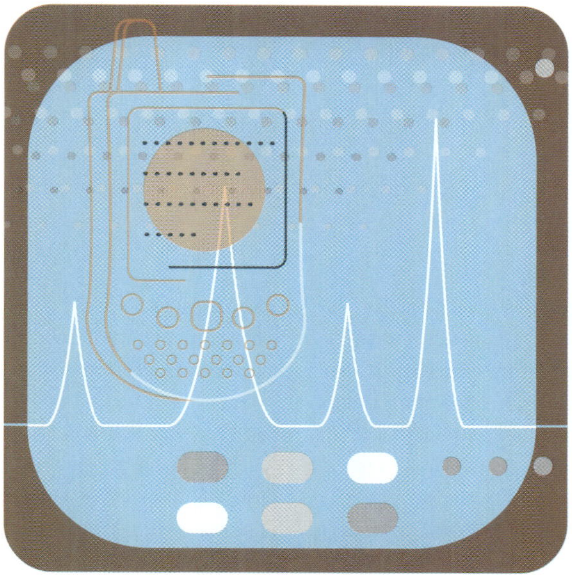

At this point, the U.K. is also ahead of many other countries in articulating a social policy for healthcare delivery and for spelling out in detail what constitutes an acceptable level of care for its citizens. Ironing out the details is a continuing challenge, but the general direction is well-established. Other countries are ahead of the U.K. in investing in infrastructure – the unglamorous, uninteresting and largely invisible information and communications technology by which the information in the EHR is stored, managed and exchanged. However, the U.K. government is involved in establishing mandatory standards for interoperability among local systems and for funding the implementation of a national network in England.

A goal of the NHS, toward which some component parts are already in place, is to make the general practitioner more central to the whole patient journey. General practitioners can stay in control of what happens to each patient, because the information is visible to them. A GP can make appointments electronically, order tests and review the results online, view the hospital discharge of patients, schedule aftercare and manage services for chronically ill patients.

Challenges

In the U.K., as in the U.S., getting physicians to adopt and use an EHR and its associated computerized functions is difficult. Adapting to a computer-based environment is not a technical issue; the challenge is managing change. The EHR must be designed and offered in such a way as to ensure that clear benefits are achievable for physicians and other clinicians, and those benefits must more than justify the learning curve and the occasional inconveniences of communicating electronically. Clinical staff need to become involved early in establishing practice guidelines and standards of care. System designers and implementers must work with physicians and other clinical stakeholders to develop advantages early to build up momentum for change. It is counterproductive to try to force doctors to behave in certain ways. Rather, physicians need to collaborate with other stakeholders to support policies and practices they recognize as acceptable levels of care. All stakeholders need rewards and motivations aligned with the success of the EHR.

The existence of an EHR bends the envelope of privacy rights. Though different countries have different standards of privacy, the need to define a standard of privacy and adhere to it is universal. In the U.S., HIPAA precludes the use of a patient's Social Security number as an identifier. In the U.K., the government has adopted the policy of standard identifying numbers for every patient. This simplifies the process of matching the patient to his or her medical, demographic and financial information. An EHR is evidence of the value of joined-up information and equally a target for those uncomfortable with the concept that their information is not in their immediate control. The same levels of sensitivity don't seem to be applied to banks which know about our money, schools which know about our children or loyalty card companies which know about our lifestyles. The irony is that the people most concerned about patient information security are people who are healthy. Sick people are less concerned about information security. They want to get well. The debate about security and confidentiality is driven by informed, healthy people.

As a practical matter, not all services are available in every hospital and every geographic region. A standard that calls for referring a patient at a certain point in treatment to a physical therapist is not applicable if the community lacks the specified resource. Localization of national policies and standards is necessary for an EHR to be useful. As an approximation, though it is not desirable for every hospital or physician to reconfigure the EHR, the system must be flexible enough so that providers serving local communities can use at least 70 percent of the system that applies universally and modify up to 30 percent to local needs.

Patient and Population

The overall health of a population is well-served by a successful EHR. An EHR is a good tool for discovering the best possible health outcomes for tax dollars. It gives quick access to a large amount of patient data and tools that can compare and analyze these data to inform decisions on a population level. Imagine that every hospital and every general practitioner in the country has access to a nationwide EHR and that every patient has a unique identifying number. Using only those numbers – leaving out patient identities – patient information can then be simply aggregated into a large, valuable database, which grows larger and more current daily because every day people have more and different health-related activities. It's then possible to track what medications patients are on, what hospitals they're in and what their health outcomes are. Interrogating such a database could tell us that there are 3,000 diabetics in the London area, for example. It could tell us how often they were admitted to hospitals and for what conditions. It could tell us how long each patient stayed in the hospital and whether that patient was re-admitted within the next year. If there are variations from region to region or physician to physician, investigators could work out the extent of the variations and potentially determine what caused them. They could discover, for example, whether improved outcomes were tied to different medications, different treatment options or other factors. This information and analysis can help direct how to spend public money to get the best possible outcomes. Right now, treatments can only be tied to surrogate markers – activities which indicate the condition of the patient's health. Eventually mechanisms tying medical interventions to quality of life will further enhance the value of population studies made possible by an EHR.

They could discover, for example, whether improved outcomes were tied to different medications, different treatment options or other factors.

A Long Journey

Implementing an EHR on any reasonable scale is a complex and expensive undertaking; too challenging to make false starts. It would be madness to switch off existing systems and start at square one. Start where you are. It matters little which technology you choose, because none are perfect. Start by changing how you treat patients; change it until it looks close to what you think you want to offer as a service. Join together service components and processes, even if the supporting technology is old, cobbled together, supplemented and patched up. What's vital is to establish a direction of travel and migrate gradually to a set of services which are robust, integrated and based on a single platform and single logic. The commitment is to the migration and to never again invest in products or services that are inconsistent with the journey's architecture and direction. This is a change in strategy from implementations based on products that are complex, proprietary and built on vertical logic. An integrated solution, scalable, flexible and based on horizontal logic, is a much better migration objective and more reflective of the patient's journey.

Summary

The single point of logic for an EHR has to be the experience of the patient. Previously the single point of logic in hospital systems was the experience of the physician. As recently noted in a speech by Professor Richardson of the Great Ormond Street Hospital for Sick Children, physicians today are gatekeepers at the temple of medical knowledge. They decide who to let in and what information to share with patients. In the future, physicians will be more like guides or advisors, sharing access to information and assisting patients in making better, more informed choices about their medical care.

The EHR must facilitate that evolution. It must support the experience of patients who will accrue the health benefits. Otherwise it's an interesting diversion not worth the expenditure of tax dollars.

The EHR is an expression of what we as a society believe healthcare should be today. Its practices and technology should exemplify those beliefs and evolve towards what we hope healthcare can become tomorrow. It must enshrine the changes we chose to make. ■

Endnotes

1. *Health at a Glance – OECD Indicators 2003 briefing note (United Kingdom).*
2. *An Information Strategy for the Modern NHS 1998-2005, A national strategy for local implementation; NHS Information Authority 1998.*

6

Roles & Perspectives

As a collaborative initiative, EHRs need commitment and involvement from a variety of stakeholders in the healthcare industry. Through interviews, leaders of government, business, consumers groups, and hospitals share their opinions about the specific objectives they have for EHRs, as well as their views about the rate of adoption and the barriers to implementation.

Newt Gingrich Advocates the Creation of A 21st-Century Intelligent Health System

Accelerating universal adoption of health IT is fundamental to creating a safer and more affordable health system.

[Newt Gingrich, Center for Health Transformation] [David Merritt, Center for Health Transformation]

What Are the Goals And Objectives of EHRs?

The Center for Health Transformation advocates the creation of a 21st-century intelligent health system. Our vision is of a health and healthcare system that is centered on the individual, not the provider or hospital. Prevention and wellness are fundamental priorities. Care is driven by outcomes, not by volume. Consumers own their data and have a right to know cost and quality information. Innovation is rapid. The dissemination of knowledge is in real time. All of this must be built upon an electronic system. It cannot happen with paper.

Paper kills – it's that simple. Instead of saving lives, our current system is taking them. With as many as 98,000 Americans still being killed by medical errors every year, ridding the system of paper-based records and quickly adopting electronic health records (EHRs) will save lives and, at the same time, save money.

This is not just a theory. Health information technology (HIT) is vital to making American healthcare the safest it can possibly be. Already we can witness the benefits. Indiana Heart Hospital in Indianapolis built a new facility that is totally paperless. They reduced medication errors by 85 percent. If we could get the same results nationwide, we'd save at least 7,500 Americans, since medication errors kill nearly 9,000 citizens every year. Indiana Heart also reduced physician administrative time by 30 percent. This means that doctors can now spend more time with their patients and provide them with higher-quality care.

There are plenty of programs working today that may serve as examples of how a technology-enabled health system can save lives and save money. For instance:

- Danville Regional Medical Center in Danville, Va., utilized Siemens Medical Systems' electronic prescribing system and prevented more than 1,200 wrong drugs or dosages, saving countless deaths and untold suffering, as well as nearly $750,000.
- Central Utah Multi-Specialty Clinic, the largest independent multi-specialty group in the state of Utah, with 59 physicians and nine locations, implemented an electronic medical record built by Allscripts Healthcare Solutions. The clinic saved $1 million in the first year through direct spending reductions and revenue increases. They anticipate saving more than $14 million over the next five years.
- PeaceHealth is a six-hospital system in Alaska, Washington and Oregon. Working with IDX, they created the community health record, an electronic record for every one of their 1.4 million patients. The community health record is totally online, HIPAA-compliant and can be accessed by all the stakeholders: hospital doctors and nurses, independent physicians, specialists, health plans and patients. The results are phenomenal: adverse drug events cut by 83 percent; for diabetics, A1C levels less than seven jumped from 44 percent in 2001 to more than 60 percent in 2004; for patients with cardiovascular disease, LDL levels of less than 100 jumped from 28 percent in 2001 to 52 percent last year. Their patients are healthier and their quality of life is dramatically better.

The urgency of adopting HIT cannot be overstated. We must build a 21st-century intelligent health system that brings healthcare into the information age. HIT is one of the vital levers to accomplish this worthy goal.

What Are the Roles of Various Constituent Groups?

Everyone in health and healthcare must make modernizing the system the top priority. Hospitals, providers and insurers cannot wait for interoperability standards to coalesce before investing in

Newt Gingrich, former Speaker of the House of Representatives, is founder of the Center for Health Transformation. **David Merritt,** a project director at the center, is an expert on health information technology.

HIT. We will lose far too much time if they do that. The private sector must aggressively move on HIT because it is a matter of life and death. The Centers for Disease Control and Prevention recently reported that only 31 percent of hospital emergency rooms, 29 percent of outpatient departments and 17 percent of doctors' offices have EHRs to support patient care. That is shamefully low. Facilities like PeaceHealth, Danville Regional and the Central Utah Clinic did not wait for the rest of the industry to make up its mind. They implemented cutting-edge technology and saved lives and saved money. Everyone should use this approach.

Patients must also get engaged. A majority of Americans do not take responsibility for their own health or healthcare seriously, and the debate over interoperability and electronic health records is meaningless to most. If individuals began seeking out providers who used electronic records, the adoption rate would no doubt begin to accelerate, driven by consumer demand. Americans are key to changing the healthcare marketplace, but to do so they must become informed advocates for their own health and well-being.

One thing every individual can do is sign up for an iHealthRecord, a new online personal health record available to anyone. The service is free to individuals but does charge a monthly fee to physicians. Approximately 100,000 doctors have signed up to use it, and it has been endorsed by the American Medical Association, the American Heart Association and dozens of medical societies and other groups. Individuals can use an iHealthRecord to send a secure email to their doctor, research medical conditions, treatments and healthy lifestyles and store vital health information. In addition to using an iHealthRecord for regular care, an ER doctor can use this information in an emergency away from home. It could save someone's life. Getting individuals and doctors accustomed to using an online health record is imperative to building a 21st-century intelligent health system.

The private sector must take decisive action to realize the full potential of HIT, but government will play a critical role as well. Congress and the Bush administration should make funding HIT a top priority – on par with national security. Millions of lives are at stake. Dr. David Brailer, President Bush's national coordinator for health information technology, has said that HIT could save the healthcare system upward of $140 billion a year. These savings could be used to expand coverage to the nearly 45 million Americans who have no health insurance. The savings could also be used to find solutions to the diabetes and obesity epidemics that are overwhelming our nation. Despite projected budget deficits for years to come, the federal government should dedicate 1 percent of all federal spending to HIT. Seven billion dollars a year is a lot of money, but the return on this investment cannot be overstated. We would save hundreds of thousands of lives and hundreds of billions of dollars.

One solid step in the right direction is all of the momentum on Capitol Hill and in the Administration. Secretary Leavitt has been out in front of this issue since day one, and his leadership will make a difference. There are also at least seven different proposals on HIT pending in the House and Senate. From Congressmen Tim Murphy, a Pennsylvania Republican, and Patrick Kennedy, a Rhode Island Democrat, to Senators Bill Frist and Hillary Clinton, these bipartisan bills will play an integral role in modernizing healthcare and moving our system into the information age. Most of the proposals provide financial incentives for doctors to invest in HIT, and allow local hospitals to supply the doctors in their community with the infrastructure needed to electronically exchange patient information. It is another indication of how backward our current health system is that this practice is presently forbidden by law.

Most of the proposals provide financial incentives for doctors to invest in HIT, and allow local hospitals to supply the doctors in their community with the infrastructure needed to electronically exchange patient information.

These bills also encourage private-sector innovation through federal grants to regional groups that are trying to electronically connect patients, doctors, hospitals and insurers. In addition, these bills will promote accelerated transformation by requiring that those regional organizations adopt common technology standards, meaning that variant systems from diverse locations must be able to communicate with each other.

weblink

Read how computers need to be able to act on data from other computers in "Interoperability."

Beyond these bills' commitment to health transformation, it is imperative that the federal government take decisive action to promote widespread HIT adoption. Changes to the administration of public health programs could accelerate adoption – the Medicare and Medicaid programs, for instance, could make HIT an essential component of healthcare delivery by creating financial incentives for providers who use it. In addition, federal agencies should coordinate on federal HIT strategy and on the interoperability of their own implementation, rather than continuing to operate in silos.

How Does Your Approach Differ From Other Proposed Solutions?

First, we believe that what is needed is transformation, not reform. Rather than focusing on small changes or reactionary fixes to pieces of the system as many groups do, we focus on transformation of the entire system. It's like the difference between passing legislation requiring doctors to write legibly and passing legislation requiring doctors to use e-prescribing. One is a small (not to mention unlikely) change to the current system and the other creates a whole new system. We focus on – and have the reputation of being as good as about anyone at – discovering, creating and impacting key leverage points that will accelerate the transformation of the entire system.

Second, we believe that you have to involve a broad coalition of stakeholders. Our members represent a very wide spectrum of stakeholder groups, many of whom are not accustomed to working together. We bring together provider groups, hospitals, health plans, employers, technology vendors and patient and issue advocates, as well as government leaders at the state and the federal levels. It makes a huge difference to have both the perspective and the influence of leaders across the board when trying to accomplish the level of change we're advocating.

Third, related to the second point, we are a collaboration of leaders. Both words are important. We think the only way it's possible to transform the system is by building a critical mass of leaders who collaborate to get it done. One person or one stakeholder group – or one political group for that matter – can't do it alone.

Fourth, we are vision-driven. We have a clear vision of a 21st-century intelligent health system in which knowledge saves lives and saves money for every American. While our members may not agree with every one of our strategies and while some may be competitors in the marketplace, they come together at the Center because they share a larger vision of a better future. That vision and our vision principles create a common ground, bringing us together and helping drive and guide our activities.

Fifth, we are focused on solutions, not problems. We are constantly learning, constantly searching and constantly creating new solutions and new policies, which we then work to drive through the system as rapidly as possible. One of our key rules with regard to being solution-oriented is to always say "yes, if ..." not "no, because ... " It's amazing how much that one habit can do to help a group work together to create solutions rather than bickering about problems.

What Are Some of the Implementation Challenges?

One challenge is reaching an agreement on interoperability standards for EHRs. Many companies develop EHRs, and they are built on technology platforms that differ from one system to the next. If these products cannot talk with one another, the goal of building an interconnected system will never be realized. The EHR Vendors Association, physician groups, standards-developing organizations and others should converge upon one standard. Duplicative standards would be inefficient and delay adoption indefinitely. Every day that we waste bickering over proprietary interests and which standard to use we kill countless Americans. The industry and lawmakers must reach agreement on a single standard and move forward.

Stark and anti-kickback statutes are also barriers to rapid HIT adoption because they prevent hospital systems from providing HIT to physician offices and clinics. Laws such as these are part of a larger question: Who is going to pay for the investment in health IT? Until Congress makes HIT funding the top priority it should be, the private sector must make the investment.

One solution is for large hospital systems and other entities to provide the IT infrastructure to surrounding physician practices and clinics. While many hospitals, medical groups and other organizations would be willing to do this, current Stark and anti-kickback laws stand in the way. The Government Accountability Office (GAO) concluded as much in a recent study. These laws were

Many companies develop EHRs, and they are built on technology platforms that differ from one system to the next. If these products cannot talk with one another, the goal of building an interconnected system will never be realized.

meant to protect patients from fraudulent and corrupt referring arrangements. But by preventing the rapid adoption of HIT, they are not protecting patients – they are endangering them. Congress should create new HIT exemptions giving hospitals the ability to fund HIT for community doctors, but they should come with an important requirement: The technologies provided must be interoperable once data standards are announced by the Secretary of HHS. Such a requirement would allow doctors to use the technology to refer their patients to any hospital, not just the one that supplied the technology. This would embrace the spirit of the laws while allowing the private sector to move ahead.

Finally, to address one major challenge, Congress must reform the way legislation is "scored." Currently, the Congressional Budget Office and the Office of Management and Budget view HIT as a cost, not as an investment. They miss the point that after an initial investment, HIT will ultimately save a significant amount of money. The Center for Information Technology Leadership estimates $78 billion in annual savings from sharing electronic patient data. The GAO noted recently the "proven benefits to implementing health IT." An earlier GAO report cited dozens of examples where HIT brought significant savings. For example, the Mayo Clinic invested in a total overhaul in its clinical information systems and now saves more than $21 million every year. Why do CBO and OMB refuse to score such savings? The fact that investing in HIT will often pay for itself through avoiding duplicate tests, automating chart pulls and review, and eliminating unnecessary hospital admissions and office visits is lost on them. This approach is so short-sighted that it inhibits any serious discussion of meaningful legislation.

What Is on the Horizon for Electronic Health Records? Will There Be Widespread Adoption in the Next Five Years?

EHRs are one piece of an even more powerful system. We call this a "personal health knowledge system." This system is not an isolated passive record in the 20th century sense, but it is instead a dynamic, interactive and real-time exchange of knowledge.

Through this online system, individuals, providers, insurers and others will exchange four types of information. First, they will exchange clinical information, such as home diagnostic reports, treatment updates, diagnoses, lab results and other details. Individuals will have home health kits that will measure blood pressure, cholesterol, heart rate, glucose levels and other key indicators. The results will be automatically uploaded into the personal health knowledge system where providers will be able to review and monitor the information. When depersonalized, this information would provide an enormous amount of data to mine for emerging trends in treatment and patient care.

Second, a personal health knowledge system will be used to share general information on health and healthcare. Through their system portal, individuals will access websites like MedLinePlus from the National Library of Medicine when they have questions about their health. Individuals will be able to research healthy lifestyles, best practices, treatment options, quality measures, provider performance and other information. Based on the latest research, providers and insurers will send information through the system tailored to an individual's particular illness, treatment or condition. This is an essentially an "information prescription."

Third, a personal health knowledge system will be used to exchange administrative information, such as appointment reminders, prescription refill requests, scheduling, address changes and new insurance coverage.

Finally, a personal health knowledge system will be used to exchange information on benefit coverage and insurance information. Based on an individual's specific insurance coverage, providers and insurers could offer options in care, such as brand name versus generic pharmaceuticals.

A powerful, sophisticated system like this will dramatically improve health and healthcare in America. Giving the research world a wealth of non-identifiable data to mine for best practices that will improve their health and receiving tailored information from their doctor and other sources puts individuals firmly in charge of their health and healthcare. Attaining such a system should be the long-term goal for current EHR vendors and their technologies. It is possible, and we can and must build it.

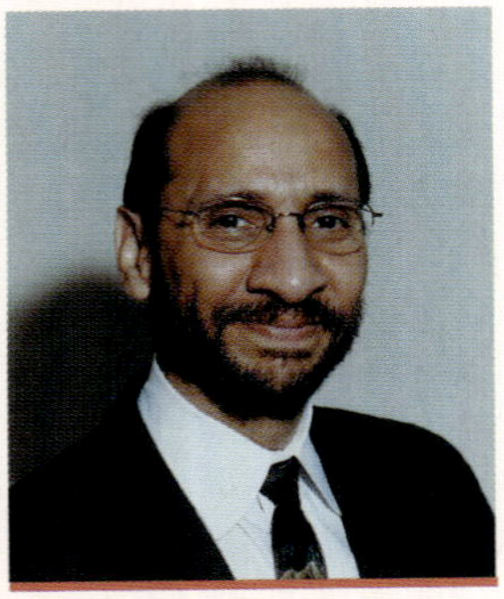

John Lumpkin
Senior Vice President
Health Care Group

John Lumpkin, M.D., M.P.H., is the senior vice president and the director of the Health Care Group. He is responsible for the overall planning, budgeting, staffing, management and evaluation of all program and administrative activities of the Robert Wood Johnson Foundation Health Care Group.

Q&A With Dr. John Lumpkin

The leader of the Robert Wood Johnson Foundation explains how EHRs provide patients with critical information as well as efficient and effective care that costs less.

Healthcare Technology: *What do you think are the goals and objectives of electronic health records (EHRs)?*

John Lumpkin: I think a key goal of an EHR is improving quality of care and patient safety. I'd like to quote something Daniel Masys said at an Institute of Medicine meeting in 2001: "Current practice depends upon the clinical decision-making capacity and reliability of autonomous individual practitioners for classes of problems that routinely exceed the balance of unaided human cognition." The rapidly expanding body of medical knowledge essentially means that people can no longer provide high-quality care unassisted. And one of the roles, one of the key roles, of EHRs is to provide them with the information they need to make the right decisions.

EHRs can also provide patients with critical information. The chronic disease model that was developed by Ed Wagner envisions that the best interactions between a patient and a physician occur when the physician and the caregivers are part of a team that's prepared and responsive, and that the patient is engaged and able to participate in the decision making. And so the ability of an EHR to populate personal health records would enable the patient to be a more active participant in their care. So these are all the enabling areas under quality.

Another key goal of EHRs is to provide efficient and effective care that costs less. For example, an antibiotic would be selected because it is the most effective for what the patient needs, not because it was the most recently detailed by a drug company. You can go down the whole list of rows of treatment, so in some instances where there's overuse you'll be able to use

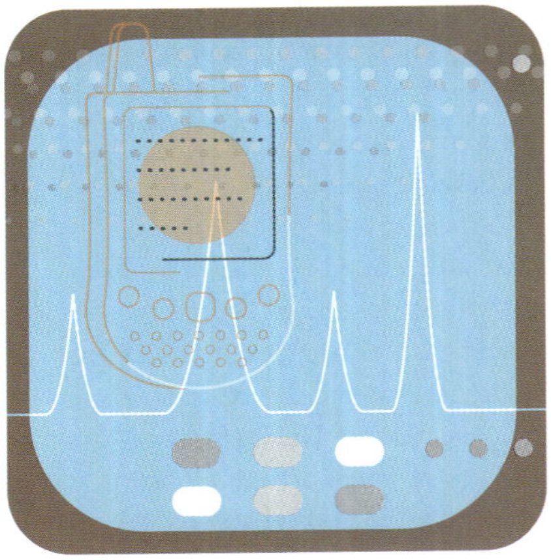

resources more appropriately. In other areas there's under-use, and this under-use tends to lead to higher costs, not necessarily in each individual encounter, but in the overall system. So if you don't give a patient aspirin after a heart attack, then what you're going to find is that down the road they are going to have more complications. And as a result, costs for that individual are going to be more expensive.

HCT: *We're trying to understand the roles of different stakeholders in making EHRs happen. What do you think about the roles of various groups, business coalitions, physicians, hospitals, payers and consumer groups?*

JL: Well in order to answer that question, it is important to understand the basic economics of EHRs. We have seen from some of the earlier studies that there is a mismatch between who pays for EHRs and who profits from them. The costs for EHRs where they've been implemented have primarily been borne by the individual providers – physicians, other caregivers, hospitals, etc. However, the savings that are yielded, the cost savings, don't actually accrue to them. The savings basically go to those who are paying for the care: the patient, the insurance companies and those who buy the insurance. And so for EHRs to happen, that mismatch needs to be rectified. We can rectify this through a system that enables clinicians to be able to afford and have EHRs. This system would include pay-for-use and pay for performance – those things that really reward clinicians for the outcomes that would result from using EHRs: better adherence to clinical care guidelines and better quality of care.

HCT: *What are some of the implementation challenges?*

JL: There continues to be implementation challenges associated with standards. We've made a fair bit of progress with adoption standards that started with HIPAA. The next important step in developing standards was the adoption of the Consolidated Health Informatics Initiative between the Department of Defense, the Department of Veterans Affairs and the Department of Health and Human Services, which identified standards in 24 different domains. The next phase of important standards adoption is what is being put forward by Connecting for Health, which is identifying standards for health data interchange. Not having a common set of standards and architecture is a major obstacle and creates tremendous challenge. The key part of that challenge is the fact that the true benefits of EHRs will not be yielded until there is an interconnecting system of EHRs. People don't see just one provider, they see multiple providers, through distance, through time and through different illnesses. If we are to deliver consistent quality care, it's important to be able to provide clinicians with the information they need to make the right decisions.

> ... now we're seeing various state governments across the country also trying to create environments where inter-connectivity of EHRs will occur through the adoption of legislation that's supporting the development of statewide networks.

HCT: *Do you think we'll have widespread adoption in the next five years?*

JL: I think that there are a lot of very positive trends that will lead to adoption. Number one is the belief that EHRs are possible. And this has really been driven initially by Secretary Thompson. Secretary Levitt, if it were possible, has eclipsed Secretary Thompson's zeal and enthusiasm for EHRs. And then of course the push that has been put on by the president. And now we're seeing various state governments across the country also trying to create environments where interconnectivity of EHRs will occur through the adoption of legislation that's supporting the development of statewide networks.

The second important trend is the initiative by the Certification Commission for Health Information Technology. One of the problems in the field is that no one knows exactly what to buy. The promise of CCHIT is that it will put the purchasers of these systems in a position to make reasonable decisions in implementing those systems. So I think that that's a very important development.

The third is the rise of disease-specific personal health records systems. Here you see individual patients, starting out with those with chronic diseases, who want to be active partners in the delivery of their care and have their medical information available to them. As a result of either health plan or individual provider pressure to provide this electronic information to their patients, they're recognizing the need to adopt EHRs. Finally, a growing commitment to improving quality of care paired with an increased recognition that EHRs are valuable tools for tracking treatment and standardizing care.

So I think that there are a lot of trends that would indicate we're entering the logarithmic growth phase of adoption of EHRs over the next couple of years.

HCT: *If you had to give a percentage, what percentage of adoption do you think we'll have in five years?*

JL: In five years? If current trends continue, I would predict adoption in the 60 to 75 percent range. ■

Q&A With HealthCare Partners

Three executives describe the challenges and rewards expected of electronic health records.

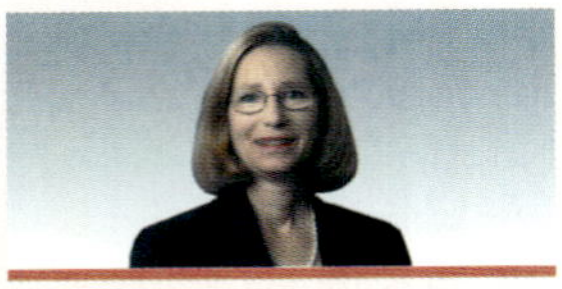

Melayne Yocum
Chief Operating Officer

As HealthCare Partners' chief operating officer and executive vice president, Ms. Yocum's responsibilities include operational oversight of all medical group care sites and hundreds of IPA offices for HealthCare Partners in the Los Angeles area.

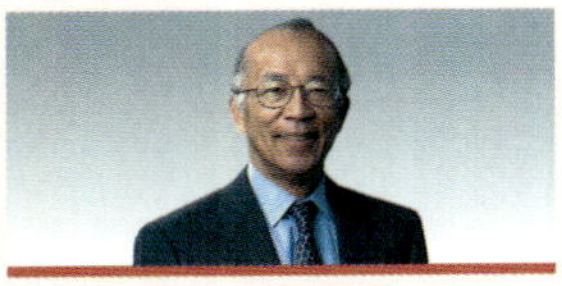

William Chin, M.D.
Executive Medical Director

William Chin, M.D., is one of the organization's founding partners. As executive medical director, Dr. Chin heads the Office of Medical Director. Under the clinical oversight of this office, HealthCare Partners continually improves its quality of patient care and its clinical processes.

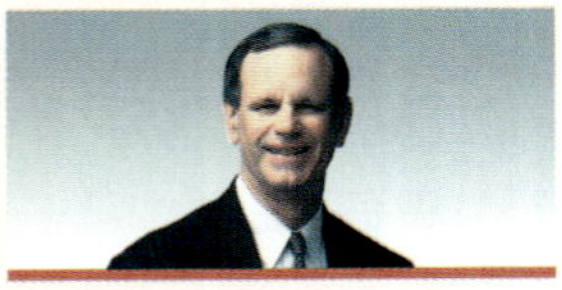

Zan Calhoun
Chief Information Officer

Formerly president of OAO HealthCare Solutions, Inc., Zan Calhoun, CIO of Healthcare Partners, has a distinguished history in healthcare information technology in both payer and provider segments of the industry.

HealthCare Partners Medical Group (HCP) and its affiliated independent physician associations (IPAs) serve over 500,000 managed care and fee-for-service patients in Southern California. The organization's group model division provides medical services in 30 offices and four urgent care centers throughout greater Los Angeles. Its IPAs provide care through hundreds of other offices around Los Angeles and Orange County. It is the second-largest medical group in California.

HCP's business model provides medical services funded by capitation from the health plans. The model supports a variety of clinician, hospital and ancillary contracts, as well as the agreements, partnerships and relationships with various health plans.

Driven by its vision – "Dedicated to the well-being and respectful compassionate healing of our patients and communities" – HealthCare Partners has long been involved in strategic process improvement initiatives to improve patient care. The most recent, and most exciting, undertaking is a multiyear process improvement program: the Clinical Information System (CIS) project. The goals of CIS include:

- Enabling clinicians to improve the outcomes for chronic diseases, to achieve preventative care goals and to increase safety for their patients through decision support, disease management programs and safety programs.
- Empowering patients by improving communications between patient and physician, and providing access to their medical record, laboratory results, medication lists and other clinically important information.
- Expanding clinical trials programs by linking the patient base of data.
- Leveraging technology to enhance relationships with contracted physicians, hospitals and other vendors.
- Creating and identifying highly efficient outpatient care processes and clinical guidelines.
- Prescribing medications more effectively and safely.
- Improving communications between primary care clinicians and specialists to reduce inappropriate referrals, and provide better satisfaction and efficiency.
- Improving communications between primary care clinicians and hospitalists/specialists to reduce admission and re-admission rates.
- Improving the organization's ICD-9 and CPT coding.

A key component of CIS is the implementation of the Allscripts™ TouchWorks™ product, a Web-based electronic medical record system. Here three of HealthCare Partners' senior executive team discuss the company's motivation, the challenges and expected rewards of electronic health records (EHRs).

HCT: *What are the goals and objectives of EHRs?*

William Chin, M.D., Executive Medical Director: I think everyone who has used an EHR will stand by the statement that this will improve the quality of care. Some of the reasons for that statement are that there are fewer lost records, there are reminders built into the system to prompt the physician and the healthcare team to know what needs to be done for a given patient, for a given disease. From the physicians' point of view, it is a real benefit to have a tool that will allow them to provide better care, reduce frustration and improve satisfaction with the process.

Zan Calhoun, Chief Information Officer: In addition, another of the major goals of EHRs is more standardization of the data. So that what we have is more consistent data throughout the entire healthcare system, so that data can be more easily aggregated, so that data can be more easily shared. It all supports what Bill just talked about in terms of improving the quality of care. More standardization of data will support interoperability between systems and healthcare information users.

Melayne Yocum, Chief Operating Officer: A word that I many times hear associated with the EHR is "enabling," because it does enable physicians to have more data at their fingertips; it enables sharing of that information across a wide range of healthcare entities and providers. And it enables patients to be more participative in their healthcare, to take on more decision making and be a true partner with their clinician and their care team.

HCT: *What is the role of physicians in making EHRs happen?*

WC: The physician plays a key role in that if they don't use it, if it isn't intuitive for them, then the system is not valuable. So the physician must play a leadership role in this whole process.

ZC: There are several roles that a physician might play. The first one is as a "thought leader," providing the visionary leadership in terms of where we want to go with our use of the product. The second one is to be a "champion," which is perhaps less about vision, but more about enthusiasm and attitude: "Yes, we can make it happen. Yes, we can figure out how to do it." The third is as a "team leader." It's working more collaboratively, a "let's work things through" attitude. The fourth is a "trainer": "I, as a physician, am going to train other physicians." Lastly, the physician role is just as an individual user.

HCT: *What do you think are some of the implementation challenges?*

MY: One of the challenges that our industry has in implementing EHRs is the lack of standardization in our processes. Healthcare is more of a craft industry with many individuals who have developed their own processes to accomplish their goals in delivering care. This lack of standardized processes can make the implementation of an EHR very challenging.

ZC: Other challenges are the technical and security components of rolling out such a large system. Clearly the networks need to be enhanced to deal with the additional traffic and security needs to be a high priority issue to be addressed.

HCT: *Healthcare Technology: What's on the horizon? Do you think there will be widespread adoption in the next five years?*

MY: Yes. As we see physician organizations installing and improving their EHRs, we will then continue to reap the benefits of these systems in improved care for patients. This will lead to improved functionality and added benefits for patients and physicians alike.

ZC: I agree with that. Other issues on the horizon include significantly more focus on security. HIPAA is a first step in that process, but in the intervening few years, there will be more issues around unanticipated or unexpected divulging of health information, which will lead to much more focus around security. This will, I think, break down some of these walls that might have been keeping some out of this market. I also believe you'll see more portability of the information, where I as an individual have more control over my health information. The P in HIPAA stands for portability, and yet very few people are talking about portability. So I do think you'll see more and more discussion and action surrounding how to make our records more portable. And as we see the adoption rates climb, there will be more integration of data from more sources, and that will inherently make the value of these systems even greater, causing yet more growth in adoption rates.

WC: Everything I see is that there's going to be more adoption of the EHR, and as more and more folks are using it – the hospitals, the physicians, etc. – that in itself will drive integration. As more and more users have systems, then they want to talk to each other. ■

The P in HIPAA stands for portability, and yet very few people are talking about portability. So I do think you'll see more and more discussion and action surrounding how to make our records more portable.

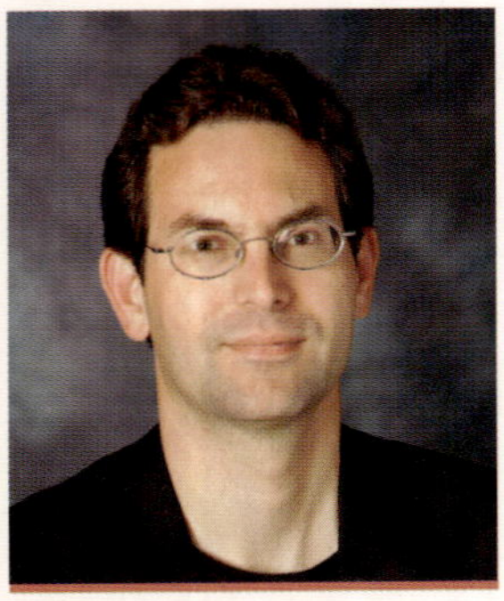

John Halamka
CIO
CareGroup Health System

John Halamka, M.D., M.S., is chief information officer of the CareGroup Health System, chief information officer and associate dean for educational technology at Harvard Medical School, chairman of NEHEN and the CEO of the RHIO for Massachusetts.

Q&A With Dr. John Halamka

The CEO of the RHIO for Massachusetts describes how they have implemented a system for sharing all of the clinical data in the entire region.

Healthcare Technology: *You are the chairman of NEHEN, CIO of the Harvard Clinical Research Institute and a practicing emergency room physician. And I understand that you have taken on a new job this year.*

John Halamka: In addition to being the CIO of Harvard, I'm the CEO of the RHIO (regional health information organization) in Massachusetts. So I'm responsible for all the clinical data sharing in the entire region.

HCT: *Last year you wrote a white paper about NEHEN, which is a standards-based approach for exchanging HIPAA-compliant eligibility transactions. This year we are hoping you can tell us what you have been working on at CareGroup.*

JH: Let me start with an example. You have the doctor's office, you have the hospital, you have the ER – you're lucky if the information is electronic but it might as well be on paper. If no one can get to it, it is just electronic data that's locked away. What we need to do is take the data where it lives today in the outpatient and in the inpatient world and make it Web-accessible in a standard and secure fashion. What we need to do is break down the barriers to care so that physicians who are authorized can know what medication a patient is on, what the patient's allergies are and what his last EKG was like.

Let me give you an example. Say it's the middle of the night, the patient comes to the hospital and you ask what he received from his outpatient doctor. He says he received a bunch of medicines: a pink one and a green one. According to the EKG he's having, his chest pain indicates a myocardial infarction, i.e., a heart attack, but it is hard to know without looking at the old EKG.

So we took the MediTech database and wrapped middleware around it that enabled our doctors to query it. We did the same thing for NextGen, GE's Centricity and other EMRs. And we did the same thing for a number of home-grown and departmental systems. We did the same thing for our PACS system.

CareWeb

The end result was a Web viewer called CareWeb. Let's say I want to learn everything there is to know about this patient without having to have 27 different log-ins and 5 different user interfaces. Let's say we were able to see all the data gathered about this patient in one place. What does that do for us?

Well it immediately reduced costs. We stopped using paper medical records, meaning that there's still a paper record out there, but now that everyone can get the data electronically, we no longer have to keep tons of paper in the hospital. We actually moved all of our paper medical records to cheap warehouse storage 15 miles away. So we ended up saving about a million dollars a year in real estate and staff costs by just dispensing with all the paper that we used to push around.

So how about the response time? It's 2:00 in the morning; I need an old EKG. Can we pull it out of the file room? Well by the time we pull it out of the file room, the patient either has a cardiac catheterization or expired. So now that all this data is instantly available to clinicians at the touch of a button, it truly enabled just-in-time good care.

Provider Order Entry

The next product that we developed on top of CareWeb was provider order entry. The

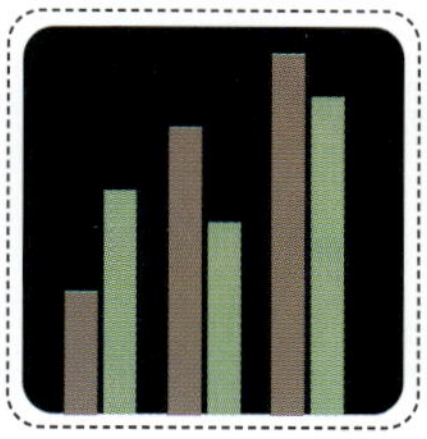

And what does that do? Well, medication error is a quality of care problem and also an economic problem. It costs roughly $5,000 per adverse event to treat a patient in a hospital.

Institute of Medicine report says we are killing 98,000 patients a year due to the misuse of medications, drug interactions, wrong dosing, transcription errors, etc. If you're going to build provider order entry, you need all the underlying data to know about the drug interactions. So we took all the data that CareWeb provided and then layered on top of it a complete ordering system, so that in 2001 we actually eliminated all the handwritten and voice orders in the entire organization.

Today we go from the doctor's brain to the patient's vein without a single handoff or transcribed piece of paper. When you think for a moment about the insane way that we wrote medication in the past – the doctor generally writes pretty badly – we wrote a medication on a piece of carbon paper. Is that a .5 or 5 milligrams? Is that Atenolol or Ativan? It goes through the carbon, then it's faxed to a pharmacist, the pharmacist re-keys it into another system and then it's given to the patient. We hope it is the right medication at the right time to the right patient.

With the new work flow, where a doctor walks up to a wireless tablet or a PDA or whatever device he would like to use; it's all Web-based. Say he is on the second floor of the west campus. He is shown a dashboard of all the patients that are around him. The doctor picks a patient by clicking on their name from a dashboard, so he is identifying the right patient; then he sees their comprehensive history, and then he goes to write an order. That medication is checked against all the other meds, all the other allergies, adjusted for any kidney or liver dysfunction and then is dosed per best-practice guidelines. And by best practice guidelines, it may be that it has range-of-sanity dose. You can't go right for a pound of morphine, you can't do something that is going harm the patients, and it checks some medications that are particularly dangerous, such as insulin or Heparin. For those types of drugs, a doctor actually can't write for a dose at all. So we've gotten to the point of now having diagnosis-based orders as part of the system for using all the data that CareWeb gathered, and laying on a whole new one, imparting almost artificial intelligence staff. So without having voice or handwritten orders, in 2001, we reduced medication error by 50 percent.

And what does that do? Well medication error is a quality-of-care problem and also an economic problem. It costs roughly $5,000 per adverse event to treat a patient in a hospital. We have 60,000 patients on average in patient volume a year. So imagine that 1 percent of them has medication errors when you use the old paper-based systems. Now 60,000 times 1 percent times $5,000 is $3 million a year; we save $3 million a year. Adjust that by 50 percent, because that's the reduction in adverse drug events we've observed. So it's around $1.5 million a year quantifiable cost reduction. And given that provider order entry only took $2.5 million to implement, it has return on investment in just over 18 months.

So why isn't every hospital in America doing provider order entry as part of their whole electronic record implementation? Because it's the hardest thing you can possibly do from an organizational change management standpoint. Doctors feel like they lose their autonomy. Doctors now have to actually go up to the computer and do the work, make the choices. They can't delegate that to a clerk or to a nurse. So to the extent that it's more work, it is lost autonomy; it requires a mouse, there's a generational component to that. For a 25-year-old fresh out of medical school, that's great. But if you're a 65-year-old chairman of the department, maybe the computer isn't so comfortable for you. And so we had to really take the entire organization and shift some mindsets to say, this is so important from a quality standpoint, that provider order entry is not an option; it is compulsory to use.

Web OMR

After CareWeb provider order entry, we implemented full Web-based ambulatory records with e-prescribing and full decision support for the outpatient community. We went live with that in 2002. The name of the product is called WebOMR (for online medical record), and it shows you all the data in CareWeb, and presents the data that is most relevant to the doctor who needs to understand the patient's needs beyond the patient environment.

One of the problems we have is there's so much data in medicine but so little knowledge. How valuable is it to know the last 10 years of labs or the last 14 X-rays?

weblink

Read how timely and accurate information improves the delivery of care in "Patient Safety."

Q&A With Dr. John Halamka

What you really want in one place is a dashboard profile that tells the physician about the patient that they are going to see in 10 minutes: their medication list, their last visit, their last labs, their last X-ray, the reason for the visit today. And that enables our outpatient environment to be much more efficient.

We knew that we needed to create communitywide exchange data. You can't take a piece of paper and share it with your neighbor very easily. So even though we have the most wired hospital in the country, it's still only 40 percent electronic. And for consent forms or procedure forms, that means, how do we go from 40 percent electronic to 85 percent electronic to ensure that every aspect of that patient's care is accessible on the Web?

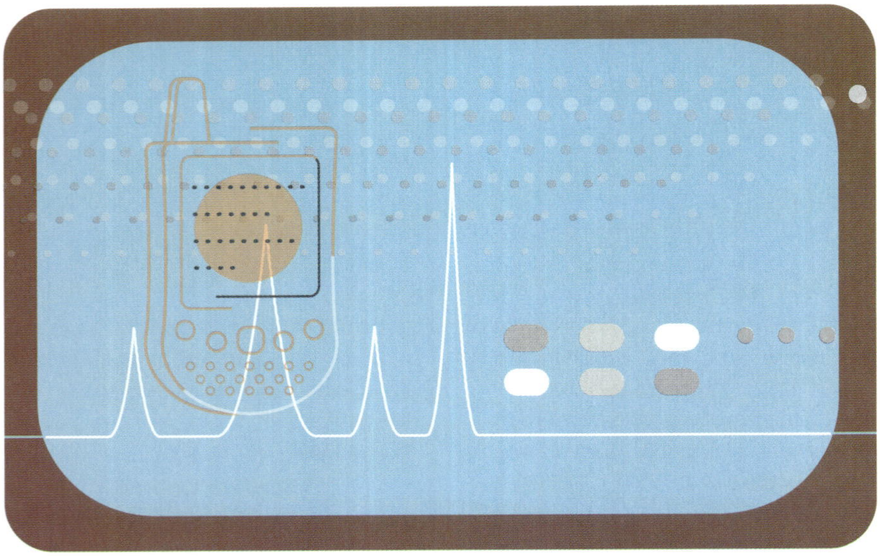

E-Forms

So this year we implemented e-forms. We partnered with Adobe, which has a smart-form capability, where we can design a form that's a PDF. They have 100 checkboxes that are actually rules. For example, you can't make both male and female at the same time. You fill out the form and say, here's the tumor-staging form. Where is the tumor; what is the size of the tumor? Based on the size and location of the tumor, I'll stage it for you automatically. The doctor signs the form using a digital pad, pushes a button and then it generates XML, which goes right into my electronic record system. I've been able to take the last mile of all this paper that's in organizations and begin the process of retiring it, by moving all the standard paper-based workloads to totally electronic workloads, using Adobe technology.

Connectivity

We have CareWeb, provider order entry, WebOMR and e-forms. So how do I solve the connectivity problem for regions of the country? To that extent, the big revolution that we're all working on now is turning everything into a Web service, building out everything that we've done in the past now as a service-oriented architecture, so it is just a Web page, an application that you have to log in and use. Web services allow machine-to-machine communication of all data in XML. This means that a private doctor's office that isn't affiliated with us, but we decide is trustworthy, can pull the information out of our clinical systems in a computer-to-computer fashion, and integrate it into their electronic record.

We've just finished some prototypes of it. We partnered with a local practice management company so they now can sell their practice management systems to a thousand local physicians and, if you're authorized and credentialed, it comes with the capability of just touching a button, and suddenly all the history about the patient is there for you in your private doctor's office, without having to go to a different application or a different log-in.

This whole notion of Web services exchange is the foundation of what we're now creating for the country, because we're building it for Massachusetts. By the end of the year, we will have a master patient index for the whole region, which would involve the record locator service. So imagine you see your outpatient person in Sausalito, and then you go see somebody at UCSF and then you're driving down the coast and you have an accident down in the Monterey area. All of the records where you visited, not your clinical data, but the records of where you visited, would be sent, with your consent, to the statewide database, which is just a pointer system. It's not a record system. We don't want to centralize data; we don't want a situation like Ameritrade where centralized databases have been hacked.

And then, if those places have electronic records, this Web service is kind of an exchange, and you can get data from them, again, in an authorized, private fashion. So we are building for the state of Massachusetts the record locator service, clinical data exchange, medications and labs and an e-prescribing gateway that routes prescriptions to every part of the state for free. ■

Managing and Delivering the *Complete* Patient Record

VIGNETTE®

Today's expensive and complex electronic medical records systems promise to make patient data readily available at the touch of a button. But the reality is that most patient information remains on paper, in the patient chart. This outmoded system creates unnecessary costs, delays and, just as importantly, security lapses in personal information.

One of the largest IDNs in North America has already reduced its chart-pulls by 87 percent with Vignette.

On average, medical institutions spend up to $11 per chart-pull request. With Vignette ProFiciency Patient, you can significantly reduce that expense while introducing business efficiencies, improving coordination of services, enhancing HIPAA compliance and increasing patient satisfaction and safety.

Vignette has developed a solution to capture, secure and manage the *complete* patient record – regardless of its format – and then makes it possible for only the right people to access the right data, when they need it, where they need it.

Introducing Vignette ProFiciency Patient: An Efficiency-Boosting Solution Designed Specifically for The Healthcare Industry

We've taken years of experience working with dozens of the most demanding healthcare providers around the world and created a specialized solution aimed at providing clinical personnel a single point of access to complete medical records.

Built on Vignette's proven enterprise content management platform, the ProFiciency Patient solution lowers the cost per chart-pull while improving patient care, HIPAA compliance and coordination of services across your provider network.

Generate Significant Economies and Efficiencies

Vignette ProFiciency Patient also enables you to digitize and manage paper-based back-office business processes and eliminate the paper while enabling new capabilities such as:

- Patient online self-service;
- Secure cross-facility information sharing;
- Care provider collaboration; and
- Integration with payer networks.

Integrates With Your Current EMR System To Both Handle Structured And Unstructured Data

ProFiciency Patient complements your current electronic medical record system and data repositories with capabilities to capture, manage, retrieve and display a total view of the patient record. The types of information handled include:

- Encounter details;
- Claim forms (HCFA and UB92);
- Charts from outside providers;
- Consent forms;
- Physician notes;
- Prescriptions;
- Outside lab reports;
- Invoices and payments;
- Photos of problem areas;
- Radiology images;
- Cardiogram video clips;
- Patient/provider correspondence;
- Audio and transcripts;
- Pathology reports;
- Discharge summaries;
- DICOM images;
- X-rays and interpretations; and
- Referrals.

Offered by a Team of Specialists Who Know Your Needs

Vignette's team brings decades of healthcare experience to bear to ensure your Vignette solution delivers efficiency, security, scalability and, ultimately, a higher level of care for your patients. Our team has packaged the best practices from our hundreds of deployments into a powerful set of solutions tailored for healthcare providers. ■

Vignette helps organizations harness the power of information and the Web for measurable improvements in business efficiency. By incorporating portal, enterprise content management and collaboration solutions, Vignette enables the capture, management, security and delivery of the complete patient record.

Thomas E. Hogan
President and
Chief Executive Officer

Conleth S. O'Connell
Chief Technology Officer

Bruce Milne
VP & General Manager,
Insurance and Healthcare
Division

Brett Bachman
Senior Vice President –
Product Strategy & Marketing

Vignette Corp.
1301 S. MoPac Expressway
Ste. 100
Austin, TX 78746
Phone 512.741.4300
Toll-Free 888.608.9900
Fax 512.741.1537
usinfo@vignette.com
www.vignette.com

Business Contact
Ron Canonico
Director, Insurance and
Healthcare Division
Phone 617.261.8422
ron.canonico@vignette.com

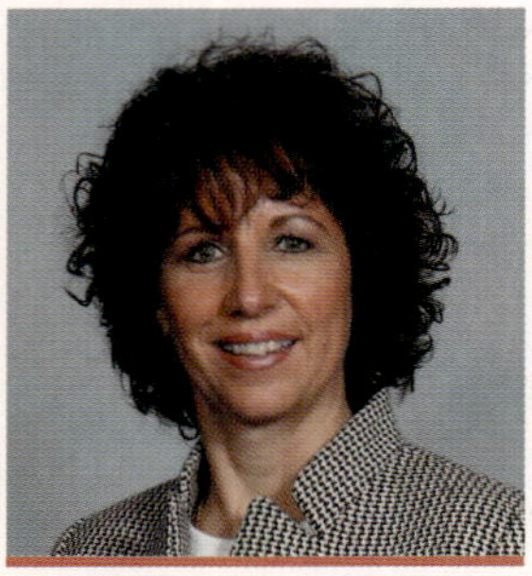

Lee Ann Stember
President
NCPDP

Lee Ann Stember, president of NCPDP, represents the council and its strategies, issues and policies through her work with government agencies, pharmaceutical and health care organizations, academia, standards development organizations and others actively involved in standards development for the pharmacy industry.

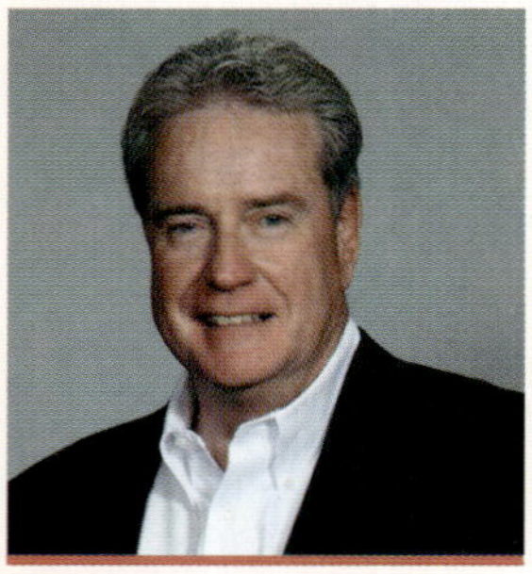

Phillip Scott
Senior Vice President
NCPDP

Phillip Scott, senior vice president of healthcare relations and development for NCPDP, is responsible for developing business and professional alliances. He has been an active member of NCPDP since 1988, and served on the board of trustees and as the chairman of the association.

Q&A With Lee Ann Stember and Phillip Scott

Leaders of the NCPDP explain why adoption of e-prescribing will be more rapid than EHRs.

Healthcare Technology: *Can you provide some background on the NCPDP?*

Phillip Scott: The National Council for Prescription Drug Programs (NCPDP) is a not-for-profit ANSI-accredited standards development organization consisting of over 1,300 members representing virtually every sector of the pharmacy services industry. NCPDP creates and promotes standards for the transfer of data to and from the pharmacy services sector of the healthcare industry. The organization provides a forum and support wherein our diverse membership can efficiently and effectively develop and maintain these standards through a consensus-building process. NCPDP also offers its members resources, including educational opportunities and database services, to better manage their businesses.

HCT: *What are the goals and objectives of EHRs?*

PS: Well the goals and objectives are those that everyone has been touting for a number of years, which would be the obvious things: patient safety, and portability of the information. For me, I guess there are two issues: electronic health records (EHRs) and electronic medical records (EMRs). The terms get used interchangeably, but I think they're actually two different things.

EHRs are the overall affirmation relating to a patient's health, and the other is very specific information related to medical adventures in their life. I think that the overall goals are that we're really looking at the opportunity to take a patient's medical experience or history out of individual silos. As it exists today, what happens in the community stays in the community. What happens in the hospital tends to stay in the hospital. And if a patient has an event or long-term care, or any of the assisted living care, what happens there stays there. It's truly three individual silos. And patient medication information, drug history and medical history all travel in a big brown envelope or in a little brown sack. For the first time, we're really looking at the opportunity to get rid of that. So that when a patient has a change in medication or has a medical adventure, it is taken from the community environment into a hospital.

Up until very recently, when it comes to drug history, it's whatever your daughter-in-law remembered to throw in the brown sack. And that is no way to run an army. So at a grassroots level, that's really what the goals and objectives of EHRs and EMRs are. A community pharmacy will tell you that when a patient is put on a new medication, when they're discharged, the pharmacy where they normally do business does not get that new information. So there's a lot of confusion. If you've got histories, or you're taking a product that is contraindicated for a new circumstance that you're being treated for in the hospital, there's no way for the pharmacist to know that. And that's a terrible set of circumstances for a patient. And now you move the patient out of the hospital straight into long-term care or to assisted living for a period of time, and something changes there – the attending doctor is not the same doctor that they saw in the hospital, because the patient went in and was treated by a cardiologist, but the patient is being treated by an internist in the nursing home. So the goal is to get that whole environment out of manual transmissions of big brown envelopes and little brown bags.

Let's say you've got an emergency circumstance at home. The EMT (emergency medical technician) comes, they do what they can to stabilize the patient, and as they head out the door they shout and say, be sure and grab all his medications that he's taking. Well, you know, folks don't always keep them all in the same place. This morning he picked up one of them and went to the phone and took it to get it refilled and left it sitting on the desk. So you only get three of the four, or whatever. Or it's not even somebody that's normally in your house and you just kind of go rummaging in and you pick up stuff, and half of it belongs to the spouse.

So there's the advantage of EMRs, if a patient is within the system and we know that it's United or Kaiser, then we are able to go in and plug in the patient's ID and, in the best of circumstances, be able to call that up and know immediately what the patient's drug history is and what their medical history is. And it's not at all unusual for someone to be going in for a circumstance where the medicine to be utilized is contraindicated for another chronic ailment that they are on. If we don't have access to this information, we can't know it.

HCT: *What do you think are some of the implementation challenges for EMRs and EHRs?*

PS: I'm not so sure that the public really is aware right now. I mean, they hear all the right stuff, so, say you're in the San Francisco Bay Area; well, when they find out that they're starting to have all of that health record information, whether they care if anybody knows or not, you know they're going to raise a big stink, right?

Lee Ann Stember: I think one of the main concerns is how all this information is going to get disseminated, and is the right information going to be given? Also where is this big database going to reside and how are we going to make sure that everything is correct? I want to make sure that Lee Ann Stember is Lee Ann Stember, with all the correct data.

PS: I think the challenges tick off like this. One, it is a standards issue. There are three standards bodies: X12N, HL7 (Health Level 7) and NCPDP. We have to continue with our initiatives around interoperability in

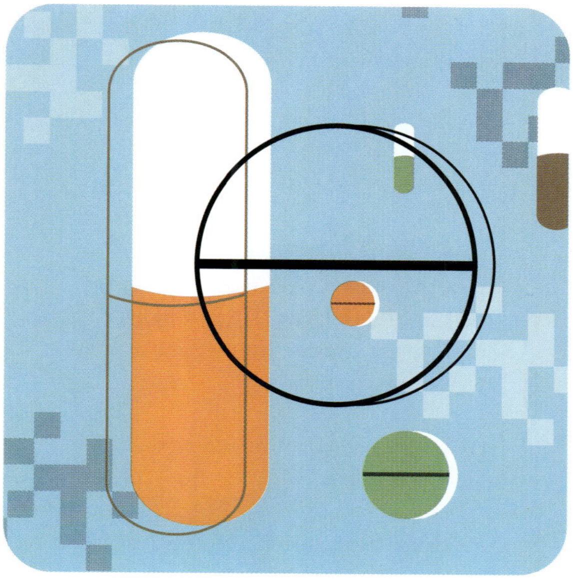

mapping the standards so that we can talk to each other across what have been existing barriers in the past. Just as we talked about the three silos earlier, with institutions, community and extended care, there are three existing silos, and that's X12, which is financial; HL7, which tends to be medical, and the hospital stuff; and then NCPDP, which is the pharmacy services sector of healthcare.

We've been fine operating within our own environment, for the most part, for the last number of years. We can't do that effectively in the future. We have to be mapping our standards so that we can speak to each other across these invisible barriers. What happens today is that the physician thinks he's doing an electronic prescription because he has the handheld system that he can do all of his stuff with inside his office, and then he hits send and it goes over to his office system, and because his office system is written potentially in HL7 language, it can only send a fax to the store that he wants the prescription to go to. So it leaves an electronic world, goes into a paper world, and then when it goes into a paper world, it goes to the exact same level of performance as a handwritten prescription does. So that's a barrier. It's got to go to, as one of our members says, all electrons all the time. Well that's maybe a little grandiose, but it's certainly more akin to what we expect to get to than it is today.

Another concern is the uptake of technology by the physician. But let me tell you, there's a level of physicians out there today that is what I would refer to as the second generation or the third generation in practice, and those are in that 40-, say 50-year-old level and lower.

A pharmacist told me about an environment where there were 10 physicians that he was dealing with in a practice and they were all less than 10 years in practice, and they didn't use paper. So the ones that are leaving school right now, they're ready. So the challenge for them is the technology being available to them as soon as they're ready for it. Then there's those that have been in practice that are 35, 40 years old, so they've been in practice 15 or 20 years and they're not as technically savvy but they're certainly willing. Then there's the ones that have been in practice who are looking to retire, and they want no part of it. The downside of that is that if it's a group practice, they're probably the managing partner. So if there's cash outlay, they're not looking to spend $100,000 or $200,000, because they're looking at that as reserves for them to divvy up when they retire in two years.

LS: That is resistance to change.

PS: So to say that physicians are technophobes, I think that that's not exactly true. But what I do suspect, and we've heard it from doctors who are in that kind of middle ground of practice, is that they found that if their life gets a lot easier in an electronic prescribing world than they would prescribe electronically, but it is the guy who is controlling the purse strings that won't make the investment. So that's a major hurdle, if you will, to implementation.

In March 2005 there was a demonstration both at HEMS and NCPDP annual in which the prescription left the patient's bedside in the hospital and through the hospital system was transmitted in a community-based pharmacy.

How do you start to figure out who to ask and what the questions are to ask, and to pursue this as a serious goal to get yourself up and running in an electronic world? It's a whole lot of trouble. And the handheld products, over the last three to five years have left a lot of doctors unsatisfied, because they'd get one, they'd get fully implemented and the company goes away.

Then they'd go off to another device, because they like it, and that company goes away after a year and a half, so some of these physicians, not only are they seeking knowledge, it also becomes a matter of, can I trust the technology, is this a solid company, what am I going to be left with if, three years from now, this device goes belly up? And those aren't issues of technology, those are the issues of business and the negative impact that happens to early adopters, you know, those pioneers out there that really move ahead early and have the idea to make it happen, but they can't get the funding to survive. I had a friend who was one of the early folks in a customer relations management system, and he tromped all over New England selling this thing and trying to get it up, and trying to get it funded. He said the first guy over the hill is the first one to get shot, but those that come after him can get over that hill really easy by crawling over him.

And so a lot of that happens: You have great ideas and great folks, insufficiently funded, and you end up leaving a bad taste in a practitioner's mouth because they've tried three times. Now why are they going to waste their time and money on that again?

HCT: *Do you think there will be widespread adoption in the next five years?*

PS: I think that in medical records, maybe not, but I think that in electronic prescribing, we are going to have widespread adoption in the next five years.

LS: I would agree with that.

PS: Part of that is that 86 percent of the pharmacies in the U.S. are ready to receive electronic prescriptions today.

So in this EHR world, electronic prescribing is just one element, but the NCPDP standard was adopted and accredited in 1997, so the script standard for electronic prescribing has been in existence since 1997. The pharmacies have been prepared to do that and have pretty widespread implementation now for at least two years.

So it's a matter of getting the physicians ready to use that. And the federal government has encouraged that. They've named the NCPDP script standard as the base standard to use, and they've encouraged that because it's one of those early successes for them in the bigger picture. Any time you take a grandiose initiative to do something as needed and as incredible as EHRs and EMRs, it takes a long time. So I think that a five-year outlook for that is ...

LS: That is very optimistic.

PS: Very optimistic around that element of it, for sure. And I think that the other elements of medical records are going to start to move a lot faster as well. For example, the task of mapping from HL7 to NCPDP has been going on since September 2004, and while that initiative is not completed, there is a significant amount of work that is happening. In March 2005 there was a demonstration both at HEMS and NCPDP annual in which the prescription left the patient's bedside in the hospital and through the hospital system was transmitted in a community-based pharmacy. So now it's the back half of that that we're working on, which is the communication, the ticket from the pharmacy back to the hospital and then all of the information that has to occur in between. So I think there's a bright outlook for this, really a bright outlook. ■

Cost-Efficient Healthcare Transactions and Information Access for Every Constituent

A New Lifeline to Help Cut Costs And Streamline Operations in Today's Ever-Changing Healthcare Environment

Is it possible to cut costs, improve productivity and deliver on the promise of consumer-directed healthcare? First Data Corporation says "Yes!"

First Data's history is rooted in helping industries overcome similar challenges that plague healthcare today, including:

- Manual processes that can increase costs, frustrate consumers and potentially lead to inaccurate transactions;
- Regional-based systems;
- Increased regulation governing privacy, security and data integrity; and
- The need to apply technology and interoperability in an environment filled with countless endpoints and hundreds of millions of constituents.

"First Data helped set the standard for safe, secure and efficient information exchange in the financial and credit card industries," said Beverly Kennedy, president of First Data Corporation's Healthcare division. "And we are doing the same for healthcare with a nationwide universal network that connects payers, providers and patients at the point of care."

Improving the Patient Experience

With the consumer at the center, First Data is using proven solutions for both multi-use healthcare cards and point-of-care transactions to deliver on the promise of reducing healthcare expenses through process automation. Given the continued growth in consumer-directed care, First Data's healthcare solution creates a more user-friendly experience – one that mirrors most other retail consumer transactions.

- A patient presents the provider an insurance ID card that will verify – in real time – insurance coverage and benefits.
- The ID card allows the provider to access patient demographics and public health record (PHR)/electronic medical record (EMR) information.
- After the patient has received care, the provider electronically submits an instant healthcare claim.
- Within seconds, the payer returns a fully repriced and adjudicated claim, complete with patient responsibility and reimbursement details.
- Patients are asked to pay for their portion of the costs and can even use their ID card to access tax-advantaged healthcare accounts (i.e., FSA, HSA, HRA) or an alternate payment method.
- Funds and the necessary forms are electronically exchanged between the patient, provider and payer, and the process is complete.

A Future of Opportunity

The foundation for First Data's solution lies in First Data's Universal Network, which will interconnect all constituents with real-time access to healthcare information. The result will be reduced administrative expenses, streamlined payment/reimbursement systems, a more satisfying experience and lower healthcare costs by reducing the redundancy in healthcare.

Specifically, First Data's Universal Network will:

- Provide the industry with a nonexclusive national switch used to securely transport and exchange virtually any type of healthcare information;
- Serve as the infrastructure enabling connectivity among all healthcare participants – patients, payers, providers, hospitals, laboratories, pharmacy benefit managers and third-party administrators;
- Combine healthcare data such as EMR/PHR, clinical and lab information with financial data to deliver an end-to-end solution for the industry; and
- Maintain stringent security and privacy protocols, using the latest technology to ensure patients are in control of their information.

Real-Time Solutions Today

The process of automating healthcare and financial transactions will require flexible solutions to meet the needs of all constituents. With proven tools already in market, and the resources to provide a universal network already in place, First Data provides the infrastructure to deliver on the promise today. ■

First Data provides the resources to reduce administrative expenses, streamline payment/reimbursement systems and enhance the patient experience by connecting healthcare constituents at the point of care.

Charles T. Fote
Chairman and CEO

Jim Schoedinger
President, Card Issuing Services

Beverly Kennedy
President, Health Care

First Data Corp.
6200 South Quebec St.
Greenwood Village, CO 80111
Toll-Free 888.565.5990
Fax 402.222.5588
first.data.marketing@
firstdatacorp.com
www.firstdataclients.com

Business Contact
Robert Burgarino
Director of Marketing
Phone 402.222.4285
bob.burgarino@firstdatacorp.com

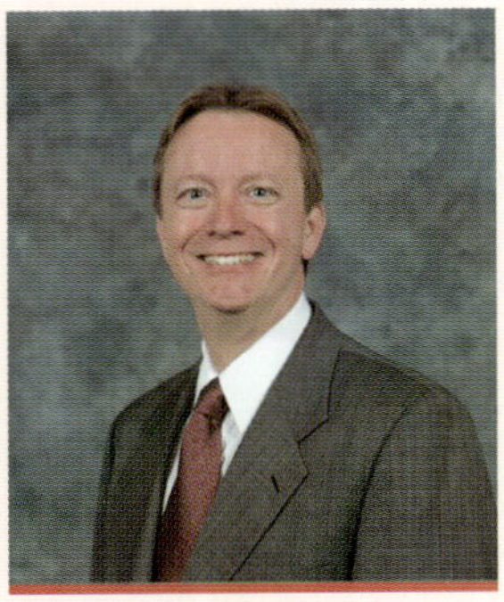

Stephen Lieber
President and CEO
HIMSS

Stephen Lieber joined HIMSS as president and CEO in 2000, bringing nearly 25 years of healthcare experience. He previously served as CEO of the Emergency Nurses Association (ENA) and as vice president of the division of personal membership groups with the American Hospital Association. In 2005, *Modern Healthcare* magazine recognized Stephen Lieber as one of the Top 100 most influential people in U.S. healthcare.

Q&A With Stephen Lieber

The president of HIMSS explains the role of hospitals in making EHRs happen.

Healthcare Technology: *Can you please give us a bit of background on HIMSS?*

Stephen Lieber: HIMSS is a blended individual and corporate member organization with about 17,000 individual IT professional members who work at several levels and with a variety of specializations in IT. We also have about 275 companies that belong to the association – therefore the blended membership. Primary focus areas for the organization are around four major strategic areas. One is industry intelligence; our second major area is public policy and advocacy. We're engaged in activities around standardization; interoperability, electronic health records, privacy and security. Our third strategic focus area is around professional development, and our fourth strategic area is around the area of IT communities.

HCT: *What do you think are the goals and objectives of EHRs?*

SL: There are two primary goals: one has to do with quality and the other has to do with cost. A primary quality objective of an EHR is to improve the care delivered to Americans through safeguards in terms of early identification and alerts around allergies, drug interactions, as well as other types of clinical decisions. It's important to ensure that the right kind of care is delivered at the right time and to the right patient. An EHR will impact quality by enhancing the continuity of care. As a patient moves from provider to provider through natural referral, it's important that subsequent providers have the information from the earlier providers to ensure that the next regimen of treatment is consistent with and compatible with what was provided before.

The second objective is around cost. EHRs can eliminate unnecessary tests in terms of having more information available to the practitioner; therefore additional tests may not be necessary because of information that is already in the record. Unnecessary tests are different than duplicate tests because unnecessary testing is a savings that comes as a result of being able to pull information from other tests directly out of the record, whereas an EHR also can provide cost savings by elimination of the duplication of tests. The patient goes in, tests have been run because the data is not there, so the tests are repeated – again at a significant cost.

HCT: *What do you think is the role of hospitals in making EHRs happen?*

SL: In their own network and their own system, hospitals have a primary responsibility. Hospitals are a place where, on a dollar basis, about half of the care in healthcare is delivered. There are fewer incidences of care than you find in a doctor's office, but hospitals account for nearly half of the expenditures in healthcare. So clearly hospitals have a primary responsibility as it relates to their own record keeping to move toward the EHR for those very reasons which I identified as the objectives. I think they also have a responsibility beyond their own networks, beyond their own facility, because they are a place where there is more technology expertise than you find in other places. Obviously a large healthcare facility or system is going to have a fairly significant IT department and therefore has expertise, knowledge and capabilities that could be of assistance to others in the community who are moving toward an EHR. Unfortunately federal regulation and legislation in place right now really prevents hospitals from providing that sort of support to non-affiliated entities at anything less than full market price.

Therefore hospitals that might be in a position to help out within the community, such as assisting individual physician practices, and do things at a cost that those small clinics could afford, actually cannot do so under federal law at the present time. So I think organizations like HIMSS and others need to get the federal government to recognize that there is an opportunity here for large hospital systems to help out in the community and at the same time not violate the provisions that were designed in this legislation to prevent self-referral and kickback types of arrangements that would undermine an open enterprise competitive market. But if we can set up systems to protect against that negative outcome while encouraging those with the capabilities to help out small physician group practices, then I think that's another role that hospitals can play. So I think hospitals have a responsibility as it relates to their own house, and I think there is great potential in helping others as well.

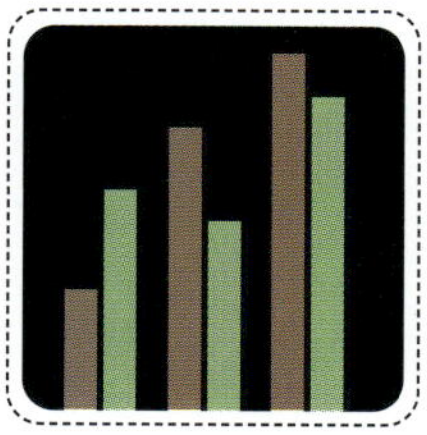

True interoperability, where one doctor's EHR application will actually transmit data and be received by another one, doesn't really exist today if they are using different vendors' products.

HCT: *What do you think are some of the implementation challenges?*

SL: Well the first is I think financial. A large hospital has the financial resources to invest in technology, and they're doing that already; probably anywhere from 20 to 30 percent of American hospitals already have EHRs. But you see a much different picture in small physician offices and group practices, where the estimates are more on the order of about 10 to 15 percent that have installed EHRs. So the availability of capital to invest and make the purchase is a problem, especially in those physician offices and in hospitals that are financially strapped, particularly inner-city hospitals and rural hospitals where they simply are not doing all that well from a business standpoint and therefore don't have the capital to invest in the technology.

Related to this, another financial barrier is that the reimbursement system that we operate under now doesn't provide sufficient incentives for the adoption of IT. There are pilot projects both in Medicare and among some of the private payers to try some models that do pay incentives for the adoption of technology, but those are just pilot projects – it's not widespread. So right now that's a real challenge to a physician – to invest the $20,000 or $30,000 necessary to automate their practice – because the financial return for that is not always evident.

I think there's also a technology barrier that exists in that we still do not have true interoperability, we do not have true standardization and so the buyer is a little bit hesitant to go out and make a decision around an EHR. They're uncertain – and again this is primarily in doctors' offices more than it is in hospitals – but they're uncertain as to where the market's going, which are the providers of the systems that are going to survive and thrive, which ones are going to be able to actually transmit data from one physician's office to another's. True interoperability, where one doctor's EHR application will actually transmit data and be received by another one, doesn't really exist today if they are using different vendors' products. And until we can break down those barriers of different standards used by different applications, there's going to be a real holdup in terms of widespread adoption.

HCT: *Do you think we'll have widespread adoption in five years?*

SL: Again, depending on where you're measuring it. You'll certainly see widespread IT adoption in the hospital setting within five years. We're already a third or so of the way there. In physician offices, we're starting to see some percentages of physicians starting to adopt this technology despite these barriers. You're still in the phase where the early adopters are the ones who are simply more focused on the technology and more comfortable with the technology and so the five-year timetable in physician practices may be a little bit on the early side.

However, the five-year horizon could be met with just a couple of things happening. If payers and Medicare and Medicaid introduce reimbursement changes that provide incentives for the adoption, you'll see a huge move relatively quickly. If we can solve the standardization issue and get the vendors to all agree to a common set of standards so that your application talks to mine and we can get on the computer and send records back and forth easily, again, you'll see a quicker rate of adoption. So I think the five-year horizon is likely. I think to be on the safe side I'd say maybe seven to 10 years on the ambulatory side before we truly have universal adoption without other changes to speed it along. ■

6

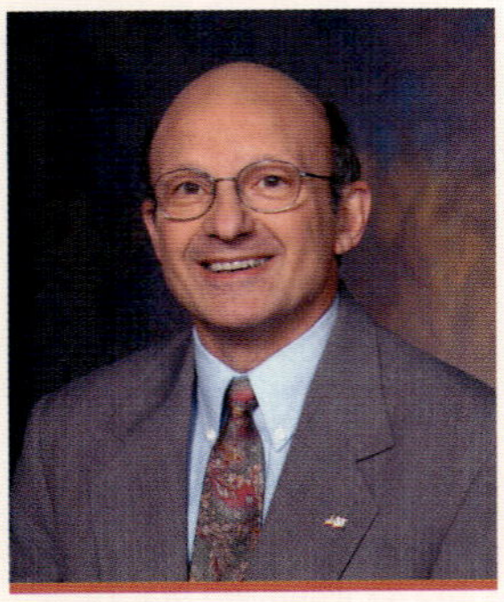

Bill Novelli
CEO
AARP

Bill Novelli is CEO of AARP, a membership organization of over 35 million people age 50 and older, half of whom remain actively employed. Prior to joining AARP, Mr. Novelli was president of the Campaign for Tobacco-Free Kids. Previously he was executive vice president of CARE, the world's largest private relief and development organization and co-founded and was president of Porter Novelli.

Q&A With Bill Novelli

The CEO of AARP describes the benefits EHRs offer people over 50.

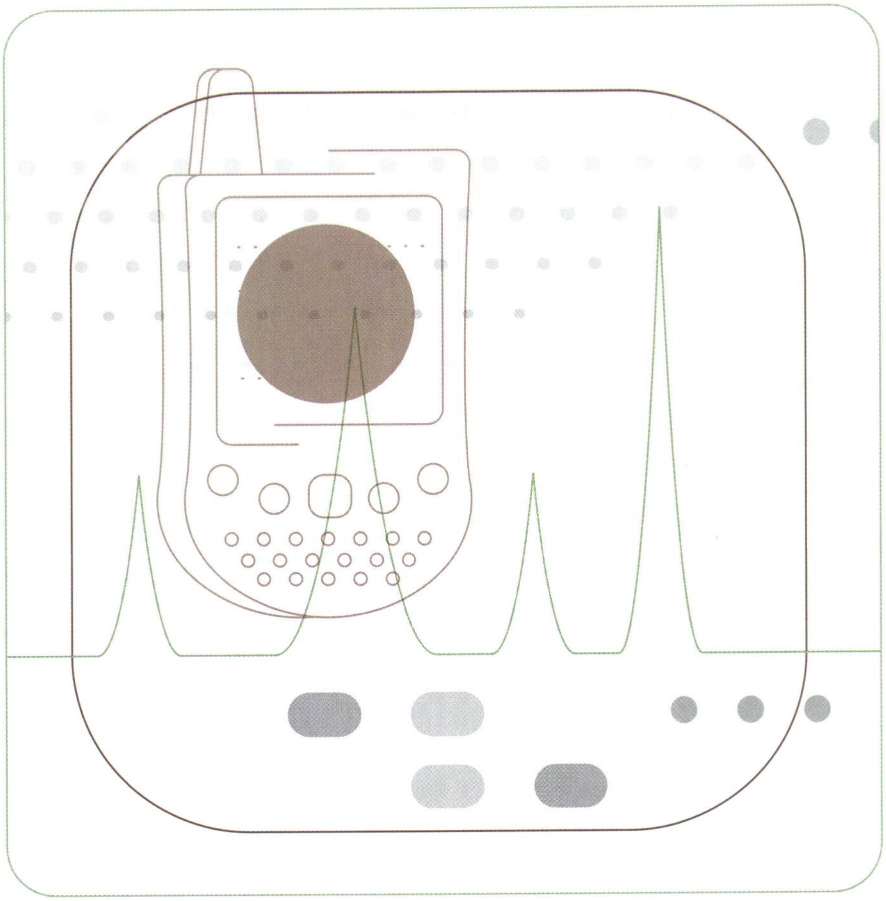

Healthcare Technology: *Can you provide some background on AARP?*

Bill Novelli: AARP is a nonprofit, nonpartisan membership organization that helps people over 50 have independence, choice and control in ways that are beneficial and affordable to them and society as a whole. AARP produces *AARP The Magazine*, published bimonthly, *AARP Bulletin*, our monthly newspaper, *AARP Segunda Juventud*, our bimonthly magazine in Spanish and English, *NRTA Live & Learn*, our quarterly newsletter for 50+ educators and our website, www.aarp.org. AARP Foundation is our affiliated charity that provides security, protection and empowerment to older persons, with support from thousands of volunteers, donors and sponsors. We have staffed offices in all 50 states, the District of Columbia, Puerto Rico and the U.S. Virgin Islands.

HCT: *Why are EHRs important for your constituency?*

BN: AARP's interest in health information technology stems from our conviction that healthcare quality in the U.S. must be improved. Ultimately we hope that improved care will also lead to cost containment. Americans only receive about 55 percent of recommended care; patients are too often at risk because of avoidable medical mistakes; and scarce resources are wasted through the inappropriate or unnecessary application of technologies or treatments. Health information technology can help play a vital role in addressing these concerns. EHRs can offer clinicians decision support with prompts to conduct tests and treatments based on evidenced-based guidelines, help in monitoring their patients' progress and they provide timely reports of laboratory and X-ray results. They also can help reduce error by improving the accuracy and legibility of patient records, help to enhance coordination by facilitating shared use of records and expedite access to medical information and knowledge about medical advancements.

In addition to the potential of improved clinical care, patients benefit from the convenience of online appointments, secure email communications with their clinicians and rapid access to test results. They can also have access to and control of their own medical information, which will empower them to become more engaged in their own care. Ultimately this will contribute to better health outcomes. In particular, EHRs offer people with chronic conditions significant opportunities for self-management of their conditions.

Finally, EHRs can help promote quality improvement by easily and efficiently capturing information that will enable us to use medical-encounter data to measure and benchmark performance, design interventions for improvement, promote public accountability and realign payment methods.

HCT: *What is the role of consumer groups in making EHRs happen?*

BN: Consumer groups can help stimulate the demand for EHRs by advocating for improved healthcare quality and public accountability of the healthcare system and educating their constituents about the need for improvement, making informed healthcare decisions, accepting appropriate responsibility for their own health and engaging in healthy behaviors. AARP believes that stimulating the demand side will encourage clinicians and healthcare institutions to seek cost-effective and efficient ways of responding and will lead to more rapid adoption of EHRS.

HCT: *What are some of the implementation challenges?*

BN: There are many formidable challenges to overcoming barriers such as cost; the lack of interoperability; the absence to date of a common nomenclature or standards for data aggregation, storage and communication; provider and practitioner resistance; and more. From a consumer perspective, the major implementation challenges relate to designing consumer-centric care standards that will permit a focus on patient outcomes. In addition, many consumers may be suspicious of the connectivity that comes with EHRs in the healthcare setting. Therefore a standardized health information infrastructure that will ensure the protection and security of patient information is key to address these concerns. Without such assurance, patients will not have confidence in EHRs.

HCT: *What is on the horizon for EHRs? Will there be widespread adoption in the next five years?*

BN: Of course it is difficult to predict precisely when widespread adoption of EHRs will occur. In my view, five years may be optimistic. However, we do know that it will take leadership from a wide range of stakeholders who will champion the importance of improved healthcare quality and recognize that health information technology is an essential component to improvement. This means that, in addition to the healthcare community, consumers, public and private purchasers, regulators, accreditors and others must participate in a full-scale effort to achieve the Institute of Medicine's six aims of the 21st-century healthcare system: safe, effective, patient-centered, timely, efficient and equitable. It is highly unlikely that these aims can be achieved without applying healthcare technology to healthcare. ■

A standardized health information infrastructure that will ensure the protection and security of patient information is key to address these concerns. Without such assurance, patients will not have confidence in EHRs.

Bank of America
Higher Standards

Banc of America Leasing Healthcare Finance provides financing for medical equipment, telecom systems, information/energy management systems, and hospital furniture/fixtures.

Banc of America Leasing Healthcare Finance
2059 Northlake Parkwy.
Ste. 400
Tucker, GA 30084-5399
Phone 770.270.8400
Fax 770.723.2121
www.bancofamerica.com/leasing

Business Contact
M.J. Klimas
Healthcare & Institutions
Phone 724.933.3106
mj.klimas@bankofamerica.com

Banc of America Leasing Brings Specialized Expertise to Medical Equipment Financing

Companies in equipment financing are often labeled as either "relationship driven" or "transaction driven" based on the way they do business. Banc of America Leasing Healthcare Finance takes a different approach. We believe that a good relationship is a continuing series of well-executed transactions. Our goal is to do our job so well that we become your most highly valued financing partner.

Healthcare Finance works with acute care hospitals and affiliated services to meet the challenges of a changing healthcare marketplace. We can finance all of your equipment including medical, telecommunications, information and energy management, furniture and fixtures and more. Whether you need one lease or a turnkey solution for a complete facility, we can make it happen for you.

Our healthcare focus, equipment expertise and unrivaled financial resources give us the financial depth to offer you far-reaching options and the most competitive rates in the industry.

Experience

Is your hospital just like every other? Of course not, but to many people all hospitals look alike. What about leasing companies – do they look alike to you? Healthcare Finance is different because we're specialists: We provide equipment financing solutions for healthcare organizations. Our ongoing success proves we meet our clients' needs.

Financial Product Knowledge

Financing solutions range from very simple to enormously complex. Some clients get greater benefits from operating leases, others from capital leases. No two organizations are the same, and Healthcare Finance structures each transaction to meet individual client needs. You may even benefit from selling us equipment you own and financing it back, all in one seamless transaction. We have the dedicated staff and resources to apply the universe of financing options, and we can recommend the ideal solutions for your needs.

Service

Our job, quite simply, is to get things done for you. When you choose Banc of America Leasing Healthcare Finance, you effectively outsource the equipment acquisition process. We handle the PO, invoicing, delivery, acceptance, setup and integration. Need a deal done in one day? We've done it. Need help accessing the capital markets? Our syndication team has successfully arranged financings for over a billion dollars. This extraordinary track record and capability allows us to say "yes" to many of our clients. Need help selling the equipment you're replacing? We can help. The quality of our relationship comes down to how well we do our job. Our goal is to delight our clients and exceed their expectations.

What's the bottom line? Our people are financing professionals with specialized expertise in healthcare equipment and related assets. We have over 325 hospitals as active clients and have closed more than 5,000 deals. Healthcare Finance wants to become your expert ally by providing you with ideas and solutions to fuel your growth and drive your success. ■

> Our job, quite simply, is to get things done for you.

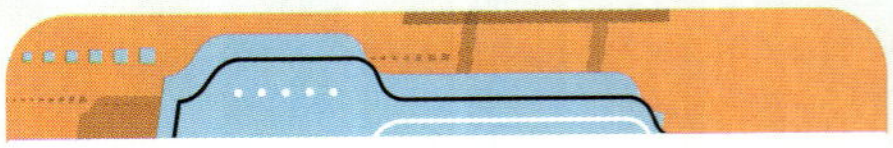

Leases Are *Not* Loans

Leases provide 100 percent financing with payments largely driven by equipment values, not just interest rates. And unlike a loan, a lease can be structured to help your balance sheet. Both nonprofit and for-profit healthcare organizations can benefit from leasing as a financing method, and Banc of America Leasing Healthcare Finance can structure the best solution for you.

7

Local Health Information Infrastructure Initiatives

Through conversations with leaders who have implemented communitywide projects, we learn how initiatives develop and how diverse healthcare stakeholders work together and overcome the roadblocks that they encounter. A national EHR system will be achieved through a series of independent, local systems that are implemented in a phase-by-phase process.

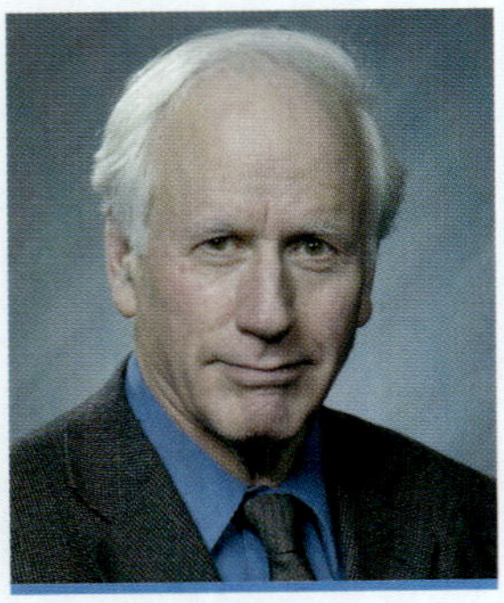

Clem McDonald
Director
Regenstrief Institute, Inc.

Clem McDonald is the director and research scientist for the Regenstrief Institute, Inc., a Regenstrief professor of medical informatics and a distinguished professor of medicine at the Indiana University School of Medicine. He is a leader in medical informatics, physician order entry systems randomized trials of medical computer systems and a pioneer in electronic medical record systems for institutions and communities.

Q&A With Dr. Clem McDonald

The director of Regenstrief explains how the longest-standing continuously running EMR system was developed.

Healthcare Technology: *Can you tell us a little bit about your work at Regenstrief?*

Clem McDonald: The Regenstrief Institute has invested in medical information systems since 1972, when we began to build an electronic medical record (EMR) called the Regenstrief Medical Record System (RMRS). It grew over the years, continues to operate today and is one of the largest EMR systems. Regenstrief has organized a consortium of the five major hospital systems (15 separate hospitals) in Indianapolis called the Indiana Network for Patient Care (INCP; all of five of these systems contribute information to the central INPC database. However, it's not a single database in the center; it's a federated database, so each of the institutions that contribute the clinical data has its own separate physical file system.

For a number of purposes, the data can be combined for one patient across many institutions for display and care. We have stored 700 million rows of discrete clinical observations, 14 million narrative reports (like discharge summaries) and 45 million separate radiology images from these five different systems. One hundred and twenty message streams deliver 90 million Health Level 7 (HL7) messages per year. For at least five years, ER physicians have been able to access the combined data from all INPC hospitals for use in emergency care. The access by physicians in any one ER is limited to the patients who have been checked into their ER for 24 hours from the time of checking. So the access is controlled very tightly. We now have agreements in place to provide the same kind of access to hospital physicians while patients are in the hospital. So while a patient is in their hospital, they will be able to access data, e.g., laboratory tests, radiology reports, operative notes produced at any of the participating hospitals and view it as though it came from a single medical record. But a physician at hospital A will only be able to see the full INPC medical record for patients who have checked in to hospital A.

The INPC also assists public health activities. For example, it examines laboratory results as they are delivered to the central database, looking for reportable cases according to predefined rules. When it finds evidence for such a case, e.g., a positive culture for cholera, it ships information about this report to the public health department in an encrypted form. Finally, INPC assists many kinds of important medical research.

HCT: *Regenstrief was ahead of its time.*

CM: Regenstrief has a strong track record in medical informatics. The RMRS is the longest-standing continuously running EMR system. Regenstrief investigators published the first randomized trial of computer reminder systems in 1976; deployed the first smart order entry system in 1984; and the first (and possibly only) randomized trial of computerized physician order entry versus manual order entry in 1993. We began investing in standards in 1984 because we realized that the cost of interfacing electronic data sources to electronic medical records would prevent the widespread adoption of such systems. We wrote the first consensus clinical message standard (ASTM 1238) and contributed to the first and succeeding HL7 message standard. (We wrote the chapter for observations and for orders.)

This effort in standards development has had a direct benefit to us. Without the HL7 message standard we couldn't have connected the hospitals in Indianapolis and created the INPC. We have also been developing standards for naming and coding observations, measurements and reports since 1994 – the result of which is the LOINC database of universal observation codes. The LOINC codes are a lingua franca for reporting clinical observations so that when a test such as white blood cell count arrives in an HL7 message, the receiving system can store that white blood cell count in a flow sheet combined with white blood cell counts from other institutions.

HCT: *It sounds like the biggest challenge has been the standards issue.*

CM: Well there are challenges everywhere. However, HL7 was up and running at all of the hospitals when we began the INPC project – a windfall to us. Such standards are a *sine quo non* for success. Challenges do remain. One is the fact that observations (e.g., laboratory tests, pulse rates) are identified in the HL7 message by local and idiosyncratic codes. Most institutions have not yet adopted LOINC codes so our biggest effort is to map the local codes that identify tests and measurements in HL7 into a common code system – LOINC – so that a glucose from one laboratory can be equated with a glucose from another.

HCT: *Do you think that we'll have EMRs implemented nationwide in five years?*

CM: Well first I would like to make some distinctions between the functions included in the rubric of EMR. The first is the repository function. The repository gathers information from many sources, systematizes and unifies it and provides tools for retrieving and displaying information about a single patient – for care purposes and for searching across patients for management or quality assurance or research purposes. These kinds of functions, though not trivial to create, are universally welcomed by clinical users and managers.

The second class of functions might be called work flow and workstation functions. These can demand complete re-organizations of the practice, and major changes in work flow and work assignments, i.e., physicians may be required to enter their orders and notes into the computer. Depending upon the kind of practice, the maturity of the system and the degree to which the computer demands more data gathering than the manual approach, these systems can require more physician time which can hurt their productivity and be considered a detriment by the physicians.

It is important to separate these two classes of functions, and be sure you have a repository function before implementing physician workstation functions. You get much value from the repository. Physicians always like having access to a repository – everywhere. It helps them to do a better job because they can always find the information they need with the computer. It takes too long to call for the chart or call the lab. The repository can also deliver reminders to improve quality and loads the database with outcomes management and research. So, I think ideally we should be thinking about EMRs as two parts, with implementation done in two steps. Put all the energy in the repository function first, and then take on the other physician workstations things – in steps. Today too often, the system is thought of as one thing.

Now to answer your question. I think you could easily have the repository function deployed almost everywhere in five years. Most hospitals, at least the hospitals and large practices, are already building repositories. But when you talk about the physician workstation functions that require retreading the office and all of the users and having everybody being online, that will take longer. Realize that it takes less physician time to shout an order or write it on their chart than to log on to a computer and navigate to the place in the computer and then enter the order. Further, regulatory demands on physician time are increasing, as are the demands to see more patients per hour. So it will take longer for this more demanding functionality to disseminate – maybe 10 years.

One last point: We should not be thinking in terms of a national database or national system, but a series of independent communitywide systems. ■

One last point: We should not be thinking in terms of a national database or national system, but a series of independent communitywide systems.

Infineon technologies

Secure Smart Card Technologies for Better Healthcare Services

Infineon Technologies AG, the world's fourth-largest semiconductor manufacturer in 2004 (iSuppli, March 2005) offers semiconductor and system solutions for automotive, industrial and multimarket sectors for applications in communication as well as memory products. With a global presence, Infineon operates through its subsidiaries in the United States from San Jose, Calif., in the Asia-Pacific region from Singapore and in Japan from Tokyo. In fiscal-year 2004 (ending September), the company achieved sales of $8.93 billion with about 35,600 employees worldwide. Further information is available at www.infineon.com.

Wolfgang Ziebart
Chief Executive Officer

Robert LeFort
President, Infineon Technologies North America

Miriam Martinez
Chief Financial Officer, Infineon Technologies North America

Infineon U.S. Headquarters
1730 North First St.
San Jose, CA 95112
Phone 408.501.6000

Business Contact
Christoph Liedtke
Director, Media Relations
Phone 408.501.6790
Fax 408.501.2424
Christoph.Liedtke@infineon.com

U.S. healthcare organizations are looking to smart card technology as a component of advanced information systems. The reasons include both regulatory compliance and benefits of smart cards as a tool to improve care. Infineon Technologies, which supplies the semiconductor chip technology at the heart of more than half of the smart cards used in the world today, has a unique view of these benefits.

Smart card features such as high security for stored data and communications, memory capacity, flexible programming and standardized interfaces make them ideal for use in electronic healthcare systems. Three major application categories have emerged since the first programs were implemented in the mid-1990s.

A health insurance card (HIC) is an administrative ID card, held by the insured person. With typical data contents that include personal identification (name, age, etc.) and complete insurance coverage information, the HIC significantly reduces paperwork and improves the speed and accuracy of claim processing. Security is based on controlling access rights to the personal data on the chip; the card must be inserted into an authorized reader at the point of patient care.

Since introduction of the first HIC in Germany in 1994, Infineon chips have been used in more than 100 million cards issued through that country's national healthcare system. It is estimated by the government and health insurers that the system paid for itself in several years. Today Germany and many other countries around the world plan to use or have already adopted more sophisticated smart card technology, typically called the patient data card (PDC) and health professional card (HPC). In Taiwan, Infineon is a supplier to the national smart-card-based health card system covering 24 million citizens.

A PDC securely stores current, accurate patient health information that individuals can carry in a secure and handy format. Only authorized health professionals can access the data, and they have the confidence that comes from knowing they are working with accurate patient data. Typical data contents include the patient's personal ID, insurance data, emergency data and prescription data. The patient PIN (personal identification number) and secure keys for mutual authentication assure secure access to and between the tools (card and reading/writing devices).

The HPC is held by individual providers. It is a secured access authorization card that defines rights to read and write information on a PDC and can also carry a digital signature for electronic authorization (i.e., prescriptions, care instructions). Patients are assured of privacy and data security by sophisticated access rules, held on the HPC, that prevent unauthorized access or tampering with stored or communicated information.

Chip-based smart cards are proven in a range of applications that require the highest possible protection of stored data from tampering and unauthorized access. These uses, including finance/banking cards and identification/access cards (i.e., for employees, students, military personnel, government workers) have helped to drive development of smart card capabilities that are particularly valuable for the healthcare industry.

Electronic healthcare cards can provide significant advantages and cost savings for healthcare providers and insurers. The technology can play a large role in compliance with the requirements of the HIPPA Act as a part of an electronic record system that assures privacy and security of patient data. Equally important, they also enable much more efficient and cost-saving storage of sensitive data and better treatment based on secure and easy access to patient data by doctors and authorized healthcare personnel. Smart healthcare cards are a key enabler to make the electronic patient record systems a reality. ■

Q&A With Marc Probst

The CIO of Intermountain Health Care describes how they are fulfilling their objective of a unified longitudinal medical record.

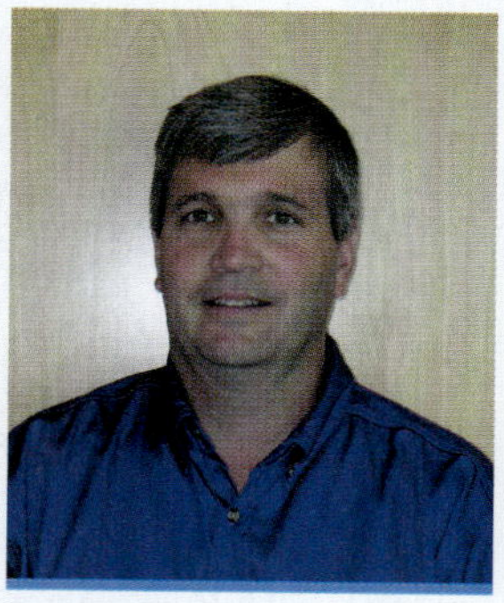

Marc Probst
CIO
Intermountain Health Care

Marc Probst has been a leader in information technology and healthcare services for the past 18 years. Prior to IHC, he was a partner with Deloitte Consulting and has served as the CIO for the nation's largest third-party administrator and as a partner for Ernst & Young.

Healthcare Technology: *Can you tell us a little bit about Intermountain Health Care (IHC) and your work there?*

Marc Probst: IHC is 22 hospitals, about a hundred clinics, with an annual revenue of about $3 billion a year. We have approximately 500,000 members in the health plan, and provide administrative services for about another 500,000 members. We have a very successful physician division, which includes about 600 physicians. All of our hospitals are in the state of Utah except one small hospital in the southern part of Idaho. Our mission is to provide the highest quality care at the lowest appropriate cost in the Intermountain region. We're currently building three new hospitals over the next three years. I am the CIO.

HCT: *We are trying to get an understanding of what's happening with local health information infrastructure initiatives as they implement EHR systems. Can you give me some background on your initiative and how it evolved?*

MP: About 30 years ago, IHC, which at the time was called LDS Hospitals, built a system called HELP that was conceived by a gentleman named Homer Warner. That was probably the first clinical information system and was primarily a clinical decision support tool. That system, although it has evolved over the years, is still in use at LDS Hospital and a couple of our other hospitals. It's relatively old, but still useful technology. It's based on an episodic medical record.

About eight years ago, Intermountain Health Care set out on an endeavor to create a longitudinal medical record which we call HELP2. We continue to

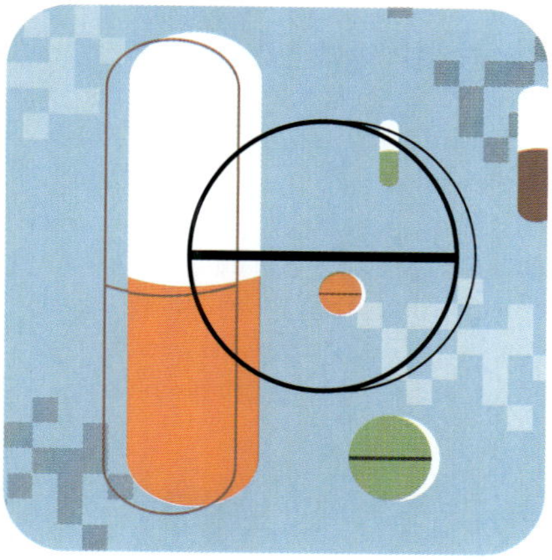

develop HELP2. Initially we focused on developing the infrastructure for the longitudinal record, including the clinical data repository, the health data dictionary, the decision support products and all the integration components. With this infrastructure in place, IHC developed an ambulatory medical record system that's used by nearly all of our employed physicians, and components of it by nearly 2,000 physicians in Utah.

Currently our primary inpatient system is the original HELP system. IHC has made a couple of attempts at developing the inpatient applications, but these were not fully successful. It was made clear to me upon arriving at IHC that a major assignment is to complete the inpatient components and implement them across all of our facilities. Last year we initiated a search to see what was available in the market, and determined that the currently available vendor offerings just didn't have all the things we needed. So we decided as an organization that we'd complete the build. We specified the budget and received approval to proceed. However, as you can imagine, this is a very large and significantly risky project.

Q&A With Marc Probst

In an effort to offset some of the risk as well as the costs, we completed a detailed review of potential partners and have decided to partner with General Electric (GE) to complete the inpatient components of our electronic health record (EHR). We will be building the system here in Salt Lake with GE.

We're also very involved in an organization called UHIN. UHIN started as a Utah claims clearing facility and is now expanding into the clinical side to become more of a regional health information organization. We're very involved in what UHIN is doing, as we see significant benefit for our community and what we're trying to do with clinical transactions.

HCT: *What are some of the objectives and who are some of the other participants?*

MP: The objective is to get a unified longitudinal medical record and standard systems to all of our hospitals. The goal is to get it done within five years. I think if you talk to GE, they want to do it quicker, but five years is pretty realistic. The other participants are GE, our providers and our business partners; we don't have any other partners beyond that. We purchased GE's pharmacy system. We also purchased ORMIS; we have MySIS in our labs. Our ancillary strategy is to buy best of breed and then integrate this into the core clinical system we are developing.

HCT: *What do you think are some of the challenges or barriers? Why hasn't it happened yet?*

MP: Certainly some of the barriers are technical and we're struggling through many, though I think we've mostly succeeded on these issues. We have approximately 5 million patients with records in our clinical data repository, which is the longitudinal record. We have 2 million active members at any given time and have complete redundancy. Obviously we've learned over time we need to have redundancy just to have the kind of reliability that we need in our system. Architecture has been a huge struggle and was a major reason for not selecting a vendor product. Although we have defined a very good architecture for the system, we still struggle with decisions such as whether to go with a thin client or a thick client, what the GUI (graphical user interface) should look like and usability.

So technology is certainly a big piece of it. User commitment also is a significant challenge. The leadership of IHC (particularly Chief Nursing Officer Nancy Nowak and Chief Medical Officer Dr. Brent Wallace) has been key to gaining the engagement of clinical practitioners. This engagement is a true key to our ability to succeed.

Other challenges include prioritizing components for development, the balance between research and development, training (we have about 25,000 users across a large geography) and balancing tactical needs while remaining focused on completing this system. We have a lot of challenges, but IHC is up to it.

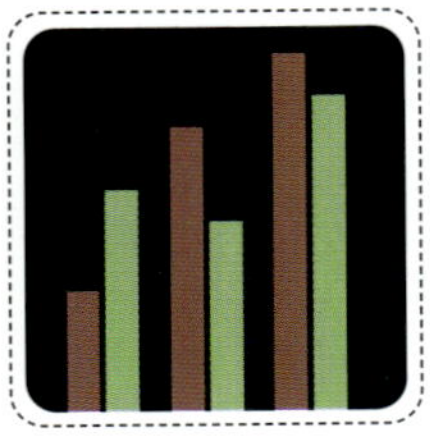

> Other challenges include prioritizing components for development, the balance between research and development, training and balancing tactical needs while remaining focused on completing this system.

HCT: *What about doctors? Do you think that physicians are technophobes?*

MP: Well some doctors are certainly technophobes. Others are techno-addicts. IHC is really blessed to have a strong core of clinicians (doctors, nurses, pharmacists, etc.) who are interested in and will spend the time to help define the requirements and test the systems we build. Additionally, IHC has a renowned core of medical informaticists that help push the envelope as to how systems can be better used in healthcare. I am much less concerned about technophobia than I am about our ability to get these systems developed and deployed.

HCT: *I think you said it would take about five years; do you think you'll be there then?*

MP: I think we'll start deploying some applications as soon as next year. We won't likely be fully deployed with the complete solutions we are striving to have, for five years. If we are complete before that, it would be a marvelous event. Right now we just need to focus on defining requirements, writing use cases, organizing teams and deploying 240+ developers on this project. ■

Wireless Bridge Links Point-of-Care Devices With Clinical Information Systems

sensitron™
WIRELESS HEALTHCARE INNOVATIONS

Information technologies help restrain the growth in healthcare costs. Sensitron delivers a very positive return on investment rapidly, while advancing paperless hospitals.

careTrends Delivers and Fulfills Healthcare Providers' Needs

Sensitron's careTrends™ system minimizes transcription errors and eliminates lag time between the reading, capture, documentation and dissemination (using machine-to-machine communication) of clinical data. This unique breakthrough system automatically captures and wirelessly transmits vital signs and other clinical data from legacy point-of-care medical devices into a clinical information system. This timely, cost-effective tool is designed to help healthcare facilities control costs and improve efficiency and flexibility, thus enabling healthcare providers to do what they do best – deliver care. This helps reduce staff time and clinical risk, and allows medical staff to maintain a higher standard of clinical care.

Sensitron's patented system works with monitors from different manufacturers, including legacy systems, and is an integrated open system – which even serves the home healthcare, nursing home and assisted living facility markets – in addition to hospitals (its major focus today). Due to automatic data transfer, transcription errors are eliminated. All data is date-and-time stamped, which creates an effective audit trail.

The careTrends system is designed to address healthcare providers' needs, including immediate access to information and reduction in paperwork. Patients' data and trends can be presented intra-hospital, inter-hospital, at a clinician's office or to any device that supports a Web browser.

Scalable System Accommodates Multiple Locations – Improving The Standard of Patient Care

The careTrends system uses a combination of standard wireless Bluetooth and 802.11b (or 11a or 11g) communications protocols for data transmission to a healthcare facility's server. Sensitron's enterprise software in the server collects the readings and records results according to clinician-set parameters before presenting data to caregivers on request at any time. The system is modular and can quickly be interfaced to the existing CIS vendor.

By combining vital signs data with other related clinical patient records, the clinician is armed with a complete view of the patient's status, thus enabling him or her to make a better assessment of the patient's overall condition. ■

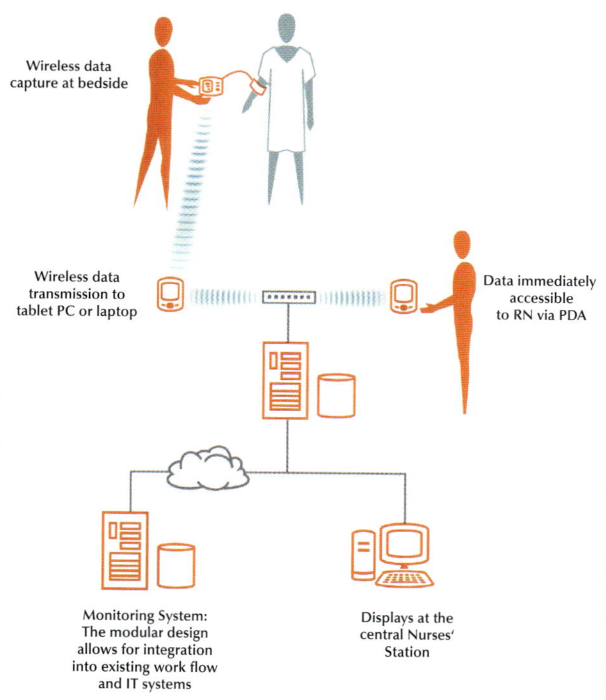

Figure 1 The careTrends® System

Sensitron, Inc. is a Silicon Valley-based wireless healthcare innovations company. Major operations began in 2000 and the careTrends product was launched and deployed in 2002. Sensitron has established itself internationally via channel partners in the U.K., Western Europe, Asia-Pacific, Australasia and Chile. By year-end 2006, Sensitron also expects to have channel partners in Eastern Europe, South America, South Africa, Mexico, South Asia and the Middle East.

Rajiv Jaluria
President & CEO

Vilnis Grencions
VP, Operations & Development

Satinder Singh
VP, System Engineering

Sensitron, Inc.
1300 S. El Camino Real
Ste. 502
San Mateo, CA 94402
www.sensitron.net

Business Contact
Samir Jaluria
Manager, Business Development & Marketing
Phone 650.232.2330
samir@sensitron.net

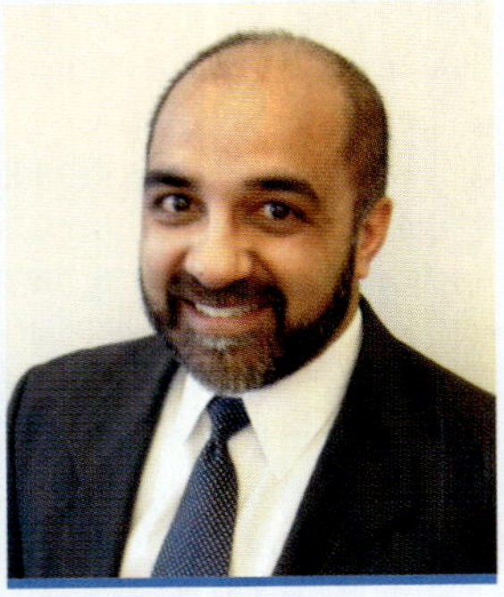

Micky Tripathi
President and CEO
Massachusetts
eHealth Collaborative

Micky Tripathi is the president and CEO of the Massachusetts eHealth Collaborative (MAeHC), a nonprofit collaboration of 34 leading Massachusetts organizations. He is also a member of the board of directors of MA-SHARE, a community utility service for statewide clinical data exchange in Massachusetts, and served as the founding president and CEO of the Indiana Health Information Exchange.

Q&A With Micky Tripathi

The best strategies for creating health information infrastructures that connect providers across the state can be determined through community initiatives.

Healthcare Technology: *Can you please tell us a bit about the Massachusetts eHealth Collaborative?*

Micky Tripathi: The eHealth Collaborative is a collaborative organization backed by 34 members of every part of the healthcare delivery value chain in Massachusetts, from healthcare professionals such as physicians and nurses, therapists, to large institutional providers such as hospitals and clinics, large clinics, payers, patient groups and ancillary health services types of organizations. They're all represented on the board. The mission is to improve quality and safety of patient care through universal adoption of healthcare technology in clinical office settings, and in particular EHRs (electronic health records), with embedded decision support in clinical settings.

The company was launched in September 2004 by those 34 organizations. It was spearheaded by the American College of Physicians, the Massachusetts chapter of the American College of Physicians that set as their No. 1 priority having universal adoption of electronic health records in all primary care physician offices in Massachusetts. They got together with Massachusetts Blue Cross and Blue Shield, which put up $50 million to fund this initiative. So the company launched in September of 2004 and I came on board the very early part of this year, January of 2005.

HCT: *Who are some of the participants?*

MT: We decided to invest the money in three pilot communities: Greater Brockton, Greater Newburyport and North Adams, which is in the western part of the state. We decided to fund pilot projects because there are a lot of barriers out there to adoption of EHRs and it's our sense and certainly the sense of all the members of the board, that before we go out and spend a lot of money we need to understand in a practical way what the best strategies are for getting that type of universal adoption of health records and the connectivity on top of it; the creation of a health information infrastructure that could connect all providers across the state. So the idea of the pilots is to get some market research on what the adoption barriers are, what the good strategies are for overcoming those barriers as well as a much clearer and hopefully more granular perspective on what the real costs and benefits are of these systems once they're implemented on a communitywide basis.

There is a lot of information out there that's been published by a number of academics who are participants in the collaborative now, like Drs. Blackford Middleton and David Bates. They have done several studies on the relative costs and benefits of EHRs, but in relatively small laboratory-like settings, one or two offices or within one provider network like Partners Network here. In terms of being able to see what it's like on a communitywide basis, no one in the country has done it on a high-profile, communitywide basis in a way that gets all the members of the community involved.

HCT: *What do you think is the greater barrier? Do you think it's privacy?*

MT: Security and privacy are obviously a huge part of it. I don't think there has been a barrier to adoption of the systems up until now, and I think that things like HIPAA define what the security standards are to protect that privacy. I think those things are more a help than they are a hindrance because they define what the rules are. When you're rolling out systems like this – I think it's much more helpful to have a set of rules that can be a touchstone that says here is at least the minimum, the widest set of guardrails that you really go outside of.

HIPAA is the lowest threshold to meet because Massachusetts state law is actually more restrictive than HIPAA. It turns out the community convention is even more restrictive than that; at least in the experiments that we've had in Massachusetts, where we have some of these community IT projects. There's one called MedsInfo-ED, which delivers medication histories in emergency departments, regardless of the source of that information. There were a number of agreements that had to be made with providers and the payers in the state to get that out there. They ended up with a set of privacy and security standards that are higher than even Massachusetts state required because the organizations said that they knew what the state law was but that their company policy was stricter than that.

The privacy part is also something that you have to engage patients in. There's an educational process that has to happen because there are a lot of distorted impressions out there of what's involved with this type of network. I think it is important to get a more balanced perspective of exactly what the changes are. Are we more secure in the future world or are we more secure now? It's one set of questions to ask.

There are also questions around what the relative costs and benefits are. Perhaps the ability to say at any given time, I don't want one provider to have this certain information because of a personal preference. Let's say you want to get a second opinion from another physician, and you don't want your first physician to know because you don't want them to feel bad about it. Well it's an invasion of privacy if the first physician is able to log on to a system that says oh, gee, I didn't know that you went to that other physician to get that test done or to get that second opinion.

On the other hand, one might argue that for best clinical care, that's valuable information for your physician to have,

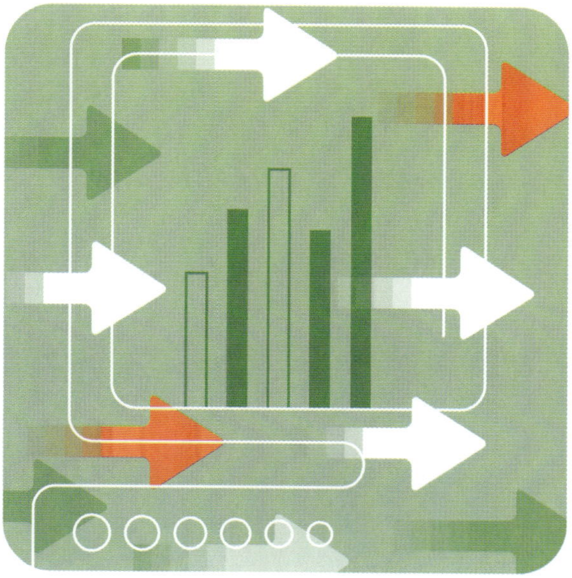

and indeed your practitioner can't give you the best care if they don't have all the information that's there; at least all the information – meaning the clinically relevant information – that's appropriate for the kind of care that the patient is asking for.

HCT: *Do you think an initiative like this is going to happen in other states?*

MT: Absolutely – it's happening all over the place. Indiana and Massachusetts are much further along than any other states in the country. California has a number of initiatives going on as well. But there are a variety of other states that just have some funding from the federal government or even if they don't have funding, they're just trying to put the groups together and just trying to move ahead with this, because it's really kind of a movement now across the country. My colleagues and I, here and in Indiana, get a number of calls from around the country asking us if we can speak here or there. Off the top of my head, Minnesota has given me a call; I was in New York last week; I just got a request today to come to Pennsylvania – I mean there are a number of states that are putting this together because it's so unique. They're really trying to forge their way in what's pretty new territory, because you're asking organizations that aren't used to working together, and they're usually rivals in the market. You're basically saying, lay down your arms and let's figure out together how we're going to work collaboratively on something that will be the tide that lifts all boats, that's not going to advantage you in a relative way versus your competitors, but it will be something that lifts everyone to a higher level for the benefit of the most cost-effective care and higher quality of safety.

I think in the next five to 10 years we're going to see a tremendous amount of activity across the country. There is a tremendous amount of activity now – there are a lot of organizational kinds of formation that has to happen and frankly more funding that have to get freed up. We're lucky because Blue Cross came forward with this money – the amount of money we have here just for Massachusetts is basically equal to what's available for health IT at a national level for the whole federal government. We happen to be in a very fortunate position and hopefully there will be a number of other states that are either able to get federal money, should that become available, or other organizations – either state government or health plans in other states – will come forward and start funding some of these activities. I think in California the California Health Care Foundation has been pretty active in funding some of these activities as well as Kaiser. ■

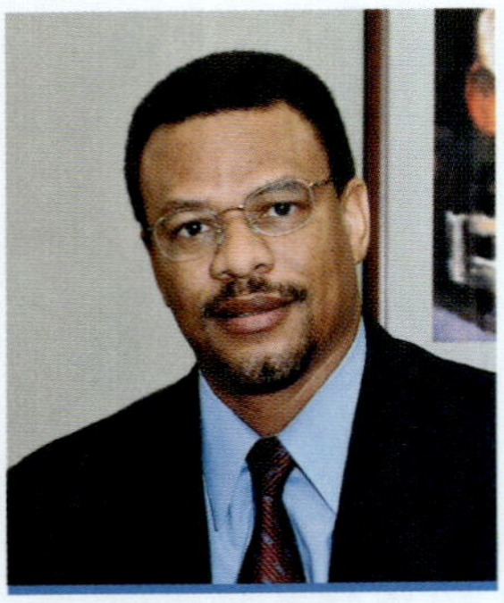

Wayne Thompson
CIO
UMDNJ

Wayne Thompson currently serves as CIO at the University of Medicine & Dentistry of NJ. His career in information systems spans 20 years and he serves on several professional committees. Previously, he served as CIO at Thomas Jefferson University and the University of South Florida.

Q&A With Wayne Thompson

The CIO of the nation's largest health science university explains the phase-by-phase process of implementing a local health information infrastructure.

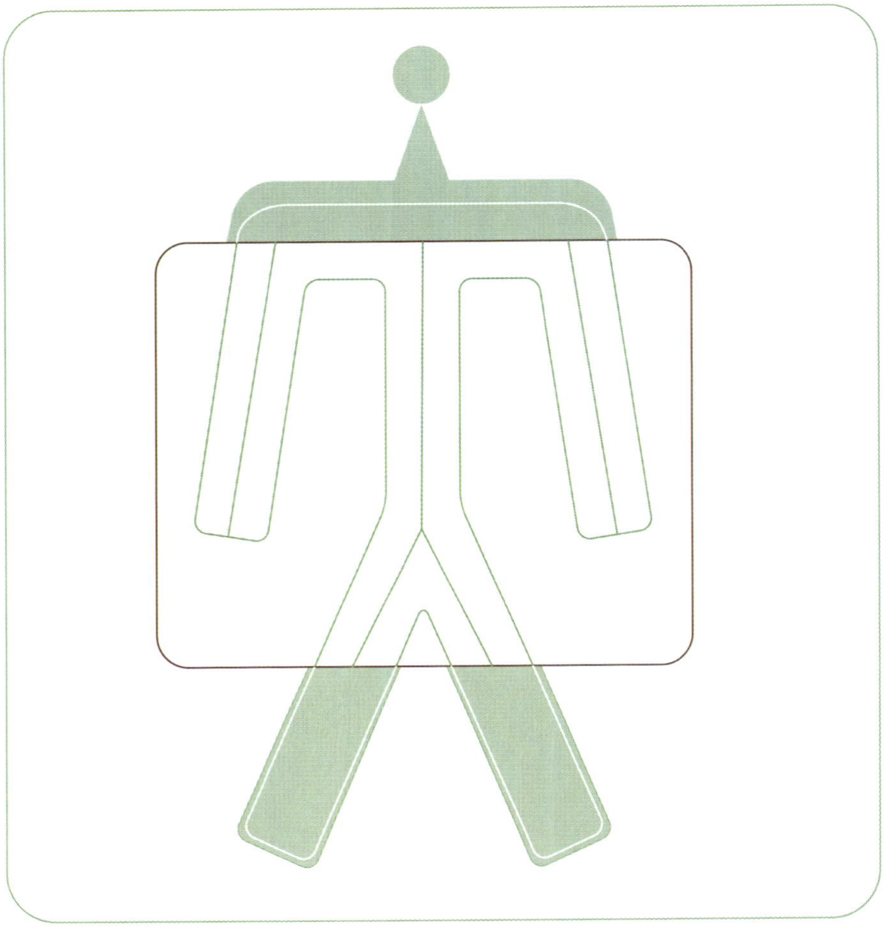

Healthcare Technology: *Can you give us some background on UMDNJ?*

Wayne Thompson: UMDNJ is the nation's largest health sciences university. We are New Jersey's statewide system of health sciences education, biomedical research and healthcare. Founded in 1970 to consolidate New Jersey's health professions education, UMDNJ has become the very core of the state's health sciences system. We have more than 4,000 students of medicine, dentistry, allied health, nursing and the life sciences, and more than 1,000 medical interns and residents. UMDNJ is the single entity responsible for statewide undergraduate and graduate medical and dental education, as well as for other health professions.

The university is New Jersey's primary source of continuing and advanced education for health professionals. Through its eight schools on five campuses throughout the state, the university provides New Jersey with a supply of top-quality health sciences professionals appropriate to meet the current and future needs of its healthcare delivery system.

HCT: *Can you give us some background on your local health information infrastructure initiative?*

WT: The initiative really evolved a few years ago, when there was recognition that a number of pieces of our current system needed to be upgraded or replaced. We had components close to end of life, and there was enough forethought at that point in time to consider a wider scope than just the components that were coming to end of life. That thought process evolved into the EHR initiative, so rather than just replacing a repository, which was coming to end of life, in which the vendor was sold, we decided to embark upon a larger electronic health record (EHR) initiative, of which the repository component would just be the first step, and that's basically how it began.

As far as evolution is concerned, the plan was to move from just the repository phase (phase 1) to then encompass ADT (admission, discharge, transfer), registration, scheduling and the emergency department, and we are in the midst of planning for go-live of those components even as we speak here today.

And then phase three is CPOE (computerized physician order entry), which we've done a fair amount of work on concurrent with ADT, and that phase is scheduled to take us toward the end of 2006. So there was a loose plan in place, and we've been making planned progress toward that goal, with some components taking longer, some shorter; but we've been making decent progress, and the CPOE phase, which is yet to come, is still continuing to evolve in terms of its scope.

HCT: *What are the objectives and who are some of the other participants?*

WT: Well the objectives ultimately, and these were reaffirmed last year, are really to improve patient safety and improve the quality of care and the efficiency of both financial and healthcare operations. So there are broad goals for the project, now that we've expanded the scope to include all of the components. As such, it really involves almost all of the key stakeholders within the hospital and the ambulatory environment, not just registration and scheduling and patient accounts focus, but the medical staff as well. So there are very few stakeholder portions of the environment that are not impacted and I would have to say that all of those areas have some participants in this process.

HCT: *What's the current status?*

WT: The repository is live and our interface engine has been live and up and running for some time. We are literally eight weeks away from the go-live for ADT, registration, scheduling and the emergency department, so that is definitely the next milestone. Even while we are approaching that milestone, we are in the planning stages and some continuing low-level effort geared toward CPOE, which is immediately to follow. So it's a critical time at the moment in the march toward this milestone, and we are planning for the next phase even while we're doing it.

HCT: *What are some of the challenges and what are some of the lessons learned?*

WT: The challenges have probably been those typically associated with a large, very complex project. Turnover of staff and in some cases leadership positions that were instrumental in moving the project forward have been a challenge. Maintaining focus on the end goal when it's relatively far away from your starting point, has been another typical challenge. I would also add the tendency to want to create the ideal environment as opposed to just getting a significant improvement over what your current state is. So those are some of the challenges. Lessons learned, in retrospect, you cannot spend too much time on the process of controlling scope and the discipline around that. Every large project has that, as a component, but I think that's an area that can always stand to have more effort, time, attention and formality associated with it. Our project was no different.

I think the second area for lessons learned is really communication. There's been lots of communication and there are both formal and informal pathways, but I think the formal integration of a communication plan into the project plan is probably a key lesson learned. This is opposed to having a separate communication plan with a separate group of people that might have had their eye on that. I think it needs to be key milestones with prerequisites and dependencies that do not differ from any other key aspect of the project. And I'd say that's another lesson learned. ■

... the formal integration of a communication plan into the project plan is probably a key lesson learned, [as] opposed to having a separate communication plan ...

Navigating the Maze

Health industry leaders need to navigate through a developing maze of ownership as well as technical, procedural and clinical requirements to implement EHRs in an integrated manner.

[Lewis Redd, Accenture] [John Quinn, Accenture]

EHRs offer the potential for a major transformation in the way that health services are delivered and the value derived from them both in the U.S. and in other countries. By comparison, other recent initiatives such as administrative self-service Web portals, regional service consolidations and new medical devices and diagnostic tools are merely incremental improvements to the healthcare system.

The Vision

EHRs provide a pathway for healthcare delivery systems to achieve goals that were previously unattainable: Improvements that could be achieved through the close integration of information technology that is available with EHRs: ensure that the highest quality of care is delivered to every patient, ensure patient safety and prevent medication errors, identify the best treatment for each individual's specific situation, streamline administrative processes, reduce paperwork and redundancy, avoid duplicative testing, enhance access to services, yet closer tying of provider payment to performance and predicted clinical outcomes.

The possible rewards are great. But EHRs are much more complex than any previous IT initiative in health or, for that matter, in any other industry. In order to realize their benefits, health executives must develop EHRs in an integrated manner. They must implement EHRs so that they address several different dimensions:

Setting of care. EHRs have potential applications in almost every care setting including: preventive, acute, post-acute, sub-acute chronic, long-term care, community and home care. To be fully effective, EHRs need to be integrated across the entire continuum of care.

Geography. Health leaders need to design EHRs based on local needs and practice patterns, yet integrate the information that they contain and functionality they provide across the entire country including regions, states, provinces and local cities or jurisdictions.

Patient health information. Clinical information itself contained in EHRs is a dimension of challenge to EHRs on its own. While standards exist for this information, they are not widely used, and even when used are applied inconsistently within organizations today.

Clinical specialty. Clinical information and functional needs that support specialty-specific clinical processes exist in many areas such as emergency care, laboratory, radiology, pharmacy, intensive care and medical and surgical services.

Industry sector. Diverse stakeholders in the health industry need to share and coordinate clinical information. They include: hospitals, physicians and other clinicians, payers, community and social service organizations, government/public health, and even life science companies.

Function. Clinical information must be integrated across supply chain, financial and clinical systems to better understand and control the care delivered, ensure availability of material resources both when and where needed and to monitor revenues versus costs.

Resource. Full implementation and deployment of EHRs must consider integration from people, process, technology, facilities and financial perspectives.

The Need for Integration

At the same time this country is gearing up to pursue portable EHRs for every individual, most entities are already in the process

Lewis Redd is managing partner of Accenture's Provider, Health & Life Sciences practice, responsible for all business development and service delivery to clients in North America. He has over 20 years of healthcare consulting experience, with a specialty in technology-enabled performance improvement. **John Quinn** is chief technology officer in Accenture's Provider, Health & Life Sciences practice focusing on emerging healthcare information systems technologies. He has over 29 and 32 years' experience in the healthcare and computer industries, respectively. He has participated on the HL7 board of directors since its inception 19 years ago and has served as the chair of its technical steering committee for the last 14 years.

of pursuing initiatives that involve clinical information systems. These existing initiatives have already created a "local maze" of agendas for change. All of these involve some level of significant investments in technology. This current investment underscores the ongoing role that technology already has and the even greater need for integration of information across clinical and administrative processes that will exist in the future.

Integration here covers many different agendas, and there are a number of potential integration points that health executives need to consider in their business and technical strategic plans. As always, technical integration must be an enabler to the definition of integrated operational processes and performance management.

As an example, consider pay-for-performance programs. Congress, CMS and many private payers have already pushed forward in their planning, which can have a profound impact in redesigning provider incentives for care delivery and are being considered by many countries around the world. The implications on provider behavior, care delivery, operations and financial performance are significant; the implications for technology integration are equally significant. The clinical information systems used to document and code the provision of care across the delivery system (acute, mental health, community nurse, etc.) and report the clinical outcomes will need to be significantly upgraded to collect more detailed and relevant data and then integrated with the local financial systems as well as the EHR. Accurate reimbursement for services will need to become tightly aligned with the accuracy of the clinical reporting.

Strategies for integration in the past have been comparatively narrow in focus with a very limited amount of abstracted data. New HIPAA transaction requirements and statutory requirements of the recently passed Medicare Modernization act have already put forces in motion that will ultimately require the providers to collect, integrate and then communicate far more detailed information if they expect to participate and not be left behind.

The Current Maze

At present most electronic record systems do not integrate with those of other vendors (and some systems offered by the same vendor aren't even integrated with each other). Most vendors currently offer their products on a variety of hardware and associated software platforms. Each vendor has chosen a particular approach, and no two vendors have even a similar approach, much less a detailed design. No two site implementations of any vendor's systems are the same. No two sets of interfaces are the same, and no two implementations use the same vocabularies or coding systems. In short, nothing is designed or implemented to interoperate beyond a specific implementation at a single organization or facility.

Currently vendors design their applications with a baseline assumption that their approach and architecture doesn't need to coexist and interoperate to be successful. They often support integration with external applications (i.e., those outside of those that they build) with significant differences in philosophy and detail. Moreover features that work across a vendor's own integrated applications will not always cross over foreign system interfaces in exactly the same way. And even if a hospital would like to implement a "total" vendor solution, it may not be practical on many different dimensions of time, scope, economics or provider organization politics.

True interoperability will require that all features and functions work across all applications. The term "semantic interoperability" is now being used to describe a level of integration that facilitates the movement of data and process context between systems. A practical definition of semantic interoperability is the interchange of data where not only can the information be transmitted among systems, but the receiving system can understand the data and process contexts that it was created in and reuse the information in many different contexts, across all healthcare information

> Hallmarks of successful implementations include physician and nursing leaders that bring universal provider adoption, strong solution architects who control the definition of the solution as well as leadership from a management team that keeps close tabs on critical path milestones and ensures rapid resolution of issues.

weblink

Read how to choose the appropriate vendors in "Selecting Technologies for an EHR" in this book.

application domains. This includes documents, reports and rules for decision support.

There is a high probability that any vendor chosen today will have to significantly alter their approach to internal and external integration, security and nomenclatures over the next few years. Many governments have already started to particular standards for integration and nomenclature to support portable electronic medical records. Providers will be motivated to comply. Payers and political voting influence forces are beginning to demand it.

Opportunities for Integration

When one considers the changes the programs will make in the daily operations of the care-providing organizations, the number of integration points and possibilities for further improvement begin to take shape. Some initial examples include:

- How can patient data from EHRs be used to both collect the data necessary to support identification and proactive care for patients at high risk of long-term chronic conditions and then ensure their subsequent treatment follows current best practices?
- How can EHRs be used to support and coordinate pay-for-performance programs both for the EHRs themselves and for other programs such as electronic prescribing that will both require data stored in an EHR and also interact with EHRs?
- As new EHR systems are deployed, how will we make sure that the new technology does not burden and create more work for providers but rather create incentives to change processes and enhance provider work flow?
- How can EHR systems support evidence-based medicine? How can they be used to manage outcomes?

For the above and other integration points, what service level and operational principles must be adopted among stakeholders and organizations to ensure success of the "whole system"? How will behaviors and reactions of clinicians and operational staff be positively directed throughout the transformation? How will the roles and performance management systems change?

What Next? Key Tenets of Any Integration Approach

While approaches will vary based on the stakeholders involved and the strength of their relationships, as well as the condition of their current situation, we envisage five key tenets of any integration approach.

1. **View the entire health delivery chain.** The value of integration becomes clearer with an understanding of the delivery chain for care provision across diverse organizations (government, private, local community, social care, volunteer, pharmaceutical companies, etc.). Critical aspects of the delivery chain to be understood include: Each stakeholder in the chain has a different incentive for participation and each has a differing impact on the patient's care experience; information requirements vary by stakeholder and the flow of that information to each stakeholder is different in form, timing method for delivery and legal privacy restrictions; each stakeholder's compensation models and the implications on incenting the proper behaviors across the value chain differs; and timing, political and contractual realities influencing and enabling integration for each stakeholder.
2. **Value the integration as part of the justifying business case.** Stakeholders need to acknowledge that the greatest benefits of EHR systems are not derived from technology implementation alone. Rather, integration can produce tremendous benefits in terms of patient outcomes, financial performance, better ways of working and employee job satisfaction.
3. **Secure stakeholder commitment and ownership.** Sponsorship by top leadership from each stakeholder is critical. In all cases, the buy-in of the clinical community is essential to adoption and the success of any healthcare venture including integration of services, processes, data and technology.
4. **Apply resources to define, manage and control the integration.** Hallmarks of successful implementations include physician and nursing leaders that bring universal provider adoption, strong solution architects who control the definition of the solution as well as leadership from a management team that keeps close tabs on critical path milestones and ensures rapid resolution of issues. Project management resources need to be invested in integration.
5. **Look beyond the technology.** To be effective, systems implementations at any level need to consider more than the technology changes required. Health executives need to address people and process changes as well. Only by integrating the necessary changes in associated business processes and roles can technology achieve its full potential.

Conclusion

The U.S. government continues to press ahead with its plans for portable EHRs for every individual in this country. This is an extremely complex undertaking and will prove to be an expensive one. A portable EHR, however, is one more element of how both government and the private sector are focusing on reforms to healthcare delivery. Healthcare executives need to develop their strategies, plans and budgets with a goal of integrating their efforts for EHRs with other initiatives that will, in most cases, involve some of the same information and many of the same stakeholders.

True change occurs when process and information flow consistently and efficiently across the system of care. Through integration, EHRs will offer us yet another new opportunity to add value to the consumers and providers of healthcare. ■

[Author Index]

[Author Index, cont.]

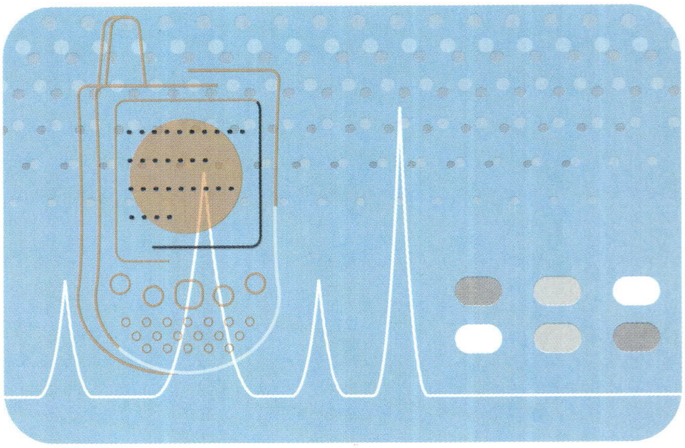

[Solution Provider Index]

[Solution Provider Index, cont.]

Panasonic TOUGHBOOK — Computers for the Outside World	Panasonic produces the industry's most reliable mobile PCs — legendary Panasonic Toughbooks®. Rugged and wireless, Toughbooks are total computing solutions for today's mobile healthcare workforces.	077
RSM McGladrey	The National Healthcare Practice of RSM McGladrey Business Consulting Services is a recognized leader in healthcare consulting. We help our clients achieve results by providing them with specialized knowledge – our term for relevant, practical and strategic business and financial information – delivered by experienced, knowledgeable and responsive industry professionals.	043
sas — The Power to Know.	SAS® software is used for a variety of applications in more than 1,000 U.S. healthcare organizations, enabling health-care leaders to turn complex data into the business intelligence needed to produce the most successful outcomes.	086
SBC	SBC Companies places a priority on delivering customized communications solutions to meet the needs of the medical industry.	133
sensitron — WIRELESS HEALTHCARE INNOVATIONS	Sensitron, Inc. is a Silicon Valley-based wireless healthcare innovations company. Major operations began in 2000 and the careTrends product was launched and deployed in 2002. Sensitron has established itself internationally via channel partners in the U.K., Western Europe, Asia Pacific, Australasia and Chile.	263
Solucient — Insight to Better Healthcare	Solucient is the leading source of healthcare business intelligence, enabling providers, payers and pharmaceutical companies to drive business growth, manage costs and help deliver quality care.	216
THOMSON	Thomson Healthcare provides health systems access to decision support solutions that help build and monitor performance and improve quality of care. The Thomson companies' Micromedex and Medstat brands marry market intelligence and clinical knowledge with actionable alerts, guidelines, reporting tools and detailed analysis to ensure efficient and effective practices facilitywide.	123
Turner Healthcare	Turner Construction Company is the nation's leading healthcare builder providing general contracting and construction management services for all types of facilities.	048
Verity	Verity provides enterprise search software that enables organizations to discover, analyze and process all the information within their enterprises. Its solutions include integrated search, classification, recommendation, monitoring and analytics, business process management and content capture solutions that deliver the true real-time process control and forward-looking visibility required by complex businesses.	068
Voltage security	Voltage's secure messaging platform provides a way to encrypt and send secure electronic patient and physician information without certificates, passwords or the complexity of PKI.	105
VIGNETTE	Vignette helps organizations harness the power of information and the Web for measurable improvements in business efficiency. By incorporating portal, enterprise content management and collaboration solutions, Vignette enables the capture, management, security and delivery of the complete patient record.	247

[Acronyms]

ANSI	National Council for Prescription Drug Programs
AWTM	American Society for Testing and Materials
CDA	Clinical Document Architecture
CMBD	Configuration Management Board Directive
CMD	Chronic Disease Management
CDISC	Clinical Data Interchange Standards Consortium
DICOM	Digital Imaging and Communications in Medicine
EHR	Electronic Health Record
EHRS	Electronic Health Record Systems
EHRVA	Electronic Health Record Vendor Association
EMR	Electronic Medical Record
GP	General Practitioner
HHS	Health and Human Services
HIMSS	Healthcare Information and Management Systems Society
HIPAA	Health Insurance Portability and Accountability Act
HL7	Health Level 7
IHE	Integrating the Healthcare Enterprise
ISO	Internal Organization for Standardization
JCAHO	Joint Commission on Accreditation of Healthcare Organizations
LOINC	Logical Observation Identifiers, Names and Codes
LOPD	Law on Protection of Personal Data
MMA	Medicare Modernization Act
NCPDP	National Council for Prescription Drug Programs
NCVHS	National Committee on Vital and Health Statistics
NHIM	National Health Information Model
NHS	National Health Service (England)
PSV	Public Sector Value
RIM	Reference Information Model
SDO	Standards Development Organization
SEIS	Spanish Healthcare Information Society
SNOMED CT	Systematized Nomenclature of Human Medicine Clinical Terms

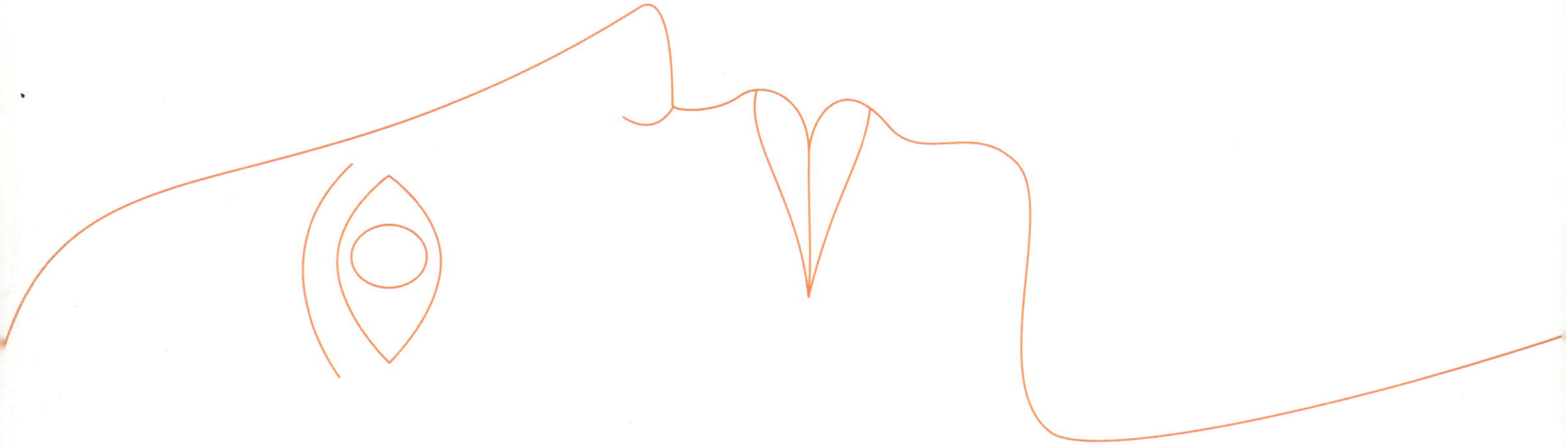